OXFORD STUDIES IN
SOCIAL AND LEGAL HISTORY

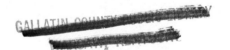

OXFORD STUDIES IN SOCIAL AND LEGAL HISTORY

EDITED BY

PAUL VINOGRADOFF

M.A , D.C.L., LL.D., Dr. Hist., Dr. Jur., F.B.A.

CORPUS PROFESSOR OF JURISPRUDENCE IN THE UNIVERSITY OF OXFORD

VOL. V

THE BLACK DEATH

By A. ELIZABETH LEVETT and A. BALLARD

RURAL NORTHAMPTONSHIRE UNDER THE COMMON-WEALTH

By REGINALD LENNARD

OCTAGON BOOKS

A DIVISION OF FARRAR, STRAUS AND GIROUX

New York   1974

Originally published in 1916 by the Clarendon Press

Reprinted 1974
by special arrangement with Oxford University Press, Inc.

OCTAGON BOOKS
A Division of Farrar, Straus & Giroux, Inc.
19 Union Square West
New York, N. Y. 10003

Library of Congress Cataloging in Publication Data

Levett, Ada Elizabeth.
    The black death.

    Reprint of 1916 editions published by the Clarendon Press, Ox-
    ford which were issued as v. 5, no. 9-10 of Oxford studies in
    social and legal history.

        1. Manors—Great Britain. 2. Land tenure—Great Britain—
    History. 3. Black death. 4. Land tenure—Northamptonshire,
    Eng. 5. Manors—Northamptonshire, Eng. I. Ballard, Adol-
    phus, 1867-1915, joint author. II. Lennard, Reginald Vivian,
    1885-   Rural Northamptonshire under the commonwealth.
    1974. III. Title. IV. Series: Oxford studies in social and legal
    history, v. 5, no. 9-10.
HC254.3.L45   1974   333.3'23'094255   73-22341
ISBN 0-374-96164-6

Printed in USA by
Thomson-Shore,Inc.
Dexter, Michigan

PREFATORY NOTE

THE part played by the great pestilences of the fourteenth century in the economic evolution of England has given rise to much discussion and has been regarded, at one time, as the principal cause of the crisis in the agrarian history of the Middle Ages : it was supposed to have led to the passage from customary services to agreements based on cash nexus. A reaction against this view became more and more manifest in later years : various writers refused to assign to the Black Death such a catastrophic influence, and thought that its action merely accentuated the general features of a protracted evolution. Miss Levett has approached the subject in the light of a minute and exact investigation of the data provided by the ministerial accounts of the see of Winchester, which range over centuries and present an instructive series of entries for the fateful years of the pestilence as well as for those immediately preceding and following them. The verdict based on this study is emphatically in the negative : as far as the Winchester estates represent average conditions, the accounts do not disclose any abrupt change as to tenure or husbandry. This does not exhaust the possibilities of further investigation,

A 2

but an analysis based on the study of groups of manors placed in different surroundings and affected by the plague in varying degrees cannot fail to exercise an influence on general conclusions as to the matter under discussion.

The late Adolphus Ballard has added a chapter to Miss Levett's monograph, treating the subject in relation to three estates taken to represent, as it were, three stages in the process of economic changes. Witney, Brightwell, and Downton are taken, not only in their fourteenth-century aspect, but in their historical growth from the time of the Conquest, and we are able to observe the greater and the lesser stress of the devastation wrought by the plague. It may be mentioned that the untimely death of A. Ballard prevented him from giving the last touches to his description. The proofs had to be read after his demise by the editor, and Miss Levett kindly verified some of the figures in the Public Record Office, though it would have been out of the question to overhaul all the details of that survey. The general results obtained by Miss Levett remain in force in the light of this concrete characterization of typical estates.

There is a positive side to these investigations : if, on one side, they reduce the importance of the Black Death as a factor of economic development, on the other they throw light on the process of

commutation by which the change from mediaeval
to modern conditions was brought about. Apart
from a quantity of incidental information as to prices,
wages, and agrarian methods, the various causes
which led to the introduction of money agreements
are disclosed and estimated in their comparative
influence. In the particular case under discussion the
cultural policy of William of Wykeham may have
suggested arrangements in commutation of labour
services and rents in kind. In other cases similar
results were connected with war expenditure and
town life. In so far the initiative in selling services
came from the class of landowners. But there
were powerful tendencies at work in the life of the
peasants which made for the same result. The most
comprehensive of these tendencies was connected,
it seems to me, with the accumulation of capital in
the hands of the villains under a system of customary
dues. When rents and services became settled and
lost their elasticity, roughly speaking in the course
of the twelfth, thirteenth, and fourteenth centuries,
the surplus of profits from agriculture was bound
to collect in the hands of those who received them
directly from the soil, and it was natural for these
first receivers to turn the proceeds primarily towards an improvement of their social condition; the
redemption of irksome services was a conspicuous
manifestation of this policy. It is only when fixity

of tenure went into the melting-pot after fixity of
service that the inconvenient side of commutation
made itself felt to the rustic population. But this
aspect of the process is not within the purview of
Miss Levett's essay. The subject of Mr.
Lennard's study is the evidence
provided for the agrarian history of a midland
county by the surveys of crown lands made in 1650
and about that date by order of the Commonwealth
Government. In some cases, e.g. in Grafton, these
surveys can be compared with earlier and later documents enabling us to trace the lines of economic
evolution with exactness and wealth of detail. In
all cases the evidence of the parliamentary surveys,
coming, as it does, from a critical period of English development, is exceedingly important for the
purpose of forming a judgement as to the course
and the turning-points of agrarian changes. The
processes of ' engrossing ' and of enclosure are
copiously reflected in these surveys while they do
not throw much light on the coming in of the industrial revolution characteristic of the eighteenth
century. Such investigations as that carried out
by Mr. Lennard are naturally limited in their
bearing on general problems on account of their
narrow local basis. Yet it is only by collecting
evidence set in concrete local surroundings that
we obtain a sure footing for tracing the con-

nexion of events. From this latter point of view Mr. Lennard's monograph is suggestive of interesting conclusions. It pleads, as it were, for the force of historical psychology against geographical fatalism. Professor Gonner has insisted in a recent book on the direct influence of geographical and geological conditions on the process of enclosures, and such a point undoubtedly helps to co-ordinate facts into a comprehensive panorama. For the historian the landscape appears to be more complex: variations and contrasts appear which cannot be accounted for on the strength of a direct adaptation of policy to geographical conditions. Such a scientific or 'intelligent' policy is not to be traced before the nineteenth century. In former centuries, especially in the seventeenth, strongly-rooted habits and sympathies militate against considerations of profit : farmers continue to cultivate arable lands for an income of 4s. an acre where they ought in sound economy to have passed on to grazing for a possible rent of 19s. an acre. The results of such conflicting tendencies are seen in the great differences of management within the territory of one county.

PAUL VINOGRADOFF.

IN MEMORIAM ADOLPHUS BALLARD

† SEPTEMBER 12, 1915

ADOLPHUS BALLARD was born in 1867 at Chichester, and was the eldest son of Alderman Adolphus Ballard, J.P., of that city. He was educated at University College School, Hastings, and at the Leys School, Cambridge, and in 1886 he took an Arts degree in the University of London. In 1890 he took his LL.B. and was admitted solicitor. He practised in Oxford and at Woodstock, and was Town Clerk of Woodstock from 1894 to the day of his death. It was in 1894 that he married Mary Elizabeth Henman, daughter of William Henman, of Islip Manor. In 1898 he was appointed Clerk to the Oxford Incorporation and Superintendent Registrar, and in 1910 Registrar of the Woodstock County Court, and he was for some years Liberal Agent for the Mid-Oxfordshire Parliamentary Division, and latterly Honorary Secretary of the Mid-Oxfordshire Liberal Association. In 1907 he was given the degree of M.A. *honoris causa* by the University of Oxford. He died on September 12, 1915, after a short illness bravely endured.

The beginning of Ballard's historical work was characteristic both of his modesty and of his tendency to find a sure basis for historical thought in the detailed study of concrete things. In 1893 he published some 'Notes on the History of Chipping Norton', which were an expansion of a lecture delivered to the local branch of the Young Men's Christian Association. Three years later came the 'Chronicles of the Royal Borough of Woodstock', and in 1898 a 'History of Chichester'. But Ballard could never have remained a mere student of local antiquities. He had an expanding curiosity which refused to be satisfied with the anecdotes of history. In 1899 he was evidently feeling his way towards the studies of his later years, for he published in the ' English Historical Review ' an article on ' English Boroughs in the reign of John '. His mind gradually took a wider sweep : the main currents of contemporary historical study influenced him more and more ; and ' The Domesday Boroughs ' (1904) was admittedly inspired by Maitland's 'Township and Borough'. From the boroughs of Domesday Ballard went on to the study of Domesday Book in general, and his volume on 'The Domesday Inquest', which was published in 1906, remains the most useful manual for a student seeking his first acquaintance with the problems of the great survey. Yet while Ballard's studies increased in range, he retained a firm grasp of concrete historical facts and a keen interest in local history. ' The Domesday Inquest ' contains a chapter on the ' typical village ' of Islip, which lay close to his home, and in the same year in which it was published he edited ' Seven Somerton Court Rolls ' for the Oxfordshire Archaeological Society, while in 1908 his very valuable study of ' Woodstock Manor in the Thirteenth Century ' appeared in the ' Vierteljahrschrift für Social- und Wirtschaftsgeschichte '. A few years later he contributed some articles to Hoop's ' Reallexikon der germanischen Altertumskunde '. But Ballard's *magnum opus* was undoubtedly his ' British Borough Charters, 1042–1216 ' (published 1913), which is not only an exhaustive summary of the authorities, but contains some interesting comparisons between English and continental institutions. ' The British Borough in the Twelfth Century ' followed in 1914. To the very end Ballard's interests were expanding as his knowledge became fuller and more ripe. A paper on ' The Theory of the Scottish Burgh ', published in the ' Scottish Historical Review ', and another on ' The Laws of Breteuil ' in the ' English Historical Review ', were written very shortly before his death, while the monograph in this volume also contains some of his latest work.

The historical writings of Adolphus Ballard as a whole would have done credit to the occupant of a professorial chair. But the excellence of his achievement can only be measured at its true worth in view of the conditions under which he worked. His daily journey from Woodstock to his office in Oxford, his work as a solicitor, the duties of the many public offices he held—these were invasions of his time so great that most men would have found neither time nor energy to spare for anything else, beyond at best a wearied dilettantism in study. Yet somehow Ballard found opportunities for thorough and long-continued researches ; and instead of chafing against the necessities of his everyday work, he rejoiced in that work and recognized gratefully that his practical legal and administrative tasks gave a quality of reality to all his historical writing. Nor were work and study the whole of his life. He was a keen politician and organized several election campaigns in the Mid-Oxfordshire Division. His opponents knew him as a man of stainless honour and unruffled courtesy. His friends recognized in his liberalism a political faith as courageous as it was free from bigotry. A sincere Christian, he was well known as a local preacher in the villages of North Oxfordshire, and English Nonconformity has lost in him a witness whom none could fail to respect. For his quiet unassuming industry was matched by the integrity and simplicity of his life, by the unfailing kindness of his affectionate heart, by the equable cheerfulness of his spirit, and by his open-minded readiness to examine new ideas.

R. V. L.

IX

THE BLACK DEATH ON THE ESTATES
OF THE SEE OF WINCHESTER

BY

A. ELIZABETH LEVETT

VICE-PRINCIPAL AND TUTOR OF ST. HILDA'S HALL, OXFORD
FORMERLY SCHOLAR OF LADY MARGARET HALL

WITH A CHAPTER ON THE MANORS OF
WITNEY, BRIGHTWELL, AND DOWNTON

BY

A. BALLARD, M.A.

TOWN CLERK OF WOODSTOCK

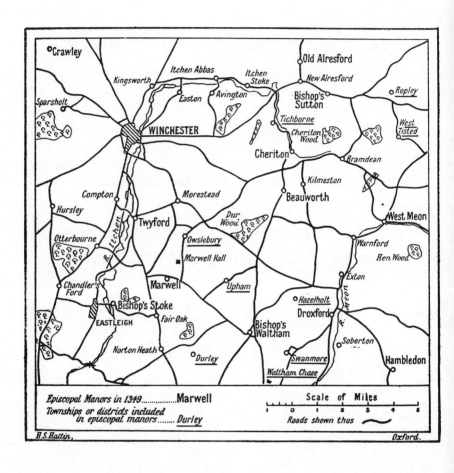

°Crawley
Itchen Abbas
Kingsworth
Sparsholt
Easton
Avington
Itchen Stoke
Old Alresford
New Alresford
Bishop's Sutton
Ropley
WINCHESTER
Tichborne
Cheriton Wood
West Tisted
Cheriton
Bramdean
Compton
Morestead
Kilmeston
Beauworth
Hursley
R. Itchen
Twyford
Dur Wood
West Meon
Otterbourne
Owslebury
Warnford
Hen Wood
Marwell Hall
Chandler's Ford
Marwell
Upham
Exton
R. Meon
EASTLEIGH
Bishop's Stoke
Fair Oak
Hazelholt
Droxford
Norton Heath
Bishop's Waltham
Soberton
Durley
Swanmore
Hambledon
Waltham Chase

Episcopal Manors in 1349 .... **Marwell**
*Townships or districts included
in episcopal manors* .... <u>Durley</u>

Scale of Miles
1 0 1 2 3 4 5
Roads shown thus

H.S.Hattin,
Oxford.

CONTENTS

REFERENCE NUMBERS

For the sake of convenience I have given my references only to year, date, and heading in the Pipe Roll, and not to the numbers by which each Roll is known. The numbers are therefore given here, with the years, from Michaelmas to Michaelmas, to which they belong.

1208–9	159270	4th year of Peter des Roches.
1274–5	159302	—
1284–5	159307	—
1343–4	159354	11th year of Adam of Orleton.
1345–6	159355	1st year of William of Edyndon.
1346–7	159356	2nd ,, ,, ,,
1347–8	159357	3rd ,, ,, ,,
1348–9	159358	4th ,, ,, ,,
1349–50	159359	5th ,, ,, ,,
1350–1	159360	6th ,, ,, ,,
1351–2	159362*	7th ,, ,, ,,
1352–3	159363	8th ,, ,, ,,
1353–4	159364	9th ,, ,, ,,
1354–5	159365	10th ,, ,, ,,
1376–7	159384	10th ,, William of Wykeham.
1384–5	159392	18th ,, ,, ,,
1386–7	159394	20th ,, ,, ,,
1454–5	159445	9th ,, William Waynflete.

TABLE OF DATES AND REFERENCES †

Old Official Reference.	Old Official Date.	Roll Date.	Amended Date.
159354	1343	11 Bishop Adam	Mich. 1343—Mich: 1344
——5	1345	1 Bishop William	9 Dec. 1345— ‡ ,, 1346
——6	1346	2 ,, ●	Mich. 1346— ,, 1347
——7	1347	3 ,, ,,	,, 1347— ,, 1348
——8	1348	4 ,, ,,	,, 1348— ,, 1349
——9	1349	5 ,, ,,	,, 1349— ,, 1350
——60	1350	6 ,, ,,	,, 1350— ,, 1351
——61 §	1351	12 Bishop Adam	,, 1344—18 July 1345‖

* The Roll marked 159361 is out of place.
† For this table we are indebted to the kindness of Mr. Hubert Hall.
‡ Prior to this the executors of Bishop Adam account.
§ From this point the series is continued in its proper order, i. e. 159362= 7 Bishop Adam=1351–2.
‖ The gap is closed by the Minister's account (Gen. Ser. 1143/17) showing that the Bishopric was in the King's hands from Bishop Adam's death, 18 July 1345, to 15 February 1346, when the Temporalties were restored to Bishop William (but see Le Neve) and the Custos was ordered to account only to 9 December 1345.

5

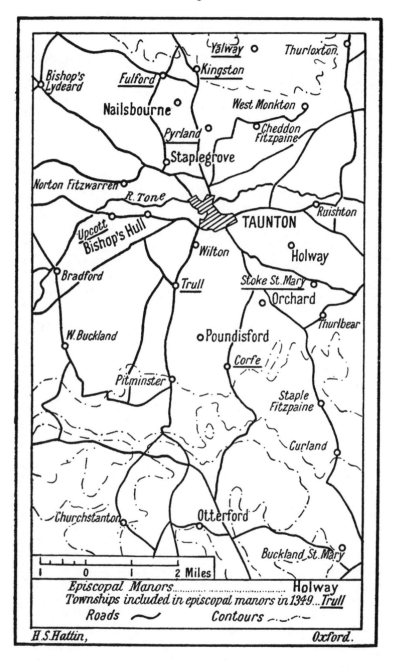

Yalway
Thurloxton.
Kingston
Bishop's Lydeard
Fulford
Nailsbourne
West Monkton
Pyrland
Cheddon Fitzpaine
Staplegrove
Norton Fitzwarren
R. Tone
Upcott
Bishop's Hull
TAUNTON
Ruishton
Wilton
Holway
Bradford
Stoke St. Mary
Trull
Orchard
Thurlbear
W. Buckland
Poundisford
Corfe
Pitminster
Staple Fitzpaine
Curland
Churchstanton
Otterford
Buckland St. Mary

| | 0 | | 2 Miles |

Episcopal Manors................................ Holway
Townships included in episcopal manors in 1349...Trull
Roads ~ Contours ‿.‿.‿

H.S.Hattin, Oxford.

INTRODUCTION

IN his ' History of a Cambridgeshire Manor '[1] Maitland
has shown what valuable material is contained in manorial
Account Rolls, and what definite and incontestable conclusions may be drawn from them, by a very direct and
simple method of examination.

In this article on the manor of Wilburton he examines
Extents, Court Rolls, and Account Rolls, ranging in date
from 1221 to 1609; the most striking evidence, however, is
drawn from the Account Rolls, which prove a remarkable
continuity in the history of the manor. Unfortunately the
records of Wilburton preserve no accounts for the crucial
years of Edward III's reign (1345–55), when the Black Death
tried to the utmost the resources of manorial organization;
thus both the changes and the conservatism of the manorial
economy are, to some extent, unexplained.

Moreover, the question remains, How far is the manor of
Wilburton typical ? Can one prove or assume that what is
true of Wilburton is true also of Southern or Midland England ?
Only a series of detailed studies can answer these questions,
and physical and local peculiarities will always make it impossible to answer them conclusively.

It is, however, possible to apply a modification of the
method to a particular problem, and this is what I have
endeavoured to do with regard to a time-honoured controversy—the results of the Black Death. The main difficulty
in dealing with the question has been the rarity of exactly
contemporary material. There is a wealth of evidence for
the period immediately preceding 1349; there is abundant
material for rural economic history ten or twenty years later.
But it is generally hard to bridge the interval. Comparatively
few manorial records of the years 1348–50 have been preserved ; of those which survive few have been systematically
examined.

[1] English Hist. Rev., July 1894 ; Maitland, Collected Papers, vol. ii.

Such a study as Jessopp's 'Black Death in East Anglia'[1] is based, as far as manorial history goes, almost exclusively upon Court Rolls, and it is perhaps true to say that a Court Roll only gives the negative side of the story. It may give the number of deaths, the number of escheats or heriots, it may show the general dislocation of judicial business, but it is no very safe guide with regard to the ordinary affairs of the manor—the continuance of agricultural operations, the exaction of rents and services, the sale and purchase of produce, the number of survivors, the fate of the vacant tenements, and, indeed, all the more strictly economic side of the manorial organization.

For the positive evidence there is no better material than Account Rolls, if they are sufficiently continuous.

An unrivalled series of such accounts is known as the Pipe Rolls of the Bishops of Winchester, which extend from the year 1208–9[2] to the year 1455, with few gaps ; between 1346 and 1356 the series is complete, as indeed it is for practically the whole of the fourteenth century. The rolls contain the accounts of some sixty manors in the south of England, in six different counties, Somerset, Wiltshire, Hampshire, Berkshire, Oxfordshire, and Surrey. Thus chronologically the material is exactly what is required, while the wide geographical range makes it more reasonable to look for some general conclusion, without being deceived by local peculiarities. The Pipe Rolls are in the possession of the Ecclesiastical Commissioners, and are deposited at the Public Record Office. For the most part, they are in an excellent state of preservation ; occasionally a section of the account is illegible owing to decay, or to dark stains, and the lower edges are sometimes torn. Unfortunately, the account for the year 1348–9 is in a worse condition than any I have seen, and in compiling tables from it I have been obliged in several cases to leave a blank, though the omissions are not often serious. The first roll extant, that for the year 1208–9, has been transcribed and published, under the editorship of Mr. Hubert

[1] Jessopp, A. The Coming of the Friars. And other historic essays. 1889.
[2] The accounts run from Michaelmas to Michaelmas ; I have therefore given all my references to the two dates covered by each roll.

Hall;[1] a valuable introduction describes what is known of
the origin and form of the Bishop's Pipe Roll, and of the
method of its compilation; the whole publication is exceedingly useful as a starting-point for further examination and
comparison.

The extreme fullness of the Accounts is the main difficulty
in extracting their evidence; I have, therefore, only looked
at a few isolated rolls before 1346, and have generally confined
my attention to the period between 1346 and 1356, and in
a lesser degree to the years 1376–81, when certain new
material is incorporated in the accounts. Geographically,
I have selected a group of closely-related manors, lying
within a few miles of Winchester, in the valley of the Itchen
and on the neighbouring downs; another group of manors
formerly incorporated in the ' classic example of a colossal
manor ', Taunton, and lying in the fertile and famous Taunton
Dean; a few manors on the Berkshire Downs and in the
Thames Valley are also quoted, either as supplementary
evidence or to mark a contrast.

It has been pointed out to me that the proximity of large
towns, such as Winchester and Taunton, doubtless affected
the development of neighbouring manors, and must be taken
into account. This is perfectly true, although my choice of
groups was not originally made with this idea in view. The
Hampshire group seemed particularly marked out for examination, because the economic conditions are fairly uniform,
and the manors are, for the most part, contiguous. The
Taunton group was chosen because it alone has a continuous
account of the ' works ' of the villeins during the ten years
1346–56. However, a choice which was largely accidental
may give some interesting suggestions as to the influence of
large towns upon their rural neighbours, but on the whole
I am inclined to believe that peculiarities of soil and physical
configuration are more important than proximity to a town.

Of supplementary material for the period under consideration there is little. A vast number of Court Rolls for the
Bishop of Winchester's estates still survive, but none of them

[1] Pipe Roll of Bishopric of Winchester, 1208–9, ed. Hubert Hall (1903).

fall within the years 1346–56. Moreover, the most valuable entries of such Court Rolls as I have examined, the Fines of Land, are more readily accessible in the Account Rolls. In looking through some forty or fifty Court Rolls for the years 1366–1404, for the manors of Bishop's Waltham, Droxford, Bitterne, and others, I have found very little indeed that throws much light upon the Ministers' Accounts.

Occasionally an ' Extent ' is inserted among the other accounts, but unfortunately I have only found one example. References occur here and there to other records, such as the Rental (cf. p. 30 n.) ; one such Rental[1] has been found for Bishop's Waltham (cf. p. 217), but its date is illegible, as well as the entries for two tithings. To judge by the handwriting, it must be assigned to the earlier part of the fourteenth century, but owing to its imperfect condition, its evidence cannot be readily utilized. Similar Rentals must have been kept locally on most of the Bishop's manors, and the labour involved in making them explains why they were not kept up to date. The Waltham Rental must be well over five yards long; it contains the names of over 600 tenements, with the quarterly rents of each arranged in four columns. An attempt has been made to note changes of tenants by altering the names.

The original Compotus Rolls, from which the Pipe Roll was compiled, have survived, to some extent, in another set of Records in the possession of the Ecclesiastical Commissioners.[2] But this collection is very incomplete, and has been imperfectly sorted and catalogued. Of some 50–100 rolls relating to any one manor, eight or ten may belong to the fourteenth or fifteenth century, while the rest are of the sixteenth, seventeenth, and eighteenth centuries. It is interesting to notice that the form of the account survived, in English, with few changes, down to the middle of the eighteenth century, though some of the items had long been completely out of date. This series of rolls would be unimportant, as they are duplicated on the Pipe Roll, but for the fact

---

[1] See Eccles. Com. Various, 159512⅑.
[2] See Eccles. Com. Various, Bundles 56–117.

that the accounts of the Labour Services are sometimes recorded on the backs of the rolls, and these entries were not, as a rule, transcribed on to the Pipe Rolls. However, these accounts of the *opera* appear very irregularly and I have not succeeded in finding any which throw much light on the Hampshire services before 1376.[1]

In one year, 1376–7, the original account sent in from Upton seems to have been bound up with the enrolled accounts; it is written in a skilled hand, similar to that of the Pipe Roll, on a much narrower strip of parchment; the account is far more conveniently spaced and arranged than the final roll.

Among the Court Rolls, also, are a few slips of parchment, only two or three inches long, containing a list of the flock, details of the corn, a list of newly-elected reeves, or a list of jurors. Some of these may have been the first written notes taken down from the tallies presented by the reeves, shepherds, or other regular servants of the manors; they are clearly out of place when sewn up with the Court Rolls. Similar notes seem to be referred to at Twyford in 1349–50, where it is stated that eighteen tenements are in the lord's hand, *ut patet per unam cedulam.*

It is unfortunate that so little parallel material should be available, but the completeness of the Pipe Roll makes the loss of less importance than it would be on less highly organized estates. Every change, however slight, left its mark upon the minute and accurate account-keeping of the bishop's exchequer; the extreme conservatism of the method, together with the scientific care of the estates, produce evidence which needs little more than much time and patience to make it available for our information to-day.[2]

---

[1] As there are perhaps some seven hundred rolls of a date earlier than 1485, I cannot claim that my search has been exhaustive, but I do not think I have missed much that is of value for the Hampshire group of manors treated in the following chapters.

[2] In view of the abundance of material, it is particularly disappointing to find it treated so inadequately as in a recent article in the English Hist. Rev. (October 1914), 'The Commutation of Villein Services in England before the Black Death' (by H. L. Gray). It is true that in this article Mr. Gray only devotes two pages to the Winchester Pipe Roll, in the midst of a survey of the question of commutation throughout England. Yet

those two pages appear to be so full of inaccuracies that it is impossible to refer to the writer's general conclusions without pointing out how frequently he is incorrect in detail. With an almost unbroken series of accounts extending over two and a half centuries at his disposal, Mr. Gray has confined his attention to the years immediately before the Black Death, has examined the roll for 1343–4, and has collated it with the preceding roll. He gives a wrong reference-number, has failed to find the imperfect roll for 1344–5, which is slightly misplaced (see p. 4), and describes the roll for the year 1346–7 as imperfect, whereas it covers a complete year of twelve months. The roll for the year 1345–6, which is imperfect, is described by Mr. Gray as missing. The method Mr. Gray employs rests upon a comparison of the value of the Labour Services, both sold and performed, with the total Rents of Assize. He admits that the rents generally include those of the free tenements, and that his comparison is thus, to that extent, inexact. I have tried to show elsewhere (pp. 16–19) how irrelevant this method is in dealing with the Winchester manors. This, however, may be a matter of opinion. There is no doubt that Mr. Gray has missed a valuable source of information in the rolls for the years 1375–6–7, which would have provided him with indispensable evidence as to the services performed on the Hampshire manors. Even in the years where he has examined the roll it is difficult to accept Mr. Gray's figures. ' In not more than eight accounts is there an entry regarding the sale of *opera* ' (i. e. in counties other than Somerset) is his clear assertion. In the roll in question (1343–4) I find the actual heading *Opera Vendita, Venditio Operum*, or *Relaxatio Operum* for nine manors only, but in twenty-eight other accounts (excluding Somerset) there are large or small sums for works sold or commuted, entered under the heading *Exitus Manerii*. These sums vary from £8 downwards to a shilling or two. They include :

(a) Sale of a few unneeded Harvest works ;
(b) Definite commutation of all the works of a virgate ;
(c) Commutation of works of a large number of virgates (e. g. twenty-two at Wargrave) for one or two quarters of the year ;
(d) Commutation of certain classes of work, e. g. Ploughing, Winter Works, Carting, part of Harvest Works, Threshing.

Thus to state that on only eight manors is there any entry of sale of works is misleading. By 1347–8 the number of manors containing the actual entry *Venditio Operum* has increased.

Again, Mr. Gray asserts that ' The threshing and weeding *opera* were always sold ' (in Somerset). As a matter of fact weeding services were employed on the demesne at Holway in 1347–8, 1348–9, and 1349–50, in very irregular numbers ; at Poundisford in 1347–8, 1349–50, 1350–1 and 1376–7 ; at Staplegrove they were uniformly sold from 1346–51 ; at Hull almost all the weeding services were performed in 1349–50 and in 1376–7 ; at Rimpton and Nailesbourne no weeding was due. The tables on pp. 89 and 180 show how irregularly most services were demanded and commuted.

The entries of wages, which might throw some light on the possibility of complete commutation, are almost entirely ignored by Mr. Gray. Trifling inaccuracies, such as the ascription of manors to their wrong counties, are not infrequent.

With Mr. Gray's conclusions I am not concerned, but it seemed necessary to make some such criticism here, to show that there is room for further examination of the Winchester Pipe Roll, on the vexed question of commutation. It may perhaps be added that this study was practically finished when Mr. Gray's article appeared.

CHAPTER I

BEFORE THE BLACK DEATH

In order to understand how the Ministers' Accounts of the Bishops of Winchester may throw light upon the results of the Black Death, it is necessary to emphasize the importance of the form of the Accounts, and of the development of that form during the thirteenth and fourteenth centuries. The introductory section of this study must therefore consist of a detailed examination of the accounts, taken heading by heading, in order to obtain a clear view of the normal working of the bishop's estates before the disturbing influence of the pestilence was felt.

Between 1208 and 1346 considerable changes had taken place in the method of enrolling the Ministers' Accounts, though in its main features it is unaltered. As in 1208, the account is divided into three main parts or schedules : (*a*) the *Income*, or assets ; (*b*) the *Expenses*, together with a balancing of the two ; (*c*) the *Stock and Corn* account : in a few cases there is added an elaborate account of the number and nature of the *opera* due during the year, and of the way in which these works had been allocated and performed.

Each of these schedules has many subdivisions, which vary slightly from manor to manor, but which preserve the same general features. Taking each of these subdivisions separately, as it stood during the normal years 1346–8, one may see what kind of information may be sought from later rolls as to the effects of the Black Death.

Each manorial entry begins with a statement of the year Date. of the bishop, dating from his consecration. The numbering of the episcopal years is not quite always correct, or consistent.[1]

The name of the reeve follows ; sometimes there are two *Prae-* reeves, possibly the incoming and the outgoing official. The *positus.*

[1] E.g. Cheriton, Taunton, and general heading 1352.

reeve might remain in office during a number of years, or might change every year. In many cases he seems to have survived the dangers of the Black Death, and went on uninterruptedly accounting for the proceeds of the manor.[1] Occasionally a ' serjeant ' was associated with or replaced the reeve for a year or two.[2]

The reeves were commonly elected, but there is a note under Staplegrove, in 1284, to the effect that the hundred of Staplegrove paid 6s. 8d. to be allowed to elect their reeve, and to have no reeve except by election.[3]

Arrera-gia.

Next follows the amount of the arrears from the preceding year, ' by one tally ', which is almost always paid off in full ; the amount always corresponds exactly with the entry *et debet de claro* of the last roll. Court Rolls for a later period (e.g. after 1380) contain evidence of considerable friction between incoming and outgoing reeves as to the payment of arrears.

Redditus Assise.

The Rents of Assize appear to have taken the place of the *Gabulum* of 1208 ;[4] both are mentioned on different manors in the thirteenth-century rolls, but by 1346 the former is the only term used.

The entry does not in itself yield much information, though valuable deductions may be drawn from it.

The amount of the rents has increased very considerably since 1208, but by 1346 it has become a fixed and conventional item in the account ; the figures in some districts hardly vary between 1346 and 1455.

Occasionally an *Incrementum* is noted ; one of the tenants adds a few yards of a path,[5] or a tiny corner of a field, or

---

[1] Staplegrove, 1348–54 ; Rimpton, 1346–51 ; Crawley, 1348–55.
[2] Beauworth, 1347–8, Michaelis de Somborne, *serviens.*
[3] This election of the reeve by the Hundred is apparently exceptional.
[4] In the introduction to the Winchester Pipe Roll of 1208–9 (edited Hubert Hall) the two are treated as if they were distinct; the difference is apparently only a difference of name. Miss Neilson (Oxford Studies in Social and Legal History, vol. i, Customary Rents, p. 46) also concludes that the *Gabulum assise* is probably only another name for *redditus assise.*
[5] The *Incrementum* was occasionally a commutation of dues in kind ; at Cheriton 1212–13 it is clearly stated that the *Incrementum Gabuli* was to be paid instead of the customary fowls.

a plot of the lord's waste, to his holding and pays an additional 2*d*. or 3*d*. in rent.

The thirteenth century, however, must have been a period of extensive enclosures from the waste, both to enlarge the demesne and to increase the holdings of the tenants. On several manors the sub-heading *Incrementa* is followed by a long list of small encroachments; thus at Wargrave in 1284 there are thirteen small increments of rent varying from 1*s*. 3*d*. to ½*d*. for plots of land varying in size from 2½ acres down to 1 *buticus*, while one tenant paid a lump addition of 2*s*. 2½*d*. to his rent, for increments on all his lands *per cartas domini*. Witney and one or two small manors in the Thames Valley have considerable entries of Assarts, or forest-clearings (cf. p. 185); in most of the manors ' *terra pur-prestura* ' is very common indeed, and seems to be the equi-valent, in more open country, of the ' assarts ' of the wooded districts; it is possible that the ' Overland ' of Somerset and Wiltshire is merely another name for purprestures or encroachments upon the open downs, which merely needed appropriation. It is at least certain that one manor very seldom, if ever, appears to contain more than one of these classes of land.[1]

By 1346 probably a majority of the tenants in Hampshire held purprestures, very often in compact holdings of from 5 to 80 acres; it is almost impossible, however, to calculate the proportion between such encroachments on the waste and the land of an older cultivation, especially as the encroach-ment is often mentioned simply as a purprestura, with no indication of its extent.[2]

---

[1] Assarts and purprestures occasionally occur side by side, e.g. at Bishop's Waltham. For ' Overland ' see below, p. 70.

[2] The assarts and purprestures were always held for a money-rent, and there are no traces on the Winchester manors of any attempt to exact services from them. The theory put forward by a recent writer (Tawney, Agrarian Problem in the Sixteenth Century, p. 141), that enclosures from the waste were rented as ' so many ploughlands' worth ', seems to rest on a mis-understanding. In the Crondal Records (Baigent), pp. 132–3, on which the statement is based, the following entry occurs: ' The same Hugh holds certain encroachments on payment of 3 ploughlands' worth, 3 hens and 3*d*.' The original text (p. 106) reads *Idem Hugo tenet quasdam pur-presturas. Reddendo ad dictum terminum iii vomeres, iii gallinas et iii d.*

By 1346 the movement for enclosing the waste had either ceased or further enclosures were kept in the lord's hand and added to the demesne or leased.[1] The following tables will show the periods at which changes in the rents took place most rapidly, i.e. in the first half of the thirteenth century. In Hampshire the rents are evidently almost stationary between 1346 and 1455; in the Thames Valley there is little or no change between 1346 and 1376, but by 1455 most of the manors were farmed and the rents are not always entered separately; in the Taunton group the manors are not sub-divided in 1208, between 1284 and 1347 the increase is approximately at the same rate as in Hampshire, but between 1347 and 1455 the rents are by no means stationary. This seems to be due to the much higher increments common in the district, to the continued enclosure of arable and pasture land on the downs, and to the numerous cottage-rents which were included in these sub-manors. Further search might reveal other causes in the fifteenth century.

In connexion with tables I–III an interesting point arises. If the rents remain approximately fixed between 1346 and 1455, what becomes of the theory that services were commuted into fixed rents ? It has been shown that such changes as there are between these two dates are commonly due to fresh inclosures and are noted as *Incrementa*. The usual assumption is, however, that the moneys due from commuted services were entered under the heading of Rents of Assize.[2] Thus in a recent article in the ' English Historical Review ' Mr. H. L. Gray asks, ' If commutation were definite, why carry on the *Opera* item thus specifically rather than sink it in the rent of assize ? '[3] The answer is partly, as Mr. Gray suggests, that the commutation in this case was not permanent ; partly

A ploughshare was a very ordinary form of rent in Hampshire, and there is no reason for any but a literal translation. The Glossary (p. 512) shows that the translator was very doubtful of his own rendering.

[1] The following entry shows that enclosure from the waste for arable had not ceased. Waltham, 1347–8 : ' *Minute Necessarie.* In viii acris de terra frisca super la Breche assarta pro terra arabili inde habendis xxii s. per acram.'

[2] See Tawney, Agrarian Problem in Sixteenth Century, pp. 115–17, for table of almost equally stationary rents.

[3] Eng. Hist. Rev., October 1914, p. 639.

ASSIZED RENTS

TABLE I (HANTS)

	1208			1275			1284			1346			1386			1455		
	£	s.	d.	£	s.	d.	£	s.	d.	£	s.	d.	£	s.	d.	£	s.	d.
Stoke	10	16	7½	17	0	0¼	17	2	4¼	19	12	10¾	19	13	1	19	19	4¼‡
Bishop's Waltham	42	4	1½	63	14	1	74	5	0¼	83	9	10½	83	14	7½	84	4	4½
Droxford	Not in Roll			—			23	14	9 †	25	3	9½	25	4	5½	25	4	5½
Beauworth	3	1	0	5	15	6	5	16	7	5	16	10	5	16	10	5	16	10
Cheriton	20	4	9 *	31	6	6	31	8	6	33	18	8¾	33	19	0¾	33	19	0¾ §
Sutton	36	15	6½	49	11	10	49	15	11	51	13	6½	52	0	2½	52	0	2½
Crawley	9	9	0	13	11	2	13	11	2	15	0	11	15	0	11	15	2	7
Marwell }										27	19	9¼	28	0	0	28	0	5½
Twyford }	31	16	5	43	6	9	47	8	6	26	7	11	illegible			27	5	5

* At first Ticheborne is included in this figure, but by 1386 it apparently counts as a separate manor.

† This figure includes one small sum of rent not 'assized', and one rent for term of life.

‡ On some manors the Net Rents vary considerably from the traditional sums due; the defects for vacant lands may amount to £4 or £5, or a special entry of New Rents of part of the demesne may have been added, but variations of any importance are not frequent in Hampshire.

§ By 1601 the Assized Rents were calculated at £26 8*s.* 4*d.*, and they remained unchanged as late as 1747. Cf. Eccles. Com., Various, Bundle 66.

ASSIZED RENTS

Table II (Thames Valley)

	1208–9 £ s. d.	1275 £ s. d.	1284 £ s. d.	1347–8 £ s. d.	1376–7 £ s. d.	1455
Wargrave	25 10 11½	62 15 5½	65 0 2	27 18 5	27 18 5	Farmed £53 6 8
West Wycombe	43 12 2¼	41 16 1¼	41 16 7¼	42 13 8¼	43 3 4¼	Farmed £64 *
Ivingho	Not in Roll	25 9 9½	25 11 5¼	26 13 8¾	27 0 0¾	£27 2 6½
North Waltham	Included with Overton	10 12 9	10 12 9	10 14 11½	13 5 3¼	£10 16 10½*
Culham	Included with Wargrave	?	?	4 8 0½	4 8 3½	Farmed. No Rents entered.
Morton	Not in Roll	4 13 0	4 13 0	5 1 0	5 1 1	Farmed £21.

* In these and one or two other manors of the Thames Valley group, the Rents of Assize and the Commutation of Services are given as one total, for convenience in handing the demesne over to a farmer. It should be noted, however, that the heading, Rents of Assize with Sale of Works, clearly indicates what has been done, and thus the fact does not invalidate the argument (see p. 19) that commuted services were not as a rule added to the Rents of Assize.

Table III (Taunton)

	1284–5 £ s. d.	1347–8 £ s. d.	1376–7 £ s. d.	1455 £ s. d.
Holway	62 15 7½	73 17 10¾	75 1 3¾	123 8 3¼
Poundisford	38 8 0¼	42 4 9¾	42 10 6¼	53 13 9½
Hull	20 14 10½	26 16 5½	26 17 6½	49 5 8½
Nailesbourne	21 2 6½	26 19 5¼	27 11 6¼	39 11 1½
Staplegrove	30 0 6½	44 5 0½	44 6 11	62 6 11½
Rimpton	4 18 0	5 3 0	5 3 0	6 19 4

that the accounts tended to become stereotyped (v. *infra*, p. 37 n.); partly, one cannot help thinking, because the Rents of Assize were not commonly regarded as the result of commutation of labour services. The origin of the Rents of Assize is a question which has hardly been adequately examined. Is it possible that they often represent very early money rents (*Gabulum*) which in some cases may be commutations of rent in kind ? [1] The survival of such payments as ploughshares, capons, eggs, and other commodities by villeins as well as by free tenants seems to lend force to this suggestion. Maitland speaks of an actual increase in the labour services demanded during the thirteenth century,[2] and there is some evidence for similar increase on the Winchester manors. Can it be that comparatively recently imposed labour services, when commuted, were not added to the Rents of Assize ?

A similar suggestion has been thrown out by Mr. K. C. Feiling in the ' English Historical Review ',[3] where he writes : ' This rise of rents [about 30 per cent. between 1368 and 1389] must be explained on some other hypothesis than as fixed commutation for services, which are accounted for as either performed or sold in the usual way.'

If there be any truth in this conclusion (which is clearly proved for the Winchester manors) that the Rents of Assize bear no relation to the commutation of services, then the method pursued by Mr. H. L. Gray loses much of its value. An arithmetical comparison of the rents and of the works rendered or sold throws no light upon the problem of commutation. Of course, it cannot be denied that there are cases (even in the Winchester Pipe Rolls) in which services were definitely commuted into rent, but it is not safe to assume this process without evidence. The custom of remitting rent to certain tenants who performed ordinary ' week-work ' seems to point to the conclusion that rents were prior to

---

[1] Cf. p. 14, note 5.
[2] See Maitland, History of a Cambridgeshire Manor. Cf. also Réville and Petit-Dutaillis, Le Soulèvement des Travailleurs (1898).
[3] April 1911, ' An Essex Manor in the Fourteenth Century ', p. 336 n.

some labour services. Several cases of such remission will be found under the heading *Acquittances* in these Rolls—notably at Brightwell, Harwell, and Witney.[1]

Acquie-
tanciae.

Acquittances appear to have been remittances of rents, in return for special services. The reeve is generally acquitted of 5*s.* ; the ploughman, shepherd, smith, cowman, swineherd, park-keeper, and beadle have acquittances varying from 2*s.* to 5*s.* per annum ; the amounts vary according to the time served, according to the number of ploughs, and sometimes according to the amount of stock kept.

The total amounts rebated appear to have declined after 1208 (though the scale remains unchanged), as they are generally less by 1346 ; in some cases the total rises again slightly by 1453. This method of payment cannot often have been a very important part of the manorial organiza-tion, but it is necessary to take it into account in estimating the wages of any given workman. The ordinary labour services were also remitted in return for special service as ploughman, reeve, &c.[2] On one or two [3] manors this is the form frequently adopted for commuting the ordinary labour services.

At Bishop's Waltham the usual acquittances were not made after a wholesale commutation with the whole homage had been arranged,[4] because *dominus habebit huiusmodi operarios ad liberationem et stipendia sua dum sibi placuerit.* Similar entries are fairly frequent.

---

[1] In the history of ' The Hundred of South Damerham' (Wilts) (by W. H. Black, Esq., and Sir Richard Colt Hoare, Bart., London, 1835) an abstract is given (p. 11) of a survey made in 1539 in which rents are thus distinguished :

		£	s.	d.
(*a*)	Rents of Assize always payable at the feasts of the Annun-ciation and Michaelmas	2	15	7
(*b*)	Rents of the Customary Tenants and Copyholders, with the works and Customs which by tenure of their lands they are bound to do	90	19	10½
(*c*)	Demesne Lands at farm	42	14	8

In 1341 it appears (p. 15) that the Rents of Assize had been valued for a subsidy at 100*s.* It is clear that in this case the commutation of services had not been added to the Rents of Assize, and that it was customary to distinguish between the older rents and the new.

[2] Cf. p. 24.   [3] e. g. Brightwell, 1348-9.
[4] Cf. p. 33.

At Witney, at Brightwell, and at Adderbury the acquittances are far more important ; not only were the rents of
the chief manorial servants remitted, but a similar privilege
was extended to the ordinary virgaters, semi-virgaters, and
cottars, in return for their week-work, both in winter and in
summer. The sums remitted are small, from 9d. to 1s. 1d.
for three days a week during the harvest, but the total
amount of rent remitted reaches £3 or £4. The acquittances at Brightwell were practically the same in 1208 as
in 1346.[1]

The interest of the entries is twofold. First, some information may be deduced from them to supply the lack of an
account of works on the Oxfordshire and Berkshire manors ;
secondly, the fact that rent should be remitted in return for
services rendered hardly harmonizes with the idea that rent
of villein lands is the result of commuted services. The
question arises, Had the lord tired of an early commutation ?
or was the remission a privilege granted to restive villeins ?
or is it possible that the rent was older than the services,
and that the remission is one way of making a slight payment
for more recently imposed services ? There is little or nothing
to show which is the more probable hypothesis.

The *Defects* in rent form a most important item, as it is *Defectus.*
under a secondary heading, *Defectus per pestilentiam,* that
much of the information concerning the Black Death is given.
Moreover, it is from these entries alone that one can gather
any hints as to the relation between size of holdings and
rent ; the areas from which certain sums are due are nearly
always noted, but the proportions appear to be very irregular.[2]
The total defects are commonly trifling in amount, ranging
from 2s. 6d. to £5 per annum. The variations between 1208

---

[1] In 1212, at Sutton, no fewer than 27 manorial servants and *operarii*
were let off part of their rents in return for services, but this custom had
partially died out by 1346.

[2] Sutton, 1348–9

1 virgate	½ virgate	1 acre	1 cotland
10s. per ann.	18s.	6d.	3s.
5s.	5s.		
8s.	3s.		
	2s. 6d.		

In each case the nature of the tenure is not specified.

and 1346 do not seem to admit of any one explanation, while between 1346 and 1455 the total deductions hardly change. By 1346 they had become a conventional item, which might be somewhat misleading, if the earlier records no longer existed. For example, in the fourteenth-century entries for Stoke one finds that of 8 tenements ' drawn into demesne ' 6 had already been counted part of the demesne in 1208. Again, at Burghclere, 335 acres had been added to the demesne before 1208, at a loss of 37s. (? 27s.) in rent, while the same 335 acres are still included among the defects in 1344, and in 1381, at a loss of 27s.

The only precise information as to the relation between rents, area, and services comes from an extent of the Manor of Orchard, which was held of the bishop as three-fourths of a knight's fee, and which came into the lord's hand in June 1348, owing to the minority of the heir. This extent is given here almost in full, as it is the only evidence of the kind available. The rents given for *terra nativa* vary from 7d. to 3d. per acre, but show more uniformity than is usual else-where. For example, the commonest rents for a ferlingland are 3s. 10d. and 2s. 10d. ; if one takes two of these together, the rent of a half-virgate (20 acres) would be 4d. an acre.

Terra Nativa.

	1 virgate	½ virgate	¼ virgate	1 acre
Morton	. 4s.	1s. 10d.	9d.	
Wargrave	. 2s. 7¼d., 2s., 2s. 1½d., 4s.	6d.		8¾d.
				6½d.

Terra Purprestura.

Sutton	1 acre	a Purprestura
	11d.	2s. 8d.
	1s.	3s. 2d.
	6d.	2s. 0d.
	3d.	6d.

Terra nativa thus varied from about 1s. 1d. to 2d. per acre ; *terra pur-prestura* from 1s. to 3d., though 4d. or 6d. is the most usual rent. Free land seems to vary from 2s. 4d. to 3d. per acre (see p. 23), but in this case it is clear that there is no relation between rent and area. Occasionally free land is held by a traditional rent in kind, such as the red rose at Orchard, the pepper and cummin which figure in some of the accounts, the plough-shares, or the arrows due at Farnham.

Only the irregular plots of eight or two acres show any serious variation from this rate, and the variations are to some extent balanced by heavier or lighter services.

' Overland ' varies from 6d. to 9d. per acre. The numerous tenements which were merely dwelling-houses with small plots attached seem to have had proportionately high rents and frequently owed light services as well. The number of tenants free and unfree of the manor was 38 ; at a moderate computation (5 per family) this would give a population of about 190. The acreage held by the tenants must have been about 200 acres,[1] while the area of the demesne was not less than 253 acres. In 1801 the population of Orchard was given as 131 and the acreage as 635.

ABSTRACT OF EXTENT OF MANOR OF ORCHARD, 1347–8.

In Demesne.

List of buildings—Hall, rooms, offices, pigeon-house, garden (6 acres), water-mill, 14 acres of meadow worth 2s. per acre ; pasture, 40 acres of wood ; church taxed at £3, worth £10 ; 193½ acres of arable land, worth 10d. per acre yearly.

Free Tenants.

		s.	d.	
1 messuage with curtilage and 15 acres	Rent = 1		0	yearly, with homage, suit of court, and one red rose on 24 June.
4 acres	,, = 3		0	and suit of court.
1 messuage and 9 acres .	,, = 7		0	,, ,,
2 acres	,, =		6	,, ,,
1 acre	,, = 2		4	,, ,,

Tenants ' in bondagio '.

Holding.		Rent.			Services.
		£	s.	d.	
1. 1 messuage ½ virgate *terra nativa* (=20 acres)	.		6	3	Sept. 29 to June 24. 1 work per week ½d.
2. 1 messuage 10 acres *in bondagio*	.		3	10	June 24 to Aug. 1. Mowing *or* 10d.
3. 1 ,, 10 ,, ,,	.		3	2	August 1 to Sept. 29. Reaping *or* 3s. 4d.
4. 1 ,, 10 ,, ,,	.		3	10	Plough 1 day at Winter and Lent sowing. Suit of Court and of mill.

---

[1] This figure is reached by estimating the messuages, cottages, and curtilages as containing from 2 to 5 acres each.

Holding.	Rent.			Services.
	£	s.	d.	
5. 1 messuage 5 acres *terra nativa* .		3	0	To make haystacks and be paid nothing beyond food, for all services.
6. 1 „ 10 „ „ „ .		3	10	Ditto to No. 1.
7. 1 „ 10 „ „ „ .		2	10	„ „ „
8. 1 „ 10 „ „ „ .		2	10	„ „ „
9. 1 „ 10 „ „ „ .		2	10	„ „ „
10. 1 „ 10 „ „ „ .		2	10	„ „ „
11. 1 „ 5 „ „ „ .		1	6	½ as much as No. 1, but the same mowing and haymaking.
12. 1 „ 8 „ „ „ .		3	8	Reap and bring one man for 3 days and be paid 1d. per day and food.
13. 2 „ „ „ .	*1		0	Reap 6 days with food and 1d. per day.
14. 2 acres of overland .		1	6	For all services.
15. 3 „ „ „ .		1	8	„ „
16. 1 „ „ „ .			6	„ „
17. 1 cottage with curtilage		1	0	Reaps for 3 days with food.
18. 1 „ „ „		1	0	
19. 2 daynas land . .			6	
20. 1 messuage with curtilage		1	4	Reaps one day, gives 1 cock.
21. 3 daynas land . .			6	
22. 1 messuage with curtilage			8	
23. 1 „ „ „		1	0	
24. 1 „ „ „			8	
25. 1 „ „ „		1	0	Reaps 1 day.
26. 1 „ „ „		1	2	Spreads hay, *opus* worth 2d.
27. 1 cottage „ „		2	0	
28. 1 „		1	0	1 Bedrip with food.
29. 1 „		2	0	
30. 1 messuage „ „		1	0	
31. 1 cottage 1 acre		3	8	Mows 7 days.
32. 5 acres . . .		3	0	Makes iron part of 2 ploughs.
33. 1 cottage with curtilage		1	0	
34. 1 „ „ „		1	0	
35. 1 „ „ 1 acre .		2	0	Mows 8 days.
36. 1 „ „ 1 „ 3 roods		2	0	
37. 1 „ „ curtilage		2	0	
38. 1 „ „ „ .			6	
39. 1 place . . .		3	0	
	3	18	1	Total unfree rents.

* If any of these (1–13) be reeve, he shall be quit of all services, rents, and customs.

Works owed.

						£	s.	d.
Opera Manualia	from	9 customers		.	.		13	1½
Mowing and haymaking	,,	10	,,		.		8	4
Harvest works	,,	9	,,		.	1	10	0
,, ,,	,,	8	,,	de prece	.		2	6
Haymaking	,,	1	,,	.	.			2
Smith's works	,,	1	,,	.	.		2	6

Estimated value of Manor.

						£	s.	d.
Rent of capital messuage	.	.	.	.	.		3	4
,, ,, pigeon-house	.	.	.	.	.		3	4
,, ,, garden	.	.	.	.	.		3	4
Value of pasture	.	.	.	.	.		2	0
,, ,, mill	.	.	.	.	.		13	4
Arable land	.	.	.	.	.	8	1	3
Meadow land (14 acres)	.	.	.	.	.	1	8	0
Pasture and underwood or wood	.	.	.	.		10	0
Pleas and perquisites	.	.	.	.	.		3	4
Assized rents	.	.	.	.	.	.	4	12	11
Works, 280	.	.	.	.	.	.		11	8
Haymaking works	.	.	.	.	.		8	4
,, ,,	.	.	.	.	.			2
Harvests	.	.	.	.	.	.	1	10	0
,, ,,	.	.	.	.	.	.		2	6
Smith's work	.	.	.	.	.	.		2	6
Church scot	.	.	.	.	.	.			1½
						18	16	1½

The *Issues* or produce of the manor is an item which varies *Exitus* very considerably in different manors and which tends to *Manerii.* subdivide under different headings. In 1346 it very generally includes such items as :

(*a*) Pannage, Potfald, Lactagium, &c.

(*b*) Peter's pence (occasionally).

(*c*) Produce of pastures, waste, and woods.

(*d*) Skins, eggs, milk, butter, cheese, poultry, fish, occasionally wool, locks of wool, &c., &c.

(*e*) Sale of Works (on about eleven manors in 1347).

The figures given under this head on pp. 162–177 are not very useful in themselves, as it is necessary to know whether the Issues include payments for commuted labour services, rent of pasture, incidental payments such as Peter's Pence, or tolls at fairs. At Otterford, for example, the only item given under this head is 4*s.* for the perquisites of St. Leonard's

fair; at Downton one-third of the total Issues is accounted
for by works either commuted or sold, at Stoke nearly one-
half. At Holway almost the whole amount received is for
hay; e. g. £11 out of £12 18s. 6d. in 1347–8, and £4 out of
£4 15s. 9d. in 1350–1. At Nailesbourne and Rimpton the
pasturage dues (*lactagium*)[1] of 20 cows are 'farmed' for £3, of
19 cows for £3 11s. 6d. or £4. At Rimpton the wood that is
sold is said to have been cleared for the sake of better pasture.

Venditio Pasture.   The increasing value attached to pasture as the waste
land was reclaimed seems to have had important results in
developing the system of leases. In the Somerset and Wiltshire manors, and occasionally in Berkshire or Hampshire,
a separate heading appears, *Venditio Pasture*, under which
are entered the various temporary sales of pasturage on
the demesne lands, on the wastes, along the roadsides, in
the woods, and even on the balks or around the growing corn
crops. This is generally a larger item than the whole of the
other *Exitus Manerii*, excluding corn and stock; it appears
on all the Somerset and Wiltshire manors, and gradually
came to be entered separately on most of the other manors.

The process seems to have been that pasture was sold to
the same buyer for a number of years in succession, at the
same price, and then, after a time, he is granted a 'farm' or
lease for life or for a term of years. His name appears next
year under the comparatively new heading *Firme*, and under
'Sale of Pasture' is the note '*nichil quia ad certum redditum*'.
These leases were by no means new in the fourteenth century,
but they evidently grew more common and more regular
during the years immediately before 1349. They also formed
a precedent for leasing out the arable part of the demesne
in small parcels—a slightly later development.

The 'sale of pasture' meant, of course, pasture for separate
use, though occasionally it was bought by a group of customary tenants. Occasionally a stranger paid a small fee
to be allowed ingress with his beasts to the common pasture.[2]

---

[1] It is not very clear whether *lactagium* here means pasture dues (cf.
Neilson, Customary Rents, p. 75) or literally the farm of their milk; probably the latter.

[2] Mardon, 1348–9: 'Exitus Manerii. Et de ii s. de Johanne atte Wyche

At Holway the mention of a tenement is often accompanied by a note of the number of beasts (2 or 4) which the tenant might turn out on a certain pasture.

Pasture on fallow lands seems to have been sold occasionally. ' Nothing because they were sown this year ' is quite a common entry.[1] It is not always very clear, however, whether this refers only to the demesne lands, in compact holdings. ' Nothing because the lord's beasts were pastured there ' is another usual entry, and would appear, perhaps, to confine the reference to the demesne. This is apparently the only evidence which shows that part, at least, of the demesne must have been cultivated in compact blocks and not in scattered strips.[2]

Firme. This heading is not found in any of the episcopal *Firme.* manors in 1208, nor in 1275, but by 1346 it is a regular item in the accounts of eight of the Somerset and Wiltshire manors. By 1386 it appears in the Hampshire accounts (e. g. Cheriton) and the *Firma Molendinae* is frequent considerably earlier.

The earliest of these ' farms ' seem to have been granted for mills, often with some meadow land attached ; for fish-ponds ; for small plots of meadow land ; for all the pasture in the demesne ; for small plots of pasture newly enclosed ; for *retro-pastura*[3] ; for pasture in a wood.

Although it was by no means uncommon to farm a whole manor,[4] there is no such case in the rolls for 1346, except Otterford, which was farmed to a woman. Pillingsbere had

ut possit habere ingressum in communem pasturam cum animalibus suis ex certa conventione.'

[1] Orchard, 1347–8 (cf. p. 55). The rate of payment for these fallow lands was 8*d.* per week for 43 acres.

[2] It is interesting to compare the treatment of pasture on the Glastonbury manors, where large tracts of moorland seemed to have been divided into small plots of about 5 acres, at a regular rent (*Morgabulum*) of 4*d.* per acre. The rental which describes this disposition of land dates from between 1235 and 1252. The lease system does not seem to have developed for pasture thus allotted. It would be interesting to know if the subdivision into plots necessarily involves the cutting up of the moorland by dykes, as at the present day. Cf. Rentalia et Custumaria . . . of the Abbey of St. Mary of Glastonbury, pp. 33 et seq. Somerset Record Society, v. 1891.

[3] *Retro-pastura* apparently means pasture in the hay-meadows, after mowing.

[4] Several of the Winchester manors were farmed early in the thirteenth century. Cf. Hall. Pipe Roll, p. xvi.

formerly been farmed. The leases noted under the heading *Firme* are generally for one year, the rent being payable quarterly, or for term of life. There are apparently none for term of years until after 1349.[1] Sometimes a lease of pasture was granted to a group of tenants jointly, as at Downton[2] and at Crawley, where the whole homage takes over 40 acres of pasture (*purprestura*) which had formerly been held by John of Kirkeby, for the same rent of 3s. 4d.

The rents paid for meadow or pasture land thus let on lease are interesting. In the Somerset and Wiltshire group of manors the following entries occur :

(*a*) 9s. for 2 acres 1 rood of meadow, on lease for life ;

(*b*) £1 6s. 8d. for pasture, amount unspecified, on yearly lease ;

(*c*) 6d. for a fish-pond on yearly lease.

(*d*) 18s. *De pastura novi clausi de Corfe tenentibus domini dimissa ad voluntatem domini ad quattuor terminos et pro anno futuro xx solidi sic concessa per senescallum* ;

(*e*) 10s. for all the pasture in the demesne, on yearly lease ;[3]

(*f*) 18s. for 14½ acres.

The entries generally contain a note that the pasture is to be used ' without waste ' and *tanquam annexa tenemento suo*. Apparently a fine was levied on the first occasion of letting pasture at farm.[4] Leases and sub-letting among the tenants themselves, both freeholders and villeins, were fairly common and are frequently traceable among the Fines, and in the Court Rolls.[5] Such leases were necessarily preceded

---

[1] Cf. p. 127. [2] Downton, 1346–7, *Firme*; Holway, 1347–8.

[3] Nailesbourne, 1345–6 : ' Et de x s. de Johanne Waterman ut possit habere totam pasturam in dominico domini super la Doune de Kyngestone tam in yeme quam in estate tanquam annexam tenemento suo reddendo inde annuatim pro firma eiusdem x s. et dominus colat dictam terram dominicalem ad libitum suum sicut prius consuevit.'

[4] See Nailesbourne, 1348–9.

[5] Such leases appear as early as 1275. Cf. Witney, and West Wycombe (1284), where leases between tenants for 10 or 20 years are mentioned, though it is not certain that they are customary tenants. These leases for years appear to have died out by 1346, when nearly all the surrenders are

by a formal surrender to the lord in Court, and their terms
are often recorded, as well as the amount of the Fine. The
fines payable on sub-letting appear to have corresponded
roughly with those payable on inheritance, assart land paying
more highly in both cases than villein land.

On most manors a few villeins paid an Annual Recognition [1]
of 2d. or 3d. in order to remain away from the manor so long
as the bishop shall choose ; they also came to one or two
Law-days during the year.   On some manors recognitions
were paid apparently by strangers for permission to remain
' upon the land of St. Swithin ' or ' within the liberty of the
lord ', as long as he shall please, or occasionally ' as long as
they both shall please '.   It is always stipulated in the case
of a villein leaving the manor that he is to remain the lord's
nativus as before.

Annuales Recognitiones.

The recognition is sometimes paid in capons, sometimes
in horse-shoes (*de vi ferreis pedalibus*). It is difficult to decide
whether these dues were commuted, or sold by the reeve
after payment, and entered in terms of money in the accounts.

The sale of corn is almost always separately entered, though
at an earlier and perhaps at a later date, both Stock and
Corn are occasionally included as part of the *Exitus Manerii*.
This entry generally gives exact details of the amounts of
grain sold, with the prices of each sale.   Sometimes a note
states how much is last year's crop ; at Holway and Poundisford a large proportion of the corn is sold to the customary
tenants.   Corn is also frequently bought, to the value of £10
to £30, on the same manors which sell to a similar extent ;
in many cases the corn bought was for seed.   The acreage
sown and the average returns are worked out later (*v.* p 132).
The prices given in the tables annexed roughly correspond
with those of Thorold Rogers,[2] but are often a little lower.

Venditio Bladi.

In the earlier rolls the sales of stock were almost always

Venditio Stauri.

for terms of life. Cf. Tawney, Agrarian Problem in Sixteenth Century,
p. 80, and the Crondal Records (Baigent), Hampshire Record Society, 1891.

[1] Annual gifts were customary on some manors, and are entered as *Dona,
Auxilia*, or *Consuetudines* ; they were, however, generally more substantial
in character than the Recognitions.

[2] History of Agriculture and Prices, vol. i.

included in the *Exitus Manerii* and were not of great importance. By 1346, however, it has become common to sell cattle to the value of £20 or £30 a year (£10 would be an average figure), while stock is often bought on the same manors to the value of £10 to £20. Possibly these sales were effected between different episcopal manors, and were really of the nature of exchanges for breeding purposes ; but even so, it is clear that a manor in the fourteenth century was by no means a self-sufficing and self-consuming economic unit.

Venditio Operum.   *Sale of Works.* This entry appears by 1347 in about eighteen of the manors included in the Pipe Roll ; on twenty-eight other manors the sales are given among the *Exitus Manerii*, and the total is not separately calculated. Where it is entirely omitted, the inference would seem to be that no commutation had taken place, or possibly only that the services owed were all required for the cultivation of the demesne.[1]

In about nine manors[2] a special schedule appears year by year, at the end of the Stock and Corn account, giving exact details of the Labour Services performed, excused, or sold during the year ; on some manors (e.g. Meon and Sutton) it appears in a mutilated or abbreviated form, at intervals ; in the thirteenth century it was more common. It may have been given at intervals, by way of report, from all the manors, or, more probably, the original Compotus Rolls were intended to contain accounts of the 'Works'[3] of all the manors.

In the years 1376–7 it is evident that a full account of the works was demanded, and the returns were enrolled upon the Pipe Roll. Full accounts are given for thirty-five manors besides the Taunton group, and for most of those omitted the account is entered either in the preceding or following year.

Thus so far as these later entries may be used for an earlier date, an almost complete account of the works due is available,

---

[1] Cf. p. 56. Works were sold on several manors as early as 1208.

[2] i. e. the Taunton group, together with Meon and Sutton in Hampshire.

[3] Holway, 1347–8 : ' *Messio per acram.* Et de messione xviii acras dimidia bladorum proveniente de diversis custumariis ut patet in rentale.' Poundisford, 1350–1 : ' *Exitus Manerii.* Compertum est per examinationem Pipe quod arrabunt ad semen hoc anno totidem acras de terra dominica. . . .' Cf. also Introd. p. 10.

PRICES OF WHEAT (HAMPSHIRE)

	1346–7	1347–8	1348–9	1349–50	1350–1	1351–2	1355
Stoke	—	8/8	5/–, 6/–, 3/4	8/–	10/–	14/–	7/4
Droxford	—	8/8	3/4, 4/–, 5/–	5/8, 8/–	6/8	14/–	5/–
Beauworth	—	7/4, 8/8*	5/–	9/–, 8/–	7/4, 10/–	—	8/–
Cheriton	6/–, 9/4	8/8, 4/8	8/8 { ? 5/–	—	8/8	14/–	5/–, 6/–
Sutton	—	8/8	6/– and 5/–	8/–	9/–, 8/–, 5/–	8/8, 9/8, 10/–	8/–
Crawley	—	6/8, 8/8	4/–, 5/–, 6/–	9/–, 8/–	9/4, 10/–	14/–	8/–

* To the King.

PRICES OF WHEAT (SOMERSET)

	1346–7	1347–8	1348–9	1349–50	1350–1	1351–2	1353–4
Hull	—	5/6, 8/–, 8/2*	5/6, 4/6, 4/4	8/–, 6/8, 8/10	12/2	14/2*	5/4, 6/10
Poundisford	—	5/–, 8/2*	5/–, 4/4	8/10	12/2	14/2*	6/10
Nailesbourne	—	5/–, 8/2*	5/6, 5/–, 4/8	6/8, 8/10	12/2	14/2*	6/10
Holway	—	8/2*, 8/–, 4/8	c. 5/–	6/8, 8/10	10/8, 12/2	14/2*	5/–, 6/10
Staplegrove	—	5/–, 8/2	5/6, 4/8	7/4, 6/8, 8/10	12/2	14/2	6/10, 5/4
Rimpton	—	8/–, 6/8, 5/–	No wheat sold	8/–, 4/–, 6/8	10/8	14/–	5/4
Downton	—	8/–, 8/8	4/–	6/8, 7/–, 9/4	8/–, 7/4	14/– †	6/–

* Sold to the Customers.   † Sold to the King.

and it is evident that the non-appearance of this section does not imply that in that case all services were commuted. Indeed, it is by no means clear that all services had been commuted on any of the bishop's manors ; certainly not on more than two or three, even by 1377. These custumals or accounts of works will be analysed separately, but their existence must be explained here, in connexion with the *Venditio Operum.*

The phrase ' Sale of Works ' [1] covers two distinct arrangements : (*a*) payments made by the customary tenants for surplus services, owed to but not required by the lord ; (*b*) definite and more or less permanent commutation of services for money payments. In the first case, the number of works sold would obviously vary according to various circumstances, of which the weight of the crops would be the most important. It might well happen that the lord realized a large sum from the sale of works without needing to hire any wage-paid labourers.[2] Thus to sell works is not at all equivalent to commuting them, though it is easy to see how the earlier practice led on to commutation. In the second case, the old labour services would be replaced by hired workmen, or sometimes by regular workmen elected in rotation by the homage, from amongst themselves.

Commutation took many forms ; the immediate advantage of both tenant and lord weighed more heavily than consideration of principle or of uniformity. The lord generally protected his interests by inserting a saving clause *quamdiu domino placuerit* into the new arrangement ; such a clause, however, could hardly hold its own against an unbroken custom of twenty or thirty years.

The Sale of Works also varied considerably in its nature ; sometimes it was a bargain with individuals, sometimes with the whole body of customers. It has been pointed out that

---

[1] On this see Maitland, History of a Cambridgeshire Manor (Collected Papers, ii. 371 ; English Hist. Rev., 1894) : ' There can be little doubt that they (i. e. the *opera vendita*) were sold to those who were bound to do them—that is to say, when the lord did not want the full number of works he took money instead at the rate of a halfpenny for a winter or summer work, and of a penny for an autumn work.' Cf. also Fleta, c. 72.

[2] Cf. p. 217.   Addenda.

labour services were often imposed upon the tenantry in a lump, so that repartition among them remains their private affair, while the lord demands the performance of the whole.[1] In such cases the tenants could often make a profitable arrangement with the lord, at a lower rate of commutation than was usual for the services of a single virgate. The bargains made at Bishop's Waltham are specially interesting, as they represent different types of sale and commutation on the same manor.

(a) The whole homage paid £16 13s. 4d. in commutation of all their manual[2] and carting services, with the reservation that the Lord Bishop shall have from among the said customers a reeve, beadle, woodward, shepherd, swineherd, ploughman, carter, and all other servants as he had been accustomed to have. Moreover, he reserved to himself one boon-work in harvest (*Dagbedrip*) and also *Landright, Benhurche*, and *Forhors*, as he had been accustomed to have them.[3] This commutation is expressly said to be intended to last ' *quamdiu domino placuerit* '.

(b) At Waltham there are two or three other examples of a bargain made between the lord and a group of customers. The whole 'hundred' of Waltham pays £4 16s. 9½d. for works which have been commuted, ' *quia tantum plus solebant operare* '.[4]

The homage of Droxford pay £1 for certain carting services (carrying corn to Waltham) which were formerly owed. Again the ploughmen and the shepherds (*custodes bidentium*) commuted their obligations for £1 6s. 8d., with the proviso that the lord should feed and pay other ploughmen and shepherds ' *quamdiu ei placuerit* '.

Some of the special ploughing services (*Arrura* or Landryght) were also commuted, although in the original agreement they had been reserved by the lord.

[1] Vinogradoff, Growth of the Manor, p. 319, and Villeinage in England, p. 279. Cf. Sutton, 1376-7, where it is noticed that the customers of Ropley mow a meadow for the customers of Sutton for 1s. 6d. per annum by a composition made between them *absque concilio domini*.

[2] *Opera Manualia* is a technical term, meaning undefined services of men, not involving oxen, horses, ploughs, or carts ; it does not, as a rule, include harvest-works, but cf. p. 65. In some districts the manual services could evidently be utilized for team-work, if the lord provided the team.

[3] Waltham, 1346-7, and all subsequent years. This commutation does not appear as early as 1301, but I have not discovered when it was first made. Cf. p. 217. Addenda.

[4] This bargain appears as early as 1301. Part of the demesne had been let at a money rent, hence this commutation.

(c) On the same manor the services on a certain plot of land had been remitted by charter, and the land made free.[1] The entry appears under the heading *Venditio Operum*, and the 3s. 2½d. that was paid seems to be a permanent commutation which was not added to the rents.

(d) There are also entries at Waltham under the heading *Custus Carucarum*, which show that the opposite process to commutation had also begun.[2] Small payments were made by the lord to the customers in return for labour-services, especially for ploughing and harrowing at the two seed-times; these payments were not of the nature or rate of wages, but were by way of a ' boon ' from the lord, or were probably in some cases commutations of the customary meals provided.[3] The rates of payment are interesting.

(i) *Winter Sowing.* Twenty-six ploughs plough 52 acres for 26d. i. e. ½d. per acre. It is expressly stated elsewhere [4] that one ploughing is valued at 6d.–9d. per acre. while *arrura de prece* is said to have been paid at ½d. per acre, and valued at 7½d. more. Harrowing was apparently only valued at 1d. per acre. The rates varied from manor to manor; these examples, taken from Somerset, can only roughly be transferred to Hampshire, where 6d. per acre was perhaps more usual.

(ii) *Spring Sowing.* Thirty-eight ploughs plough 38 acres for 3s. 2d. i.e. 1d. per acre. These ploughings are called *precariae*, and had, perhaps, retained some traces of having been originally *boon*-days.[5]

[1] Waltham, 1437–48 : 'Et de 3s. 2½d. de terra Totenhulle quam Willelmus Wodeloke tenuit et terra atte Frethe quam Johannes Everard modo tenet que facte sunt libere per cartam domini J. de Pontissara Wyntoniensi Episcopi ' [1282–1305].

[2] Cf. Marwell, 1347–8, where 1d. is paid at both sowings.

[3] Waltham, 1345–6 : ' *Venditio Operum*. Et de xviii s. de arrura liii acrarum quod dicitur Landryght precita et vendita custumariis hoc anno.' This commutation must have been made later than the first bargain quoted, which expressly reserves Landright.

[4] Rimpton, 1348–9 : ' Et de viii aruris estivalibus provenientibus de eisdem custumariis viii carucas habentibus ad warectam in estate per unam diem capientibus de domino 1d. vel eorum gentaculum, et tunc valet arura per diem ultra reprisam, v d.'

[5] Payment for ' *Precariae* ' at the rate of 2d. per acre appears on the neighbouring manor of Crondal (Sutton) as early as 1248, v. Crondal Records (Hampshire Record Society) pt. i, p. 77, where a Compotus Roll of 1248 is printed.

The total amount of the *Venditio Operum* at Bishop's Waltham is almost unchanged between 1346 and 1424 ;[1] it is made up as follows :

26 small items from 8*d.* to 6*s.*

2 small items from 14*s.* to 18*s.*

3 or 4 larger items from £1 upwards.

1 item of £8 from 12 carters.

1 item of £16 13*s.* 4*d.* from the whole homage.[2]

Thus the sums paid seem to have been definitely fixed and allotted, whereas on other manors the number of works sold varied from year to year with the exigencies of the lord's harvest and other work.

It is interesting to compare with the value of the commuted works the wages paid at Waltham for the same year. The items are scattered through the second schedule of the account, the expenses. Only the fairly normal employments have been taken ; casual labour in repairs, in carrying water for a few odd days, as well as the work of plumbers and builders and carpenters, has been omitted, though the rate of wages paid to such workmen is interesting. Supplementary allowances of corn and other provisions were made to most of the regular servants.

TABLE OF WAGES, 1345–6.

£	s.	d.			£	s.	d.	
	2	2	for *precariae*			1	6	for mowing Ballesmede
	2	3	,, ,,				8	,, turning hay
	4	6	,, ,,			1	0	,, mowing Mere meadow
	16	0	,, 2 ploughmen, 2 'fu-gatori'				3	,, turning hay
	8	0	,, 2 carters				4	,, mowing Crikelescroft
	2	0	,, 1 dairymaid				1	,, turning hay
	2	0	,, 1 cowherd (½ year)			10	0	,, mowing 3 meadows
	12	0	,, 3 shepherds			4	0	,, turning hay
2	8	0	,, park-keeper			1	4	,, carrying hay
	2	6	,, mowing park		5	19	1	Total
		6	,, turning hay					

[1] Additional commutations were apparently entered in the *Exitus Manerii*, and were considered to be made from year to year. Cf. Waltham, 1353–4. At Burghclere (1348–9) the commutations in some cases had been made by charter *ad terminum vite.*

[2] Waltham, 1346–7 : ' In acquietanciis bercarii, carucarii, et aliorum operariorum qui solebant operare ad curiam de Waltham nichil hoc anno quia opera eorum arentantur ut patet inferius in capitulo de vendicione operum. . . .'

Waltham was one of the bishop's residences, and its accounts are constantly complicated by heavy expenses for building, repairs, &c. In 1345–6 the following occasional wages were paid:

1s. 3d. per week to the carpenter.
2s. 3d. ,,   ,,   to the thatcher and his assistants (number not stated).
1s. 1d. per day to a *plumbator* and his assistants.

Threshing was paid at 3d. per 10 bushels for wheat, and 1d. per quarter for barley.

The harvest expenses work out as follows:

£	s.	d.	
4	2	10	harvesting 142 acres beyond the 40 acres harvested by the *Dagbedrip* (7d. per acre).
	1	2	watching corn by night.
	7	0	hiring carts.
	5	0	wages to one ripereve for 20 days.
4	16	0	

Thus the wages-bill, apart from building operations, amounted to about £11 or £12, and in ordinary years did not approach the £37 2s. 10½d. which represents the commuted services.[1]

At Droxford in 1348–9 the proportions are very different; works were sold to the value of £9 6s. 10¼d., but the wages paid amounted to £8 10s. 7¼d. (omitting quite casual employment).

There is no evidence in contemporary rolls that any

[1] TABLE OF WAGES, WALTHAM, 1350–1.

£	s.	d.		£	s.	d.	
	1	3	for *precariae*		12	0	for 3 shepherds
	1	10	,, ,,		6	8	,, keeping park-palings
	16	0	,, 2 ploughmen 2 *fugatori*				in order
	8	0	,, 2 carters	3	0	10	,, park-keeper (2d.p.d.)
	2	0	,, 1 dairymaid	1	10	9¼	,, threshing
	4	0	,, 1 cowherd	2	11	5	,, hoeing and mowing
	6	0	,, thatcher (?)	6	0	0	,, wages of the bailiff
	2	6	,, woman helping thatcher (2d. p.d.)				(the rest at Droxford)
	7	6	,, washing and shearing sheep	16	10	9¼	

The wages of the bailiff ought not to be included in comparing this table with the total for 1345–6.

services except those specially reserved (*v. supra*) were actually performed at Bishop's Waltham, but the comparatively small wages-bill would lead one to suppose that many of the customary services must have survived, although they are not mentioned. In 1376–8, however, a special return of all the labour services still due was entered on the Pipe Roll ; if it be permissible to carry its evidence backward, the subjoined table will complete the picture of the organization of a manor just before the visitation of the Black Death.

An examination of this table suggests several comments. The list shows no ploughing, but the bishop had already bargained to retain ploughmen from the customary tenants, the Landright is already accounted for among the *Opera vendita*, and the cultivated part of the demesne was comparatively small (cf. p. 133).

It is noticeable, too, that all the services retained are occasional, and, with the exception of the harvest and harrowing works, form the less essential part of the manorial economy. All the regular weekly services had been commuted for a fixed sum, while the chief permanent servants of the manor were either wage-paid, or chosen in rotation from among the customers. Although Waltham was a very large manor (it had at least ten tithings, and required six reeves) the demesne seems to have demanded little additional labour, except for the upkeep of the bishop's residence, and at times for the work of enclosing and planting hedges.[1] Again, the list of tenants who owed services (only 37 in all) shows that they were all holders of something less than a virgate ; evidently the more important tenants had commuted their works, while the smaller men were still held to theirs.[2] This is definitely stated to be the case at Farnham

---

[1] Waltham is an excellent example of the way in which an item in the manorial accounts became stereotyped, and when it was necessary to change or to add to the total, the change was made under some different heading. Thus additional commutations, after the sum of £37 2s. 10½d. had been fixed for the *Venditio operum*, were added to the *Exitus Manerii*, while the wages paid for enclosing and hedging appear under the *Custus Domorum et necessariorum*. It is not safe to assume that an entry does not exist because it is not to be found in the expected place.

[2] See p. 217. Addenda.

BISHOP'S WALTHAM, 1377–8.

	Works due.	Provenance.	Acquittances.	Defects.	Performed.	Sold.
Harrowing	27¾ acres	19 semivirgates 17 ferlingmen 1 half-ferlingman	1 acre	½ acre	26¾ acres	35½ opera*
Making hurdles	50½ opera		2 opera	1 opus	12 opera	
Enclosing park	126½ ,,		7½ ,,	—	118½ ,,	
Moving sheep-fold	64 ,,		2 ,,	2 opera	60 ,,	
Carrying bushes	104 ,,		3 ,,	86½ † ,,	12 ,,	
Wood-cutting	86½ ‡ ,,		—	—	All	
Shearing sheep, &c..	101 ,,		4 ,,	—	97 ,,	
Mowing and turning hay	26¾ acres		1 acre	—	25¼ acres	
Hay-carrying	172 opera		5 opera	120½ opera §	47 opera	
Stacking hay	145 ,,		—	—	All	
Hoeing and weeding	101 ,,		4 ,,	2 ,,	97 ,,	
Precariae Autumpnales	145 ,,		4 ,,	—	145 ,,	
Opera Autumpnalia	1060½ ,,		247 ,,	21 ,,	18 ‖ ,, (sic)	
Stacking corn	20 ,,		—	—	All	

The remaining services were generally owed by different combinations of the 37 customers who owed the harrowing services, with one or two inconsiderable additions.

* Not asked for.   † Because tenants have no ploughs (sic).

‡ This service is a substitute for the carting lacking in line above.   ‖ Et equat (sic).

§ Because the tenants have no horses or carts.

(1346), where 12 cottars and 6 lesser cottars were not allowed to commute the wood-cutting and carrying services, of which the holders of 146 virgates were quit for a lump sum of £29 4s. 6d. for all their works.

The early commutation of the services of *bordarii* and *cottarii* is well known, and its reaction upon the virgaters has been noticed,[1] but the converse would seem to be at least equally true on the manors of the Bishop of Winchester. Especially where the lower tenants owed *Opera Manualia* (unspecified services of a man, without horse or cart) their services tended to survive, because the lord could turn the undefined works to account in any new development of agriculture.[2] Wherever the commutation of services appears to have been particularly favourable to the customers, as it was in most of the collective bargains, one may expect to find that it applied mainly to the holders of a full virgate, the weightier members of the village community, and that the smaller tenants remained burdened with such services as the lord wished to retain.

The same principle seems to hold good between free-holders and villeins; the free tenants were often bound to do ploughing or carrying services, but in some cases they were not called upon[3] if the work could be done by the customary tenants without additional help.

When the smaller tenants could not perform the services due, because they had no horses or carts, they were either let off or were allowed to substitute other services. Certain works, such as the making of hurdles or the washing of sheep remained somewhat indefinite in amount; a fixed number was owed, with a condition that if the lord required more, more should be forthcoming. In these cases, if less was required, the surplus works were not generally sold, but simply excused.

[1] Vinogradoff, Growth of the Manor, p. 353.
[2] Cf. the tables on pp. 89–96.
[3] Burghclere, 1345–6. *Exitus Manerii.* The free tenants were allowed to pay 3s. for their ploughing services at Michaelmas, because the villeins ploughed for the winter sowing and the fallow. The same entry is repeated in 1381–2.

The information at Bishop's Waltham is unusually full
and varied, but similar details may be gathered from many of
the other manors. Nowhere else, however, does the collective
bargain appear on so large a scale,[1] nor is the sale of works
at a permanently fixed rate elsewhere.[2]

A sharp distinction has been drawn by Mr. T. W. Page, in
his study of 'The Disappearance of Villeinage in England',[3]
between the *Spanndienste* and the *Handdienste*, the services
requiring horses or oxen and those requiring only manual
labour ; the former, he thinks, had been almost entirely commuted by 1350, while the latter remain practically unchanged
on the majority of manors. It is difficult to find any confirmation of this distinction in the Account Rolls of the Bishops
of Winchester. Commutation and sale of both kinds of work
are common on almost all the episcopal manors by 1346 ;
that is to say, there are notices of individual commutations
on almost every manor (i. e on 43 in 1343–4), but these commutations affect only a very small number of the tenants.
The ' sale of works ' on the other hand probably affected
almost every unfree tenant at different times, though in
varying degrees from year to year. Not only are the ploughing-
services still performed on a large number of manors[4] in 1346,
but surplus ploughing-services were owed and often sold, while
ploughing done as *Precariae* (or *Arrura de Prece*) was allowed
a small gratuity in money, sometimes as at Downton
amounting to 2d. per acre. On some manors a more elastic
system prevailed ; ploughing and harrowing were still owed,
but part of the ploughing was sold, while additional harrowing
was provided by the customers owing *Opera Manualia*.[5]

---

[1] Farnham perhaps excepted. See above. An interesting example of
a collective bargain is found at Wield in 1349, v. *Walda* 1348–9 *Venditio
Operum*. ' Et de xi s. i d. de tota villata (vill') pro herciatura eis relaxata
quia dominus herciabit pro eis Deustland.'

[2] Except at Droxford, which was very closely connected with Bishop's
Waltham, if indeed it was not originally part of the manor.

[3] Page, T. W., The Disappearance of Villeinage in England. New
York, 1900.

[4] There is evidence that it was done on all the first 16 manors that I
examined ; there is no evidence that it was not done on most of the others ;
indeed the wages-bill makes it clear that very little ploughing could have
been paid for. Cf. p. 59 for further evidence.

[5] See tables on pp. 89–96.

The greatest difficulty in dealing with the question of commutation is to discover on what principle the services were valued. When works were sold the prices ranged from $\frac{1}{2}d.$ each for manual works in winter to $1\frac{1}{2}d.$ or $2d.$ per day for harvest works, while ploughing was sold at from $6d.$ to $10d.$ per acre. The definition of a work evidently varied on different manors. At Holway it is stated that one work meant the work of one man for half a day; at Wargrave a work is half a day in winter and one day in summer; sometimes the day lasted till the ninth hour. A harvest work might mean the work of the whole family except the house-wife. At Stoke a work in mowing-time meant mowing three swathes of grass each 12 feet wide, in some of the meadows, while in the park, which was estimated at $31\frac{1}{2}$ acres, the three swathes were only to be 4 feet in width. Threshing was valued at from $2d.$ to $5d.$ per quarter. The *Averagia* were valued at $6d.$ each at Brightwell. At Rimpton threshing 1 quarter of wheat was reckoned as 4 works; 1 whole day harrowing with a horse counts as 4 works; sowing 1 bushel of beans as 2 works. At Wargrave an '*opus*' meant half a day from Michaelmas to August, a whole day from August to Michaelmas. At Itchingswell reaping half an acre constituted one *opus*.

The services due from a virgate differed also very considerably on different manors; it is not clear, however, why virgates on the same manor paid at such different rates. The varying estimates seem to suggest either that the land was originally very unevenly burdened, even within the same manor, or that the commutations took place at very different dates. Possibly some of the differences are due to the confusion of classes which undoubtedly followed the Norman Conquest. Lighter economic burdens may point backwards to a higher social or legal status for some of the villagers now lumped together as *villani*. Again, there seems to have been a tendency during the thirteenth century for the lord to insert an extra day of week-work in the totals required from his tenants. Some commutations evidently date from the very early years of the thirteenth century, probably

from the twelfth, and these would almost certainly have
escaped with a lighter valuation. Services relaxed by charter,
often as a personal favour, may have been lightly reckoned.
The size of the virgate is another factor to be taken into
account.[1]

The fact, however, remains, that virgates paid at very
different rates, and that the amount of money derived from
commutation is no clue whatever to the area of land freed,
nor to the amount of wage-paid labour required. The
following table will perhaps make this clear:

VALUATION OF COMMUTED WORKS.

Manor.	Area.	Works commuted.	Valuation. s. d.
Sutton . .	1 virgate	all	4 6 *
,,	,,	,,	2 0
,,	,,	all, with church-scot	16 7½
,,	1 cotland	,, ,, ,,	1 6¼
Marwell .	1 customer	all	4 0
,,	,,	,,	6 8
Crawley .	,,	,,	6 8
Wield . .	1 cottage, 10 acres	,,	2 6
Wargrave .	1 virgate	,,	c. 3 0 †
,,	,,	,,	2 0
,,	,,	,,	3 3½
Waltham St. Lawrence	,,	,,	3 0 ‡
,,	,,	threshing	c. 0 4½
Culham .	,,	all	3 6 §
,,	½ virgate	,,	1 0
,,	1 coterellus	,,	0 9
Burghclere .	1 virgate	,,	7 0
,,	1 cotland	all, and church-scot	6 8 ‖
Itchingswell	1 virgate	,,	7 1
,,	,,	,,	6 8
,,	1 cotland	,,	3 6
,,	½ ,,	,,	0 6
Meon . .	Land of Wm. Fisshere	80 works [carting and harvest]	2 2 ¶

---

[1] See p. 50 for note on the measured acre and the customary acre.

* All these holdings are in the hand of Roger Haywood; the commutation is said to have been made ' *quia nullus tenere voluit* '.

† Here 32 virgates pay equally.

‡ 23 virgates pay equally.

§ 5 virgates pay equally.

‖ Commuted by charter *ad terminum vite* (3 lives).

¶ 26 tenants pay 2s. 2d. in commutation of works from land formerly
held by Wm. Fisshere.

At Sutton it is possible to compare the value of the works of an *operarius* with the rates paid as commutation by a virgate. The *operarii* in 1349–50 owed 81 week-works, and 37 harvest-works between August 1 and Michaelmas; these appear to have been uniformly sold at the rate of 1½*d*. each, and thus each *operarius* owed services to the value of 14*s*. 9*d*. per annum. If it is safe to carry back information given under the date 1376–7, one finds that some of the virgaters and semi-virgaters owed ploughing services (4 acres per annum and 12 acres per annum) which must have been worth 2*s*. or 6*s*. a year at a very moderate estimate, to say nothing of all the other services owed by them.[1] Thus when it is stated that all the works of a virgate were commuted for 2*s*. or 4*s*. 6*d*. it is evident that the valuation must have been based on 'beneficial' calculations, even admitting that the commutation may have taken place at a very early date. The valuation of works in the Taunton district will be treated later, as the evidence is separately and clearly entered under the schedule of ' Works '.[2]

These facts about commutation, inconclusive as they are, show the difficulty of basing any theory upon the growth of the item *Opera Vendita*, and the misleading nature of any attempt to deduce the necessary expenditure on wages from a comparison of the sales or commutation of services. Again, they may show how difficult it is to decide whether the services on any manor have been entirely, or half, or inconsiderably commuted, or whether one can safely adopt any such classification.[3]

However, with this tentative examination of the evidence, the way is cleared for search into the results of the Black Death on the process of commutation, but the clearing of the way serves mainly to disclose the many pitfalls into which it is only too easy to fall.

Fines and Marriages. The entry *Purchasia Curiae*, which is used in 1208, has by 1346 subdivided into 'Fines and Marriages ', and ' Perquisites of the Court '. The latter entry *Fines et Maritagia.*

---

[1] Cf. p. 110.   [2] Cf. p. 62.

[3] Cf. p. 149.

appears to contain all the ordinary judicial dues of the Court, while under the former the normal payments of tenants are included.

The chief items given are :

(a) Tithing-penny.

(b) Fines on entry upon lands held in villeinage.

(c) Reliefs on entry upon free lands.[1]

(d) Fines on sales or leases between villein tenants.[2]

(e) Fines on leases from the lord bishop*; also on pasture let ' at farm '.

(f) Fines on exchanges between villeins.[3]

(g) Fines on both parties in suit for possession of lands.[4]

(h) Fine for marriage of daughter within the manor.

(i) Fine for marriage of daughter without the manor.

(j) Fine for marriage with an heiress of land.

(k) Fine for taking over wardship with land.[5]

(l) Fine for inheriting annual rent.[6]

(m) Fine for reversion to grantor of land let for term of life.

(n) Fine on first relaxation or commutation of works.[7]

(o) Fine for converting land from one status to another.[8]

The rates at which the fines are levied are most difficult to ascertain, if indeed they were not purely arbitrary. There appears to be no support whatever in these accounts to the assertion that a fine was roughly equivalent to a year's rent.[9] Perhaps each holding had a traditional fine, which bore little or no relation to its area. In one case it is specially noted that a man would not pay a ' reasonable fine ', which his mother afterwards paid, but this fine was certainly unusually heavy,[10]

---

[1] Downton, 1349–50. Sutton (Tychborne) 1350–51. Sutton, 1348–9.

[2] Sutton, 1348–9. Cf. Tawney, Agrarian Revolution, p. 80.

[3] Sutton, 1346–7.

[4] Holway, 1347–8.

[5] Droxford, 1351–2.

[6] Sutton, 1349–50.

[7] Brightwell, 1349–50.

[8] Holway, 1350–1. Cf. p. 52, n. 4.

[9] T. W. Page, op. cit., p. 28.

[10] Staplegrave, 1347–8 : ' Et de vi li. vi s. viii d. de Matillda que fuit uxor Johannis de Tonbrigge pro 1 mesuagio et dimidia virgata terre native

and the circumstances were complicated. The part played by the sworn customers in deciding the final allocation of the land is noteworthy as illustrating the village acting in its communal capacity.[1] This half-virgate of land in Tonbrigge must have been profitable to the bishop, for a year later we find it surrendered by the said Matilda to another woman, and a second fine was paid,[2] slightly heavier than the first.

On one occasion, at Bitterne, a very large fine was repaid because it was proved by inquest and examination of the Pipe Roll that the land in question was not 'finable'.[3] No clue is given as to the reason for such an exemption, save the fact that fines had not previously been paid. It should be noted, however, that this is no ordinary tenement, but a house, water-mill, and pigeon-house, with a few acres of moor and marsh. Fines were paid on many other tenements in Bitterne and Fawley, though the tenements were generally small and irregular, and the fines unimportant in amount. There is, therefore, nothing to show why this particular holding was not 'finable', but it is possible that it was a free tenement. In 1376–7 another holding is definitely stated to be *terra finabilis*. The Court Rolls also show this distinction, but give no explanation.

in decena de Tonbrigge que fuerunt dicti Johannis viri sui ex concessione domini Episcopi retinendi licet dictus Johannes viii acras terre tenementi praedicti Johanni filio suo alias reddiderit pro quibus idem Johannes filius rationabilem finem dare recusavit, et tunc quia compertum est per xxxii custumarios juratos quod dictus Johannes pater tempore reddicionis morti fuit praeoccupatus nec aliquid pro victu ejusdem Matilldae ordinatum fuit dicta reddicio [omnino ?] adnichilatur.'

[1] Cf. p. 68.

[2] Staplegrave, 1348–9: 'Et de vii li. de Johanna filia Johannis Oseborn pro i mesuagio et dimidia virgata terre native in decena de Tonbrigge ex redditione Matilldae que fuit uxor Johannis de Tonbrigge habendis.'

[3] Bytterne: 'Et de vi li. xiii s. iiii d. de Johanne Langeforde et Cecilia uxore ejus pro i mesuagio i columbario i molendino aquatico viii acris more et marisci in Fallee ex redditione Johannis filii Radulfi Mounselowe habendis sibi et rectis heredibus dicti Johannis de Langeforde et postea compertum est quod dicta tenementa non sunt finabilia ut plenius patet in pede istius compoti.' A partially illegible note appears to the effect that scrutiny of the Pipe Roll, inquest, and other methods of proof were employed.

The varying amounts of the fines may be illustrated by the following table.

TABLE OF FINES.

Manor, and Amount of Land.	Description.	Occasion.	£	s.	d.
West Wycombe : *1 virgate	villein	marriage with heiress .	4	0	0
Knoyle : *½ virg. (2 acres assart land)	villein	*per totum homagium electus*			6
Meon : *10 acres	?	lease for life from his son .		1	8
Waltham : 1 rod land	?	on lease . . .		4	0
Staplegrave † : *½ virg.	villein	taken up by widow .	6	6	8
,, *5 acres	villein	recovered in suit .	3	6	8
,, *5 acres, 4 dayns of 1 virg.	'over- land'	previous tenant a felon .	3	6	8
,, *1 virg.	villein	marriage with heiress .	8	0	0
Holway : 4½ dayns	over- land ?	recovered in suit . .		1	8
Poundisford : *½ virg. 1 rod	villein over- land }	lease for life . . .	6	13	4
Downton : *1 virg.	villein	*ad hoc compulsus* . .	1	0	0
Downton (1349) : 1 toft, site of fulling mill ; 3 pieces meadow ; 10 acres in Wyne ; 1 croft containing 36 acres ; 6 crofts of lord's waste ; 19 acres of bord- land		? from father on condition of re-building mill, and taking lease for life at 20s. per annum		1	0
Nailesbourne : 2 mes. 2 fis- acre land (?) (fifacre land ?)	villein	? . . .		2	0
Rimpton (1349–50) : *5 acres	,,	not inherited . .		6	8
Rimpton (1349–50) : *1 virg.	,,	? .	4	10	0
Rimpton (1349–50) : *½ virg.	,,	not inherited .	2	13	4
Rimpton (1347–8) : *1 virg.	,,	marriage with heiress .	10	0	0
Droxford (1350–1) : *½ virg.	,,	lease . . .		13	4
Droxford (1351–2) : *1 ferling	,,	? wardship . .		10	0
Twyford (1354–5) : *½ virg.	,,	*electus per homagium* .		10	0
Beauworth (1381 ?) : *1 virg.	,,	from mother ; mother's second husband had forfeited it after her death	1	0	0
Sutton (1348–9) : *1 virg.	,,	from husband . .	1	8	4
Sutton (1348–9) : 5 *solidi*	,,	from uncle . . .	1	8	0
,, ,, 1 *denarr'*	assart land	,, . .		1	0
,, ,, 22 *denarr'*	assart land	from father . . .		3	0
,, *1 virg.	villein	,, . . .	3	0	0
Sutton (1348–9) : *½ virg.	,,	from cousin . . .		10	0

* All the tenements marked thus included a messuage.

† If the 4*d.* per acre rent which was common at Orchard prevailed on the other Taunton manors, these fines will be seen to amount to from 12 to 40 years' rent.

That the very high fines mentioned above (p. 44) were not infrequent nor merely local may be shown by the following table, which has been compiled simply by selecting the highest fine paid on each manor in the year 1345–6:

	Fine.			Holding.
	£	s.	d.	
Holway . . .	1	0	0	1 messuage, 2 acres and 1 dayn of overland ; 5 acres villein land ; 2 acres villein land.
,, . . .	1	6	8	1 mes. and 13 acres villein land.
Nailesbourne . .	Nothing above 8s.			
Poundisford . .	2	0	0	10 acres of overland.
,, . .	6	0	0	1 mes., 1 virgate 1 ferling villein land ; 2 dayns overland.
,, . .	9	0	0	for marriage with the heiress of the above lands.
Staplegrave . .	6	13	4	1 mes., 1 virg., and 1 cottage; 1 ferling villein land.
Hull . . .	Nothing above 6s. 8d.			
Rimpton . . .	Nothing above 2s.			
Downton . . .	2	13	4	1 mes., 1 virg. villein land.
Knoyle . . .	Nothing above 10s.			
Fonthill . . .	None.			
Bishopston . .	,,			
Upton . . .	,,			
Twyford . . .	1	3	4	1 mes., 1 virg. villein land.
Stoke . . .	1	10	0	1 mes., ½ acre villein land.
Burghclere . .	7	0	0 (marriage with heiress)		1 mes., 1 vir. 3 rods, 1 acre assart land.
Ashmansworth . .	5	10	0	1 mes., 1 virg., 14 acres assart land.
Itchingswell . .		16	4	mill, mes., cotland, 8 acres assart land [a woman retains this complex tenement ' eo minus etate, quia lxxii annorum et plus '].
Woodhay . . .		10	0	
Overton . . .		10	0	
North Waltham .	None.			
Witney . . .		13	4	
Adderbury . .	5	6	8	8 acres (unspecified) ; 3 acres meadow.
Harwell . . .		3	4	
Brightwell . .	8	0	0 (marriage with heiress)		1 mes., 1 virg. villein land.
,,	7	0	0	1 virg. villein land.
Ivingho . . .	1	13	4	1 mes., 1 virg. villein land.
West Wycombe .		6	8	
Morton . . .	3	6	8	1 mes., 1 virg. villein land.

	Fine. £ s. d.	Holding.
Wargrave . . .	10 0	
Waltham St. Lawrence	10 0	4 acres assart land.
Culham . . .	None	
Warefield . . .	6 8	
Billingsbear . .	None	
Crawley . . .	15 0	1 cottage with curtilage.
Mardon . . .	1 11 8	1 mes., 1 ferling, 12 acres assart land.
Bishop's Waltham .	2 0 0	1 mes., ½ virg. villein land ; 1 ferling assart land.
Droxford . . .	1 1 8	?
Meon (manor) . .	8 0 0	1 mes., 1 virg., 1 water mill.
,,	3 3 4	1 mes., 1 virg.
Fareham . . .	2 0 0	,, ,,
,,	1 7 0	1 mes., 4 acres.
Meon (*ecclesia*) . .	1 11 0	1 mes., ½ virg.
Brockhampton . .	3 0 0	1 virg.
Hambledon . .	1 3 4 (Relief)	30 acres.
,, . .	1 2 0	(Size unspecified.)
Sutton . . .	1 0 0	
Alresford . . .	8 4	Size not noted.
Wield . . .	None	,, ,,
Beauworth . .	3 4	,, ,,
Cheriton . . .	None	,, ,,
Bentley . . .	15 0	,, ,,
Esher . . .	2 6	,, ,,
Highclere . . .	10 0	,, ,,

The following table shows that not only did most manors contain some highly ' fined ' tenements, but that some manors demanded a large number of high fines :

LIST OF FINES AT HARWELL IN 1348–9.

Fine. £ s. d.	Holding.		
7 0	1 cottage with curtilage.		
3 4	Licence to leave manor.		
4 0 0	1 messuage, 2 ¼ virgates villein land.		
1 6 8	1 mes., 8 acres	,,	
1 10 0	1 mes., ½ virg.	,,	
15 0	1 cottage, 2 ¼ virgs.	,,	
16 8	1 cottage, 2 acres	,,	
4 6 8	1 mes. 1 virg.	,,	
4 10 0	,, ,,	,,	
2 3 3	,, ,,	,,	Marriage with heiress.
3 13 4	,, ,,	,,	
4 8 0	,, ,,	,,	
3 15 0	,, ,,	,,	
3 10 0	,, ,,	,,	
5 0 0	1 mes., 1 virg. villein land, and 1 mes. ½ virg. villein land, and 1 cottage with curtilage of 2 acres.		

Fine.			Holding.		
£	s.	d.			
3	13	4	1 mes. 1 virg. villein land.		
5	0	0	,,	,,	,,
5	0	0	,,	,,	,,
1	16	8	1 mes. ½ virg.	,,	
3	10	0	1 mes. 1 virg.	,,	
1	8	0	2 cottages.		
4	0	0	1 mes. 1 virg.	,,	
5	0	0	,,	,,	,,
1	16	8	1 mes. ½ virg.	,,	
1	13	4	,,	,,	,,
1	0	0	,,	,,	,, Marriage.
	4	0			Marriage and wardship.
74	6	11			

The above lists of fines, taken at random from different manors, seem to show how impossible it is to arrive at any definite basis of reckoning. Obviously, the area of land had little to do with the amount of the fine ; nor can one find any consistent variations according to the occasion of the fine ; nor is the assart land treated any more regularly than the ordinary *terra nativa*.

A normal holding, one messuage and one virgate of villein land, is perhaps most frequently rated at 13s. 4d. for an ordinary fine, while a half-virgate will often pay 6s. 8d. or 10s. But even on the same manor the fine may commonly run up to £3 or £4, while elsewhere £6–£8 is not unusual for a virgate or even a half-virgate of land.[1]

If any generalizations may be ventured on, one might point out that there is a rough reasonableness about the fines ; fertility and general prosperity and situation are perhaps the only guides beyond tradition. Thus the fines on the manors round Taunton, in a district famed for its wealth, and only at a late date separated from the giant manor of Taunton, are

---

[1] At Meon in 1347–8 John Blackman paid the following fines for his various tenements :

					£	s.	d.
1 messuage, 10 acres	.	.	.	.	2	0	0
1 messuage, 1 virgate	.	.	.	.	5	0	0
4 acres	.	.	.	.	1	0	0
Unspecified	.	.	.	.	2	0	0
1 messuage, 1 virgate	.	.	.	.	6	13	4
					16	13	4 in all.

E

distinctly higher than those in Hampshire, except in a few isolated cases. Proximity to a large town might account for the high fines at Taunton, but not at Harwell (in Berkshire), while the influence of the town was evidently less felt round Winchester. The size of the virgate and of the customary acre might make some difference; a virgate at Crondal is frequently estimated at 24–26 acres, while the Taunton virgates were almost uniformly 40 acres. The customary acre, too, is small in Hampshire; on some manors four, on others two, field acres are calculated as one measured acre. The occasion of the fine may have influenced its amount; evidently the same land paid different fines for different kinds of transfer. The fines on marriage with an heiress seem to have been higher than fines on inheritance, perhaps because such a marriage meant consolidation of holdings, and a double share for the family. Collinson states[1] that Borough English was the rule even among daughters on the Taunton manors; this would help to account for the heavy fines on marriage.

Similarly, fines or lawsuits seem to have been somewhat high, and, unreasonably enough, the fine was imposed on both the winner and the loser of the suit.[2]

That the high fines were no new development may be shown from some of the thirteenth-century rolls. In 1208 the fines rarely exceeded 10s., but in the Taunton group 10s. was given for one acre of meadow. By 1275 and 1284 fines of £4 or £5 may be found in the same district, while at Harwell one fine of £10 is noted (1284).[3]

Beyond a few vague suggestions, however, it is impossible to go in explaining the fines. The lack of certainty, so great a trouble in Tudor times and long after, was the rule and not the exception in the fourteenth century. It is difficult, however, to see that any hardships were inflicted thus early by the uncertainty. Occasionally a widow refused to take

---

[1] Collinson, History of Somerset, 1791, vol. iii, p. 233.

[2] Holweye, 1347–8: 'Et de xxd. de Johanne Flehe de Haidon pro iiii daynis dimidio terre de overland in la Hamme . . . quas recuperavit versus Laurence Wodecok pro defectu recordi habendis tanquam annexa tenemento suo nativo.' A similar entry is given lower down against Laurence Woodcock.

[3] Cf. p. 217. Addenda.

up her husband's land because of her poverty, but the unwillingness in other cases is due to the services demanded rather than to the heavy fine. Perhaps if one could compare the rents with the fines, one might find that they tended to balance each other, that a low assized rent meant a heavy and variable fine, while a more economic rent was accompanied by a nominal and traditional fine.[1] But the evidence of the Pipe Rolls does not admit of such comparison, unless by chance in a very few cases.

The arbitrary nature of the fines obviously makes it impossible to ascertain whether the same rates were maintained after the Black Death as before, or whether higher or lower fines were demanded.

One entry[2] might lead one to suppose that a specially low rate was asked when a tenant was compelled to take up a vacant holding, for a messuage, half a virgate of villein land, and two acres of assart land paid only 6d. as a fine, but in an exactly similar case,[3] *after* the pestilence, a normal fine of 10s. is asked.[4]

---

[1] This suggestion is not, however, supported by a sixteenth-century Customary of Crondal (Crondal Records, pp. 375–83), where the lack of any relationship between the fixed fines and the rents is very evident.

[2] Cnoel, 1347–8 : 'Et de vid. de Thomas Hoghyne pro 1 mesuagio et dimidia virgata terre native et ii acris terre purpresture in Cnoel que fuerunt Johannis de Holleye et que Amicia que fuit uxor dicti Johannis tenere recusavit et eciam ad que idem Thomas per totum homagium electus fuit habendis.' Cf. Crawley, 1315 : 'Et de vid. de Roberto Meriweder pro uno cotagio & x acris terre in Craulye que fuerunt Willelmi Bonwoulf que devenerunt in manus domini tanquam eschaeta pro defectu tenentium & ad que eligebatur per totam decennam.' (Another similar entry follows.) Cf. Twyford, 1343–4 : 'Et de vid. de Johanne Kyne pro 1 mesuagio, dimidia virgata terre native in North Twyford que fuerunt Ricardi le Fowel et que devenerunt in manus domini tanquam derelicta et ad que idem Johannes electus est per totum homagium.'

[3] Twyford, 1354–5 : 'Et de xs. de Ricardo Wygge pro 1 mesuagio dimidia virgata terre native in Northtwyford que fuerunt Johannis Dykes et que a tempore pestilenciae exstiterunt in manu domini pro defectu tenentium licet proclamatio facta fuerit secundum consuetudinem manerii et ad que idem Ricardus electus est per homagium ad hoc compulsus habendis.'

[4] Page (End of Villeinage in England, p. 36) quotes similar cases at Brightwaltham and Woolston (Berks.), where the tenants pay sums varying from 6d. to 6s. 8d. not to be compelled to take up vacant customary land. At Cranfield (Beds.) the vote of the whole homage is replaced by the verdict of a jury of six, who report that eight villeins are *abiles et sufficientes* to take up land. See also in Victoria County History of Berkshire (Social

An interesting note is added among the fines at West Wycombe, to the effect that the lord retained his right to confiscate the land, or at least to enter upon it, if the rents and services were not duly paid, notwithstanding the fine.[1]

Land might also be resumed by the lord on account of prolonged illness or impotency, or madness, and a widow who married again without consent forfeited her holding.[2] In one case, however, the tenant was allowed to pay a recognition of 1s. in order to be quit of all services and dues ' *propter notabilem infirmitatem ut patitur* '.[3]

The lists of fines also show that exchanges between villein tenants, so common in the fifteenth century, were becoming general, though not frequent, by 1346. It is unusual to find more than two in any one year, even on a large manor ; on the other hand, one can hardly look through the fines on any of the episcopal manors for a period of ten years without finding one or two. From the close correspondence in the areas exchanged, together with the exact details as to position, it is fairly clear that the object of the exchanges was to obtain more compact holdings.[4] The fine on an exchange of

and Economic History), for a case of election and compulsion at Bright Waltham.

[1] West Wycombe, 1348–9 : ' Et de iiii*li*. de Ricardo de Wydyndon pro Agneta de Hokenden cum terra sua videlicet 1 mesuagio et 1 virgata terre native in Westwycombe habenda. Ita quod si dictus Ricardus de redditibus et serviciis a dictis tenementis debitis domino faciendo cessaverit, liceatur domino eadem intrare, et per voluntatem suam disponere fine praedicta non obstante.' Cf. Glympton. Oxon. Court Roll 1327 : ' Tenementum Johannis Bolle captum est in manu domini quia idem Johannes non sufficit pro serviciis faciendis.' (The above extract was kindly copied for me by Mr. Ballard, from the Glympton Court Roll.)

[2] For a case of madness see note on p. 86.

[3] Stoke, 1376–7.

[4] Cf. Tawney, Agrarian Problem in Sixteenth Century, pp. 164–5. At Poundisford, 1348–9, it is expressly stated that the two acres of ' overland ' and the two acres of villein meadow land which are exchanged shall also exchange their nature or status: ' Et de vi*d*. de Stephano atte Welle pro excambio ii acrarum terre de Overland in decenna de Dodelestone pro ii acris prati terre native cum Nicholo de Foxgrave in eadem decenna ita quod dictum pratum remanet in overland et dictae ii acrae terra nativa habendae.' Another entry exactly similar. Cf. also Holway, 1350–1 : ' Et de xii*d*. de Roberto Gone pro una acra terre de Overland in decenna de Holeweye facta nativa et una acra prati de cetero sit overland ' (*sic*). Cf. Warefield, 1381–2, where two customary tenants surrender to each other 1 messuage, 1 virgate (of 20 acres) and 18 acres of *terra purprestura*, both

six acres of villein land in Sutton was only 9*d.* ; the process, therefore, could hardly have been objected to by the lord. It is possible that in some cases the sales and sub-letting among the villein tenants were actuated by the same motives ; in one case we find the unusual situation of a son surrendering or leasing a messuage and ten acres of land to his father, for term of life, ' saving the reversion of the aforesaid tenements to the said son '. [1]

An interesting entry at Bishop's Waltham [2] shows the lord's intention to treat surrender of land as a transfer of exactly the same nature as the usual inheritance ; a heriot is demanded from the seller, as well as a fine from the purchaser. The heriot is paid and entered below.

A curious custom appears on the Taunton group of manors ; to ensure the succession to a tenement, a man or woman would come into court and pay a substantial fine for the purchase of one acre (or any very small amount) of a larger holding, in order to attract to himself the rest of the tenement when it should fall due (*cum acciderit*)—usually at the death of the seller.[3] A second fine was paid when the whole tene-

tenements being within the same tithing. It is evident that this is really an exchange, and a very convenient exchange, or the two parties to it would not have been content to pay a fine of 30*s.* each.

[1] Meon, 1347–8. Cf. also Meon, 1345–6, for similar case of ' concession ' to a mother.

[2] Waltham, 1351–2, *Fines* : ' Et de viiis. de Henrico Laurens pro 1 mesuagio, dimidio ferlingi terre native in Waltham Northbrook ex redditione Cristine Skynnere habendis. Ita quod dabitur de cetero heriettum tam pro redditu (*sic*) tenementi quam pro decessu tenentis si habeat averum.'

[3] Hulle, 1350–1, *Fines* : ' Et de iiiis. de Johanna filia Johannis Waterman pro una acra terre native in decenna de Hulle ex redditione Aviciae atte Walle attrahendi sibi totum residuum tenementi sui native ibidem, videlicet unum mesuagium et xv acras terre native habenda.' This is a simple case ; a more complicated one occurs at Holway in 1349–50 (*Fines*) : ' Et de cs. de Nicholo Roulf pro uno mesuagio una virgata terre native in decenna de Stoke que quondam fuit Johannis Lambert, et de quibus Johanna filia dicti Johannis dum sola fuerat pro una acra que vocatur *putair* (?) finem fecit ex redditione dicti Johannis patris sui attrahendi sibi jus dictorum mesuagii et virgate terre post mortem ipsius Johannis pro qua quidem Johanna cum terra sua videlicet una acra et jure attrahendi predicta &c. Johannes de Orchard similiter finivit qui quidem Johannes vir dictae Johannae eandem acram cum jure attrahendi residuum totius tenementi praedicti dicto Nicholo modo reddit habendam.' Other examples occur at Hull in 1354–5, Holway, 1347–8, 1350–1, Staplegrove and Poundisford, 1350–1, and again in 1376–7.

ment fell to the purchaser of the precautionary acre. In many of the cases there appears to be no tie of relationship between the two parties, and the object of the arrangement is by no means clear, except that it gave a prior claim to a tenement for which there might be many competitors.

Relevia. *Reliefs.* The reliefs paid from free lands are sometimes included among the fines, though distinguished from them, and sometimes form a separate entry. In ordinary years there are very few, or none, on most manors. The rates appear to have varied greatly, but the total amounts were very much lower than the fines. At Knoyle, in 1348–9, the separate reliefs seem to have varied from ¾*d.* for 1½ acres, up to 15*s.* 4¾*d. pro diversis terris et tenementis que de domino tenentur in feodo.* At Sutton (1348–9) a relief of 10*s.* is paid for a messuage and a virgate of free land, descending from a father, while a messuage and two virgates of free land, also inherited from a father, only paid 3*s.* 4*d.* It seems to have been quite usual, however, not to specify the amount of free lands thus relieved.[1] Occasionally it was necessary to prove in court that the land was free.[2] At Downton (1349–50) a relief of 16*s.* was paid for one messuage, one hide, and ten acres of free land.[3]

It is, however, impossible to discover from the Pipe Rolls the number of free tenants on a manor, unless under exceptional circumstances an extent of the manor is prefixed to the usual account. For example, in the roll for 1347–8, there is inserted (after Rimpton) an extent of the manor of Orchard, which had been held of the bishop as three-fourths of a knight's fee, and which now came into his hand through the minority of the heir. The extent states (see pp. 23–5) that the manor contained 6 free tenants owing rents (£13 10*s.* in all) and suit of court; 13 tenants *in bondagio,* owing services,

[1] Sutton, 1348–9 : 'Et de xiiis. iiii*d.* de Edam priorem de Seleborne pro relevio terrarum et tenementorum que fuerunt Johannis Sauntenue in Roppele.' Cf. also Tawney, Agrarian Problem in the Sixteenth Century, pp. 31–3.

[2] Meon, 1348–9 : 'Et de xv*s.* de relevio Willelmi Fisshe pro terris et tenementis cum pertinentiis in Frex' que fuerunt Willelmi Fisshe patris sui libere *tenta* per cartam domini Johannis de Pontisera quondam Episcopi per Priorem et conventum sancti Swythini Wyntoniensi in curia ostensam.'

[3] Cf. p. 217. Addenda.

and a number of other smaller tenants. Tenants of 'overland', it is expressly stated, pay rent 'for all services'. Apart from this, and an occasional notice of free tenants in connexion with services owed to the lord, practically nothing can be learned from the Pipe Rolls about the position of the free men or the free lands of the manors.[1]

The profits of the courts are generally entered only as totals, and no details are given; the amount gained at each court is entered separately. *Placita et perquisita.*

In 1209, each offence with its fine was entered in the Ministers' Accounts, and Mr. Hubert Hall says, 'It is scarcely too much to say that the Compotus Roll of 1209 enables us to reconstruct the contemporary Court Roll with the help of existing local forms of a later date.'[2] Unfortunately, no Court Rolls are extant for any of the episcopal manors between the years 1346–56.

Heriots. This entry generally follows the fines and marriages; in normal years it is of little interest, but it becomes a valuable indication of the number of deaths from the pestilence. In many manors it had been commuted into a money payment, either as an occasional substitute *quia nullum habuit averum*, or as a regular due from the goods of all deceased tenants. *Herietti.*

At Waltham the 'Heriots in pence', as they were called, were levied at the rate of 1s.; on the Somerset manors 6d. is more usual.[3] In some cases corn was sold in order to raise the heriot.[4] An attempt was made to exact a heriot from the seller of land, as well as a fine from the purchaser, but this hardly seems to have become a general practice.[5]

[1] It is suggested in the Victoria County History of Hampshire (Social and Economic History) that free tenants in the county were commonly in the proportion of about 2 to every 5 customary tenants. Judging by the number of reliefs paid, this is too high an estimate for the Winchester manors.

[2] Pipe Roll of the Bishopric of Winchester, 1208–9, ed. Hall, p. xiii. The practice of copying the Court Rolls on to the Pipe Roll had nearly ceased by 1301.

[3] Miss Neilson (Customary Rents, p. 88) suggests 2s. 6d. as the usual sum. I have found no example so high as this, except at Brightwell.

[4] Cf. Orchard, 1347–8, *Exitus Manerii.* The pasture on the land lying fallow belonged to the bishop, who had the wardship of the heir, but 'de residuo terre nichil pro bladis in eadem crescentibus que sunt catalla dicti Thome de Orchard nuper defuncti.'   [5] Cf. p. 53.

In one case a heriot of one *boviculus* was paid by Alice lady of Makkeneye, who held 2 carucates of land and 60s. of rent by military service.[1]

Schedule B. Expenses.

In the account of expenses the items are less interesting and less significant. All the expenses connected with the ploughs, carts, purchase of stock and of corn, care of the dairy and sheep-folds, the manor-house, farm buildings, and all smaller necessaries are duly noted and calculated. From among the details given one may gather the wages of a carter, a ploughboy, or a dairywoman per annum ; the wages of a carpenter or a mason or a tiler per day, or the wages of men and women for such extra work as sheep-washing and shearing. The price of a plough, or a plough-share, of a horse-shoe, of a red stone for marking sheep, of salt for the dairy, of the dairy utensils—all this is given with the utmost exactitude. Under the same heading of expenses fall one or two more weighty entries. The *Custus Parci* and *Custus Pratorum* generally furnish some information as to the cost of mowing and hay-making, and distinguish in different years whether the customary services are sufficient or whether extra men have to be hired. This section, however, throws little light on the question of commutation, as only certain kinds of work are mentioned under definite headings, and the wages paid are in most cases only a part of the remuneration earned by the workmen.

The usual framework followed in accounting for the expenses runs thus :

(a) Custus Carucarum	Includes wages of ploughmen, ploughman's 'mates', blacksmith.
(b) Custus Carectarum	Includes wages of carters ; sometimes cost of extra carting.
(c) Emptio Bladi	Cf. with *Venditio Bladi et Stauri.*
(d) Emptio Stauri	
(e) Custus Daieriae et Bercariae	Wages of dairymaid and shepherds ; sheep-shearing.
(f) Custus Domorum et necessarium	Cost of enclosure and hedging often entered here ; also building.

[1] Brightwell, 1348–9.

(g) Custus Parci et Pratorum	Wages of mowers ; cost of park-palings ; wages of park-keeper.
(h) Custus Autumpni	
i. Food, &c.	A rough clue to the number of customers working.
ii. Additional wages	Ditto.
iii. Customary payments	Often a small payment to the whole group of customers; probably a commutation of food formerly provided.
iv. Hayward	Wages almost always 6s. 8d. per annum.
v. Repereeve	Wages vary with length of harvest— about 5s.

It is, therefore, possible to collect the total amount of wages paid on any given manor, and this has been done in a few cases. But it must be emphasized that the wages paid to regular servants of the manor, such as the ploughmen, shepherds, cowherds, or dairymaids, are merely supplementary payments, not their chief means of livelihood. The cost of building operations ought to form a fair test of the prosperity of a manor, but on the Bishop of Winchester's estates, money was evidently allotted from the profits of one manor to pay the exceptional expenses of another.[1] The cost of the harvest works becomes a valuable indication of the amount of services performed, during and after the years of pestilence, especially on those manors where food was still supplied to the customers. On the Taunton group, however, this entry had become stereotyped, and evidently only included a small customary payment of some kind.

On the whole, the second schedule of the account is less instructive and does not need such detailed examination as the earlier section.

It is remarkable how very small is the proportion of expenses to income on most of the Bishop's manors; the margin of profits is not nearly so narrow as, for example, on the Cambridgeshire manor examined by Maitland, or on the college estates quoted by Thorold Rogers.

The following tables will illustrate this point:[2]

---

[1] Cf. p. 169.

[2] For numerous other examples see tables on pp. 162–77. These tables will show that the bishop did not depend upon his seigneurial dues for a profit on these manors; in most cases the whole expenses could be met from the sale of agricultural produce from the demesne. Doubtless he

BISHOP'S STOKE.

					1346–7			1347–8		
					£	s.	d.	£	s.	d.
Receipts	.	.	.	.	.	78	10	7¼	70	6	4¼
Expenses	.	.	.	.	.	18	17	2½	15	9	0

CRAWLEY.

Receipts	.	.	.	.	.	111	0	0½	69	19	10
Expenses	.	.	.	.	.	13	18	3	15	14	1¼

BISHOP'S WALTHAM.

Receipts	.	.	.	.	.	218	18	3	280	6	4¾
Expenses	.	.	.	.	.	56	6	7¼	97	14	10¾

A brief summary of the expenses of one or two manors may serve to show how little was spent on wages in comparison with the receipts.

On the small manor of Stoke no less than sixteen regular workmen, holding special positions, are named (see table on p. 60), but the total annual wages paid directly in money to them are only just over £5. Money wages formed so small a part of the remuneration of a villein-labourer, that their rise or fall is very little guide in estimating the prosperity of master or man. Land, acquittances of rent, food allowances, and gifts of corn or stock must all be taken into account, as well as the money actually paid out. Moreover, the wages of the chief manorial officers, and in fact all the annual wages, were very largely traditional, and remained unaltered in some districts for at least two centuries. Day-wages fluctuated far more rapidly, and it is to the sums paid for occasional labour, such as threshing and thatching, and extra help at harvest-time, that one must look for evidences of the inter-action of demand and supply. It must be remembered, too, that not all the payments made for ploughing or harvest services were really of the nature of wages.[1] In many cases, where the work done retained something of its former charac-ter of 'Boondays', small payments were made to the custo-mary tenants. At Sutton, in 1376, as much as 2d. per acre

depended largely upon labour services, though not so entirely as has been supposed.

[1] Cf. p. 34.

Expenses

	Stoke. 1346–7 (£ s. d.)	Waltham. 1347–8 (£ s. d.)	Droxford. 1347–8 (£ s. d.)	Cheriton.† 1346–7 (£ s. d.)	Sutton. 1347–8 (£ s. d.)	Crawley. 1347–8 (£ s. d.)
Ploughs	11 10	2 10 6	1 5 5	1 8 0	1 3 11	1 6 10
Carts	12 2	2 2 8	2 2 0	1 7 8	1 10 2½	12 3
Corn bought	19 6½	26 0 2	—	1 5 7½	1 18 8¾	—
Stock	6 18 3	8 11 6	9 9 6	6 7 5	11 4 4	5 0 5
Dairy and Sheep-fold	12 6	4 1 1	1 17 3½	1 10 2½	1 13 11	2 3 4
Household and buildings	1 0 10	10 16 8	1 0 4½	1 14 10	16 5¾	1 0 5
(hedging, &c.)	—	10 1 10½	12 1	—	18 3½	—
Park	2 16 7	6 16 1½	—	Custos Molendini 9 6½	15 3 hoeing	—
Meadows	11 1	3 7 6 threshing; 1 15 9½ hoeing; 2 10 7 mill	1 9 3	—	5 0 threshing; 17 0¾	—
Autumn works	2 10 4½	6 12 2; 4 15 0(?)	5 11 10	2 18 2; Vadimonium 2 10 0	2 6 4½	1 14 0½
Total *	18 17 2½	97 14 10¾	26 9 9	19 16 10½	30 18 10½	15 14 1½

* The totals given here do not always tally with the columns of figures given above, because a few exceptional items have been omitted, to save space.

† For many of the statistics concerning Cheriton I am indebted to Mr. F. W. Cuthbertson, who kindly allowed me to use his very careful and detailed notes for this manor.

TABLE OF WAGES, 1345–6. STOKE.[1]

	Wages.	Allowances.	Acquittance.
Parcarius .	1d. per day	+1d. p.d. at Twyford	None.
Carectarius .	4/- p.a.	+16 qrs. 4 bus. barley.	
Fugator .	4/- p.a.	+4 qrs. 2½ bus. „	
Daye . .	2/- p.a.	+3 qrs. 2 bus. „	
Messor .	. 5/4 (for harvest ?)		
Cotarii . .		¼d. p.d.	
Bercarius .		3 qrs. 2 bus.	
Custos ovium .		(for 6 weeks) 4 bus.	
Prepositus .			4/- p.a.
Faber . .			1/- p.a.
Vaccarius .			2/- p.a.
Bedellus .			2/- p.a.
Carucarius .			2/- p.a.
Hayward .	6/8 p.a.		
Repereve .	6/4 for harvest		
Thatcher .	2½ p.d.		
Ballivus .	£2 0s. 0d. p.a.		

was paid to the tenants who performed the ploughing services, and similar sums were frequently paid before 1349.

However, when all allowances have been made, it is difficult to avoid the conclusion that on many of the Winchester manors the bishop could have paid double or treble the current rate of wages without converting his profits to a loss—in some cases without any serious diminution of his profits—so long as he was able to refuse to commute any more of the services actually performed.

The variations in the season, the differences in the amount and price of crops, were probably more weighty considerations than the cost of labour, and affected the profits of manorial agriculture more seriously.

Stock and Corn Account.

After the expenses follows the account of the live stock which has passed through the hands of the bailiff during the year, and of the corn. On many manors a list is also given of the *utensilia*, and of the garden and dairy produce, so far as it had not been converted into money. A few points of general interest may be gathered from this schedule, but as a rule it does not yield much.

The rate at which sheep-farming on the demesne increased

---

[1] See also p. 35 for similar list for Bishop's Waltham.

during the thirteenth and fourteenth centuries may be roughly seen from the following table :

NUMBER OF SHEEP (ALL CLASSES) BETWEEN 1208–1455.

	1208–9	1347–8	1353–4	1376–7	1455
Bishop's Waltham	920	?572	556	588	?1071
Clere	1164	{ Highclere 412 / Burghclere 427 }	403 / 529	433 / 763	
Woodhay	383	319	317	508	
Itchingswell	253	408	637	637	
Brightwell	200	{ Apparently none }	None [110 during year]	280	
Harwell	305	{ Apparently none }	306	179	
Witney	683	646	861	1240	
Downton	1764	1179	1220	1212	
Overton	775	1146	1120	1118	
Fareham	283	370	400	427	
Wargrave	190	185	230	454	
Bitterne	90	242	161	369	
Wycombe	212	323	590	1093	321 (to farmer)
Mardon	581	513	791	1232	
Farnham	498	225	199	467	
Sutton	495	733	649	909	451
West Meon	1276	1225	1562	1503	
Hambledon	533	669	937	1145	
Crawley	1063	1088 (?)	1000	1020	1897
Twyford	1627	1555	1281	1283	951 (farmer)
Stoke	None	186	209	201	
Cheriton	591	716	967	817	549 (farmer)
Beauworth	132	316	456	420	266
Wield	331	388	410	460	
Rimpton	None	None	None	None	
					1380–1
Knoyle	1048	1307	1495	1597	1727
Ivingho	—	568	488	588	734

No very striking increase is denoted for the most part, but there is enough to account for the rising value of pasture. The occasional decreases would almost always be found to be caused by the leasing or breaking up of the demesne. It should be noticed that very little evidence is forthcoming as to sheep-farming among the tenants. Of the heriots in kind which still fell into the lord's hand more will be said later. The corn account is valuable because it contains occasional mentions of threshing services, and of the 'customary' sheaves given to the harvesters; it also records the yield of different kinds of grain per acre, and the return per quarter for the amount sown. Perhaps the most useful evidence to be gathered from it is the account of the area actually sown each year; it is therefore possible to test in any given manor or group of manors the decrease in the area of demesne land under cultivation. Statistics illustrating this point are given on p. 132.

Occasionally a detailed account of the Churchscot (in corn or cocks and hens) is given; the list of tenants paying or failing to pay may be useful.

Account of Works.

This fourth schedule of the Pipe Roll probably once formed part of the accounts of each manor, but its appearance and disappearance both on the Compotus Rolls and on the Pipe Rolls is irregular and not very easy to explain on any general grounds.[1] The account must certainly have been kept locally; perhaps it was not considered necessary to send it in to Winchester each year—a comparison of the *opera vendita* with a custumal would give a rough idea of the bailiff's method of dealing with the works.

In 1208–9 there is no attempt to show in the Pipe Roll how the labour services were allocated. By 1275 an entry appears on a few manors (e. g. Meon, Sutton, Cheriton, Alresford) under the general heading of *Opera.*

By 1346 it was usual to give a complete account of the works on all the sub-manors of the Taunton district (i. e. Hull, Holway, Staplegrove, Poundisford, Nailesbourne), and also at Rimpton and Meon (incomplete). No general heading is given, but after the corn account the scribe goes straight on to the *Arura, Herciatura,* &c., ending with the *Opera Manualia.*

The evidence of these entries has been tabulated and will be found on pp. 89–96. Here it may suffice to notice in a more general way the disposition of the labour services in the normal years before 1349.

[1] Cf. p. 10.

The entries show the amount of service owed, the number of tenants and the area of land from which the services were owed, and the final allocation of the services. Taking each class of work separately, the following information may be gathered.

Threshing. Threshing and winnowing services were owed from the five Taunton manors, but are not mentioned at Meon and Rimpton. Some virgates owed threshing for seed for one acre at the winter sowing and one at the Lent sowing; others owed threshing for seed for 4 acres. The 17 virgates at Nailesbourne which owed threshing services were held by 48 tenants, who apparently had subdivided the work among themselves. Threshing and winnowing wheat was valued at 4*d.* per quarter, oats at 1*d.* Most of the threshing services were 'sold' at this value, some were excused to the reeve or other officials, and a few were performed.

Ploughing. Ploughing services were subdivided into *Arrura per acram* and *Arrura de prece.* The former, for which no pay was given, varied from 54 to 174 acres on the different manors, and was almost always sold, at a rate varying on different manors from 6½*d.* to 9*d.* per acre. A few acres were excused. The *Arrura de prece,* on the contrary, was actually performed, and the bishop paid ½*d.* per acre for it, though it is carefully noted that it is really worth 6*d.* or 8*d.* The *Arura per acram* is known as Need-earth, in contrast presumably to Boon-earth.

Harrowing. The *Herciatura* is almost always performed; very occasionally part of it was sold. But as a rule it is considered to be linked with the ploughing, and is owed by all those tenants who have horses. Those who had no horses were probably allowed to substitute the mattocking, which was so great a feature of the Taunton methods of agriculture.[1] Generally a virgate was held to owe ploughing,

[1] Cf. Norden, The Surveior's Dialogue, 1610, Bk. V, p. 192. At Tandeane, the 'Paradise of England', 'they take extraordinary pains in soyling, plowing and dressing their lands. After the plowe, there goeth some three or four with mattocks to break the clods and to draw up the earth out of the furrowes that the land may lie round, that the water annoy not the seed, and to that end they most carefully cut out gutters and

harrowing, weeding, and mattocking for as much arable land as had been sown with the seed threshed by a virgate, i. e. 2 or 4 acres.

Harvesting. The reaping is also divided into *Messio per acram* and *Messio de prece.* Both are generally required upon the demesne, but the former is occasionally sold (at 3*d.* per acre), while the latter is occasionally not asked for. Each customer, as his *Messio per acram,* reaped, bound, and shocked as much corn as grew upon the land he had already cultivated. The *Messio de prece* consisted of two *precariae* from each customer, who, besides receiving a nominal payment, were *ad cibum domini.*

Waterlette. A special service known as Waterlette was owed at Staplegrove, but was always sold.

At Rimpton (Somerset) the only services accounted for are the *Arrura de prece* (4 acres per customer) and the *Opera Manualia*; the latter appear to have been exceptionally heavy—four days a week throughout the year, and five days in harvest.

Meon (Hants) has a different classification.[1] *Opera Carectaria, Opera Manualia, Opera Autumpnalia,* and *Opera Autumpnalia ad Manus* make up a total of over 2,500 days owing. Of these services, only a small proportion were performed ; large numbers were sold, or excused as ' acquittances '. The *Opera Manualia* were valued at 1*d.* each.

The entry under Sutton is very fragmentary and appears only spasmodically.

Manual Works. The most interesting item in the account of works is the *Opera Manualia,* the works which as a rule did not require the use of the farm beasts, and which were left undefined. A very large number of manual works was owed on the Taunton manors, and a surprising number were sold. Thus at Nailesbourne 64 customers and 17 operarii

---

trenches in all places, where the water is likelyest to annoy. And for the better enriching of their plowing grounds, they cut up, cast and carry in the unplowed head-lands and places of no use.'

[1] In 1376–7 a number of other works are accounted for at Meon.

were responsible for 4,755 *opera manualia*; of these 3,841 were sold in 1346–7 and 3,860 in 1347–8. The importance of these figures is evident when one attempts to work out the results of the great pestilence. The most obvious conclusions to be drawn from the accounts of manual works are :

(*a*) that far more services were owed than were ever needed, for the wages-bill of these Taunton manors was small, and included practically no payments for harvest-works.

(*b*) that varying numbers of works were allotted roughly as follows :

  (i) To the bishop's harvesting.
  (ii) To other necessary occasional works, such as hedging, ditching, clearing, and sometimes enclosing.
  (iii) To Saints' days and Law-days.[1]
  (iv) In acquittances to regular servants of the manor.
  (v) Sold (i. e. to the men who should have performed the services if called upon).

It may be noticed that the episcopal estates seem to have demanded very heavy labour services;[2] three or four days a week in harvest, or every day except Saturday, are demanded from the villeins as well as the usual week-work in winter. Moreover, in the Taunton districts manual works seem to have been owed by a large number of small tenants, often holding less than a ferling of land. Thus there was always a very considerable margin of which the lord may take advantage when crops are exceptionally heavy, when the weather was unfavourable, or the Saints' days fell unfortunately, or when some change of method, such as increased fencing or enclosing,

---

[1] From six to eight important festivals fell between Lammas-tide and Michaelmas. The festivals observed varied rather curiously from manor to manor.

[2] Cf. Staplegrove, 1349, where a note is given to the effect that it was found that the customers had been unjustly burdened by Adam of Draycote, formerly Constable of Taunton, with 96 works ; henceforth these works are remitted in the account. The mistake appears to have arisen because eight (named) tenants had arranged themselves into four couples, each of which held half a virgate *conjunctim*, and ought to have done only the works for half a virgate, namely one work per week.

F

caused an unprecedented demand for labour. This fact has been made clear by Maitland, who asserts that only about half the labour services owed were actually demanded; it has been quoted by various writers [1] on economic history, but apparently no one has gone on to show its bearing upon the labour problem created by the Black Death. It seems clear that while the regular workmen of the manor might early commute their occasional services and develop into wage-paid labourers, the process of commutation would be very grudgingly applied to the *opera manualia*, for which there would be a brief but sharp demand, not easily met even by the expedient of paying good wages. The detailed examination of this entry for the years immediately before 1349 throws much light on the alleged disorganization of the manorial economy during the years following the Black Death.[2]

The following account of the *opera manualia* at Nailesbourne in 1345–6 is very significant, especially when compared with the same entry for the year 1349–50 (cf. p. 89).

Total number of *opera* owing		3845
Acquittances to Reeve and Beadle	98	
„ „ ploughman	24	
„ „ 10 *operarii* for festivals . . .	70	
Total number of *opera* acquitted		192
Reaping, binding, and shocking corn on demesne by 62 customers	248	
Mowing, spreading, and carrying 12 acres hay . .	96	
Mattocking demesne for winter sowing . . .	40	
Sowing	4	
Harrowing	28	
Making ' grips ' [3]	6	
Mattocking demesne for Lent sowing . . .	48	
Sowing	4	
Harrowing	42	
Reaping the lord's corn	100	
For one rook-herd	8	
Work at the mill	6	
Total number of *opera* performed		630
Works sold (for £6 11s. 7½d.)		2708
„ „ after account was made up . . .		315
		3845

[1] Cf. Cunningham, Growth of English Industry and Commerce, 5th ed., vol. i, p. 332. Page (T. W.), End of Villeinage in England, p. 74, quotes the case of Warboys, Hunts, where 4,216 *opera* were owed; in 1380 2,785 were performed, and in 1390 as many as 2,407 were still required.

[2] Cf. p. 87.   [3] See note on p. 89.

A very similar account is that of Holway for 1345–6 :

Total number of *opera manualia* owing . . .		6803
Acquittance to Reeve	49	
,, ,, 3 ploughmen	108	
,, ,, 1 Beadle	86	
,, ,, ,, ...	39	
,, ,, 1 *Messor*	163	
,, ,, 1 Smith	109	
,, ,, Woodwards	78	
,, ,, 13 *operarii* for festivals . . .	91	
Total number of *opera* acquitted		723
Mowing demesne meadows (22 customers) . . .	44	
Reaping, binding, and shocking corn (97 customers) .	388	
For one rook-herd	12	
Mattocking demesne for winter sowing . . .	120	
Harrowing ,, ,, ,, . .	180	
Making 'grips'	26	
Spreading manure	8	
Mattocking demesne for Lent sowing	74	
Harrowing	64	
Making 'grips'	19	
Reaping the lord's corn	668	
At the mills	281	
Miscellaneous	100	
Total number of *opera* performed		1984
,, ,, ,, sold		3998
,, ,, ,, ,, after account made up .		98
		6803

With the 'Account of Works' the bailiff's work was done ;
inquisition had been made into every change in the manorial
organization ; every egg and even every apple had been
accounted for. An amazing amount of information is stored
up in these Pipe Rolls, but on one or two points they are
unsatisfactory.

As it has been already pointed out, they tell us practically
nothing of the free tenants of the manor ; little or nothing
of the relation of rents to area of holding ; little of the legal
status of the tenants ; comparatively little of the total
burden of works and money due from any one tenant, for
the tenants owing services are often not named, and it is
difficult to ascertain whether the men who ploughed the lord's
demesne also washed his sheep and carried his letters.

There is, however, some additional information to be
gained on general questions of manorial organization, by

considering several of the entries together, and collecting incidental references.

There is interesting though scanty evidence of the power of the whole body of villeins to act as a community. The 'homage' could lease pasture collectively, and could make general bargains with the lord for the commutation of services; it could hold itself responsible for choosing the lord's regular manorial servants in rotation from among themselves—a system which becomes increasingly common in the fifteenth century; it could make bargains with other groups of villeins to exchange services, without consulting the lord. Thirty-two sworn customers were able to decide that a surrender made by a man at the point of death was unreasonable, and must therefore be annulled. The inquest is used side by side with the examination of the Pipe Roll to show when a fine ought or ought not to be paid.

Moreover, the homage was traditionally responsible for escheated or derelict lands and could choose a new tenant from among themselves and force him to take up the vacant holding. Alternatively, the homage occasionally paid the rent and value of services for a vacant holding which they had subdivided or agreed to hold in common.

This power of acting in common and thus keeping some kind of check upon the lord's officials seems to have declined under the influence of the more individualistic methods of the fifteenth century. Indeed, the economic position of the tenants varied to so great an extent by the end of the fourteenth century that solidarity of interests among them grew steadily less.

Size of Holdings. It is difficult to obtain any clear idea as to the normal holdings of the bishop's villeins; the lists of fines will show how very widely the tenements varied in size, even on one manor, while there is also a great difference in different districts.

Most of the manors retain the usual classes of virgaters, semi-virgaters, ferling-men, and the holders of cotlands. In many cases, however, the virgates had accumulated additional fractions of a virgate, as well as considerable encroachments (*terra purprestura*, or *assarta*), which might be used either as arable or as private pasture. In other cases one tenant had evidently accumulated holdings until his share approached far more nearly a hide than a virgate. In a few cases his holding is actually called a hide of villein land.[1] The Hampshire holdings are apparently measured by the customary acre, which is often only $\frac{1}{2}$ or $\frac{1}{4}$ of the acre by perches, and thus the size of the holdings may be to some extent deceptive.[2] A few typical groups of tenements are subjoined. In 1375–6 virgates at Meon were estimated at 80 acres and 60 acres each, while others contained 34 and 24 acres.

HAMPSHIRE.

Meon, 1347–8.	Twyford, 1350–1.	Alresford, 1343–4.
1 messuage	1 messuage	2 messuages.
10 acres	6 acres meadow	3½ virgates.
1 messuage	3 virgates	17 acres assart.
1 virgate	3 acres pasture	(Held by a woman).
4 acres	7 „ wood.	
1 messuage	22 „ assart.	
1 virgate	8 „ (croft).	
	35 „ (3 crofts).	
	5 „ Snakemor.	
	(Held by a woman, but possibly a free-holding.)	

Bishop's Waltham, 1349–50.

Holding of Henry le White, inherited from his father. Fine=£5 6s. 8d.

1 messuage with garden.	1 cottage with garden.
1 ferling *terra nativa*.	4 acres in one croft called Moyses-croft.
1 „ „ „	2 acres *terra purprestura*.
1 „ „ „	5 „ in one croft called le Inhom.
½ virgate „ „	1½ „ „ „ „
5 acres in one croft called Donkes-croft.	3 „ „ „ „
20 acres *terra purprestura*.	1 mora (3 acres)
1 messuage.	1 garden.
½ virgate *terra nativa*.	1 messuage with curtilage.
1 ferling „ „	

Total (30 acres to the virgate) c. 107 acres and 3 gardens, 3 messuages, 1 cottage.

---

[1] Marwell, 1350–1.

[2] The acres of assart holdings appear to bear no definite relation to measured acres. Thus at Marwell 10 acres in la Roghehay contain by estimation 76 acres of arable land, and 6 acres of waste in the same wood contain by estimation 13½ acres of arable land and 14 acres of wood.

Somerset and Wiltshire.

Holway.   *Nailesbourne.*

Holway	Nailesbourne
8 cottages	1 messuage.
5 acres *terra nativa*	15 acres *terra nativa*.
2 ,, meadow (overland)	2 ,, meadow.
9 ,, overland	32 ,, land (?) and meadow.
4 ,, meadow (overland).	

Downton.

1 toft, site of fulling-mill	36 acres in one croft.
3 pieces meadow.	6 crofts of the lord's waste.
10 acres (?).	19 acres ' Bordland '.

Thus in the Taunton district it would seem that a double process of extreme subdivision and of considerable 'engrossing' went on side by side, though the holdings do not reach such high figures as those in Hampshire. The virgate was calculated at 40 acres and the most normal holding is perhaps a ferling-land of 10 acres. At Otterford in 1351 fifteen tenants held $3\frac{1}{2}$ virgates between them; when the extent of Orchard [1] was made in 1347–8, there were no virgaters, and only one semi-virgater; eight tenants hold 10 acres each and there are twenty-seven smaller holdings, many of them merely cottages with curtilage. About half these small tenements owed trifling services (*opera manualia*, for the most part); the others generally consist of 'overland',[2] i.e. land paying

[1] See pp. 23–5.

[2] 'Overland' was common on all the Somerset and Wiltshire manors, and almost every customary tenant held some 'overland' in addition to his ordinary holding. Probably it was land on the Downs, equivalent to the *terra purprestura* of the more wooded districts. Cf. Collinson, History of Somerset (1791), vol. iii, p. 233 : ' In the manor (Taunton) there are two sorts of lands, bondland and overland ; the bondland is that whereon there have been and commonly are ancient dwelling tenements, and is held by a customary fine and rent certain, paying heriots and doing other suits and services to the same belonging. The overland is that whereon in ancient time there were no dwellings, and is held by a fine and rent certain and fealty ; but the tenants thereof pay no heriots and do no other customs, suits, or service for the same.' In the introduction (p. lxxxvii) to the 'Surveys of Lands of William, First Earl of Pembroke' (Roxburghe Club), overland is explained as land taken from the lord's demesne, and not from tributary land. ' Bord-tenants ' are explained as holders of table-lands, who paid their rents in food for the lord's table or ' board '. The two explanations harmonize well, as ' Bordland ' and ' Overland ' are commonly found on the same manors. But otherwise the definitions hardly seem applicable to the lands of the Bishop of Winchester. The exact meaning of *Terra Bord* remains uncertain.

rent for all services. In a few cases a tenant held land in two
or more manors; this slightly complicates the attempt to
estimate either the population or the size of the holdings.
The consolidation of holdings had thus made considerable
progress before the Black Death; the increased death-rate
quickened the process for a time, and it was again hastened
by the numerous desertions which are noted in the latter years
of the century.

Having thus roughly surveyed the condition of the Bishop
of Winchester's manors before the Black Death, we are in
a position to examine closely its actual effects, as measured,
not by rhetorical lamentation or interested petition or
paternal legislation, but by hard cash and definite figures.

CHAPTER II

THE IMMEDIATE EFFECTS OF THE BLACK DEATH, 1348–50

HAVING thus examined the condition of the episcopal manors immediately before the devastations of the Black Death, it is possible to go to the accounts for the actual years of the plague, and to trace both the direct references to it, and the direct results of the heavy death-rate. The first and most striking fact is that the Accounts were continued without a break and without change in form during the two plague years. There is no sign whatever of the disuse of old methods, owing to the death of all the experienced accountants. It is true that the handwriting of the rolls changes during 1350–1, and possibly during 1349, to one which is larger, less pleasing, and apparently less skilled, but the change is only temporary, and, moreover, only denotes a change of scribe at Winchester.[1] It is evident that on all the manors there still survived an official capable of giving in the usual exact details of his administration, either by tallies, or by slips of parchment, containing brief notes.

On several manors the same reeve continued in office straight through the years 1348–52, or even longer. It is true there are no Court Rolls extant for these years, but the collection of Court Rolls for the Bishop's estates, although immense, is very incomplete. The absolute continuity of the Account Rolls is a warning of the danger of pushing the argument from silence too far. This fact may well be emphasized. On some sixty manors in the south of England, of which exactly contemporary accounts are preserved, there is no sign whatever of chaos, of complete depopulation, although they were all (or almost all) visited by the Black Death. The evidence here is on so large a scale, and is so widely distributed that it must be very carefully weighed

[1] Cf. Hall, Pipe Roll of Bishopric of Winchester, 1208–9, Introduction.

against the rhetorical statements of chroniclers, or the more precise but isolated evidence drawn from the accounts and Court Rolls of other single manors in the same districts.

Dislocation of the ordinary system is certainly indicated ; on some manors the reeve receives an extra payment by the precept of the Seneschal, *pro magno labore*, and it may well be that his labours were greatly increased by the unprecedented mortality. Nevertheless, he went on doing his work, and on the whole, doing it well. Only on a very few of the more remote manors is there any hint of the peculation in which he might easily have indulged.[1]

It would be easy to draw from the Account Rolls a dark picture of the loss and misery caused by the plague. Incidental references to it abound in the rolls for 1349 and 1350. Again and again one reads the curt note, ' Nothing because he was dead '. So great was the multitude of heriots that extra labour was required on several manors to attend to them ; extra hay and straw had to be bought ; certain pastures returned nothing because of the lord's heriots pastured there ; at Staplegrove extra hedges were needed because of the heriots. It must indeed have been disconcerting for the ordinary manorial servants to find that they had on their hands 46 horses instead of 9, 60 cows instead of the usual 20, or an additional 20 oxen beyond the ordinary teams. On one manor the oxen had to be put out to keep, while nothing could be obtained for milk. At Cheriton it is noted that 10s. for the *Chivinagium* (? *Cheminagium*) of itinerant carts passing through the lord's pasture was not paid, because there were no itinerant carts. At Brightwell the tenants somewhat naturally refused to do their carrying services (*Averagia*) either to London or elsewhere. Extra help was commonly needed for washing and shearing the sheep, ' beyond the customers ' ; women were often hired for this, and were paid 2d. per day. At Witney corn was sold standing in the fields at harvest time. At Bishopston and Downton and Twyford old houses were pulled down and the timber sold.

---

[1] v. p. 150. Cf. Page, Disappearance of Villeinage in England. (New York, 1900.)

In some cases the cost of the harvest meals declines considerably, because of the fewness of the customers, while for the same reason extra men have to be hired. The sale of works is affected because eighteen tenements are in the lord's hand, and there are no works to sell. Often the entry is simply, ' Nothing this year, because of the pestilence ', the exact effect of the pestilence being left to the imagination.

Again and again comes the entry, among the fines, that proclamation of a vacant tenement was duly made, according to the custom of the manor, and that as no one ' of the blood ' had made claim, the tenement fell into the lord's hands as an escheat. Whole families had evidently been swept off. Very often, too, the land escheated to the lord because the heir died before he could ' make Fine '. The mere length of the lists of fines and heriots shows how sharp was the visitation of the plague.

But to obtain this gloomy picture one must put together evidence from a large number of manors and thus produce a composite impression ; moreover, the picture is frankly impressionistic. It has no outlines, no exactness, little or no proportion. A much stricter analysis is needed before results can reasonably be discussed.

As a starting-point one may ask, What are the questions to which one really seeks a reply ? What problems may one hope to answer ? Briefly, the chief questions are these :

[Population.] What proportion of deaths occurred on each manor ? Is the death-rate evenly distributed ? Could one hope to discover an average rate for the whole of southern England ?

[Vacant tenements.] What proportion of tenements were thrown on the lord's hands, i. e. how far were whole families exterminated, and how far was the existing population capable of filling up the gaps in the ranks of the manorial tenants ? Are there any cases of villages swept absolutely bare ? Does the rural depopulation of the fifteenth century really date back to 1349 ?

[Labour and Wages.] How far is there a serious dearth of labourers ? How does the decrease of labourers affect the question of commutation ? How far is the rate of wages lastingly affected ?

How were the landlords affected ?

Can one trace the influence of the Black Death on the growth of the system of ' Farms ' and leases ? Do the methods of agriculture undergo any striking changes ?   Does sheep-farming or enclosing make any notable advance immediately after 1349 ? [Leasing and Farming.]

Can one trace a direct connexion between the ravages of the Black Death and the discontent of 1381 ? [The Peasants' Revolt.]

' The most striking and immediate effect of the mortality was to bring about nothing less than a complete social revolution,' says Gasquet.[1] ' It seemed as if the agriculture of the country was completely ruined ' is Cunningham's judgement.[2]

No one who had looked through one of the Winchester Account Rolls for 1349 or 1350 and had compared it with a similar roll ten years earlier or later in date could possibly endorse either of these statements. A strong impression of continuity in method and in prosperity is left on one's mind after such a cursory examination, and the more closely one compares details, the more fully is the impression borne out.

Each question that arises can be answered in some sort by actual figures, and although any one set of figures may be misleading, the total result is generally consistent and reliable. Taking the groups of questions as suggested above, the first problem appears to be that of population.

It is almost impossible to arrive at an estimate of the population of a manor from the information given in an Account Roll ; none of the entries provide the material for such a calculation. From Court Rolls it might be possible to arrive at a *minimum* number of tenants, but even such an unsatisfactory estimate is not possible where no contemporary Court Rolls exist. In one case only, the *Extent* of Orchard,[3] the number of tenants can be ascertained, but this is precisely a manor which does not occur in the accounts in ordinary years. Again, on those manors which give an account of

---

[1] Gasquet, The Great Pestilence, 2nd ed., p. 227.
[2] Cunningham, Growth of English Industry and Commerce, 5th ed., vol. i, p. 332.
[3] Cf. p. 22.

the ' Works ' a rough estimate may be made, but this is possible only on the Taunton Group, before 1349, though similar figures may be given for the Hampshire manors in 1376–7. Occasionally the item Harvest Works (under Expenses) may give a clue, but as a rule it is not possible to distinguish the number of customers working from the total number of days' work done by them. I have therefore worked out a *minimum* estimate of population for a few manors,[1] taking each able-bodied tenant as representing a family group of *five* (probably a very low figure, as many of the virgaters and ferlingmen may have had under-tenants or ' squatters ' on their land, as well as large families).

More light, however, is thrown on the question by the entries of Fines and Heriots, and it is impossible to treat the questions of tenants and tenements separately.

The following tables aim at showing how much land was thrown on the lord's hands during the years of pestilence, how long it remained in his hands, and, to some extent, the number of deaths on each manor. Thus in the year 1348–9 many tenements paid no rent, and on many manors still more were vacant in 1349–50. It is remarkable, however, that Rimpton, Crawley, Droxford, Harwell, and Brightwell show no vacant holdings whatever in 1348–9, while Rimpton, Crawley and Harwell had none in the following year. The number steadily decreases in almost every case, until in 1353–4 only two Somerset manors show a clear loss of rents ; the tenements cultivated by the lord's reeve on his behalf also show a decrease in number between 1349–50 and 1350–1, but the latter year was disastrous to all kinds of crops, and there is little change observable by 1353–4. It is worth noticing that where the *number* of tenements left vacant is the largest (i. e. in the group of manors around Taunton) the size of the holding is frequently very small.[2] In this district there were very few virgaters, but even the ferlinglands were not often left tenantless ; the bulk of the ' Defects ' belong to cottages with curtilage, crofts, and plots of one or two acres in extent, and from 1*d*. to 1*s*. in rent. (Cf. the tables

[1] Cf. p. 81.   [2] Cf. p. 70 and p. 82.

on pp. 162–177, where the total value of the 'defects' is given, with the number of defects here noted.)

Where the rents are raised on the produce, it is generally found that the lord reaped a small profit as well, though this fact is partly obscured by the fact that many tenements were taken up at Hocktide, and thus part of the rent counts as a 'defect'. It is evident, too, that when the rent was raised from the produce, the lord must have been able to procure the necessary labour to cultivate the vacant holdings, or at least to act as shepherds or cowherds if he decided to use them for stock. Occasionally tenements which had been let at a yearly rent without services were entered among the *Exitus Manerii*, and it is thus difficult to distinguish whether the 'Issues' denote these temporary rents, or the usual sale of produce. But the ordinary entry is quite clear.

With regard to the light thrown by this table upon the number of deaths due to the plague, one cannot be very confident. The number of heriots paid is the best guide, if each man's land paid only one heriot; but it is quite possible that when a villein engrossed holdings, a heriot might be paid for each.[1] This fact does not appear, however, to affect the figures above to any considerable extent. Here and there two heriots were paid from one tenant, but this is the exception. At Nailesbourne, where 51 heriots in pence were paid, an examination of the names shows that they are paid by 51 different persons; of 179 heriots paid at Poundisford at least 106 are paid by tenants of different surnames; at Bishop's Waltham, where 83 heriots in pence are noted, there are only three cases in which the same surname recurs; at Rimpton, among 20 persons paying heriots, there are only three cases of a recurring surname.

If all tenements were 'heriotable' it is clear that the number of tenements in the lord's hand, plus the number of fines, would give one approximately the number of heriots, and would check the calculation of the number of deaths. On

---

[1] Cf. Surveys of Lands of William, First Earl of Pembroke (Roxburghe Club), where many of the manors in Wiltshire seem to have demanded the *three* best beasts as heriots.

TABLE OF VACANT TENEMENTS.*

Name of Manor.	1348–9.				1349–50.			
	Tenements Vacant. No Rent paid.	Rent raised on produce.	No. of Fines.	No. of Heriots.	Tenements Vacant. No Rent paid.	Rent raised on produce.	No. of Fines.	No. of Heriots.
Hull . . .	25	—	40	c. 66	25	32† 8‡	61	16 in pence 1 beast.
Poundisford .	53	—	94	104 in pence 75 beasts	75 +	c. 20	104	39 in pence 3 beasts.
Nailesbourne .	c. 36	—	c. 60	51 in pence c. 30 beasts	39	16† 30‡	34	1 beast.
Holway . .	25	—	c. 100	c. 84 in pence 91 beasts	c. 11	28† 3‡	c. 88	32 in pence 2 beasts.
Staplegrove .	18	—	c. 72	76 in pence 59 beasts	c. 15	29† 6‡	74	12 in pence 5 beasts.
Rimpton . .	None	None	c. 22	4 in pence 15 beasts	None	None	3	None.
Downton .	To value of £4 0 0¼	To value of 10 6 9½ [49 tenements]	78 +	108 beasts	36	40† 30‡	64	,,
Stoke . . .	3	1	c. 67	35 beasts +	3	—	23	2 beasts.
Crawley . .	None	—	24	26 beasts +	—	7† 2‡	15	None.
Bishop's Waltham	2	—	c. 240	c. 241 (83 in pence)	6	—	88	1 beast.
Droxford . .	None	—	85 +	c. 67 beasts	7	—	10	1 beast.
Beauworth .	8	—	4	10 ,,	—	19 §	2	None.
Cheriton . .	24	—	18	53 ,,	—	38 §	25	1 beast.
Sutton . .	44	—	46	60 ,,	—	49 §	45	3 beasts.
Marwell . .	11	c. 20	19	c. 20 ,,	—	31 §	14	None.
Twyford . .	49	—	37	30 ,,	—	47 §	15	,,
Brightwell .	No entry	—	25	9 in pence 14 beasts	—	5 §	20	,,
Harwell . .	No entry	—	27	12 beasts	None	None	10	,,

* Many of these figures are approximate, because the MS. is torn or illegible ; but the inaccuracy is generally slight.

† Rent wholly raised on produce of tenement.

‡ Rent partly raised on produce of tenement.

§ Including tenements on which no rent is paid and tenements on which rent is partly or wholly raised.

TABLE OF VACANT TENEMENTS.

Name of Manor.	1350–1.				1353–4.			
	Tenements Vacant. No Rent paid.	*Rents raised on produce.*	*No. of Fines.*	*No. of Heriots.*	*Tenements Vacant. No Rent paid.*	*Rent raised on produce.*	*No. of Fines.*	*No. of Heriots.*
Hull . . .	11	2	46	10 in pence 1 beast	—	10	19	4 in pence. 1 beast.
Poundisford .	19	4	59	13 in pence 2 beasts	—	22 ‡	31	14 in pence. 6 beasts.
Nailesbourne .	13	2	36	16 in pence	—	22 ‡	15	2 in pence.
Holway . .	4	3	65	19 in pence 4 beasts	13 §	—	19	4 in pence.
Staplegrove .	7	6	55	19 in pence 1 beast	10 §	—	32	8 in pence. 3 beasts.
Rimpton . .	None	None	2	None	None	None	2	
Downton . .	—	58 *	27	None	—	41 *	18	
Stoke . . .	2	—	12	—	—	1	11	1 beast.
Crawley . .	—	3	5	—	—	2 † 2 ‡	2	
Bishop's Waltham	—	—	49	15 in pence 1 beast	—	—	23	9 in pence. 3 beasts.
Droxford . .	—	—	10	2 beasts	—	—	2	1 beast.
Beauworth .	6	3 † 8 ‡	1	—	2	10	3	—
Cheriton . .	13 (?)	4 † 15 ‡	12	—	—	23 §	6	—
Sutton . .	—	25 §	12	—	1	24 †	7	1 beast.
Marwell . .	—	22 §	2	—	—	20 §	5	—
Twyford . .	—	26 §	16	—	2	12 † 15 ‡	15	—
Brightwell .	1	—	11	1 in pence 1 beast	1	—	2	—
Harwell . .	None	—	4	1 in pence	—	—	2	1 beast.

   * Includes a few on which no rent was raised.
   † Rent wholly raised on produce of tenement.
   ‡ Rent partly raised on produce of tenement.
   § Including tenements on which no rent is paid and tenements on which rent is partly or wholly raised.

some manors one finds this correspondence in figures,[1] but it is evidently not to be relied on. Many small tenements probably did not owe heriots, and a tenement consisting entirely of overland did not pay a heriot. It is more significant to notice that while the heriots give the approximate death-rate, the fines give the number of able-bodied men and women who survived.[2]

Thus taking as an example Bishop's Waltham, where 241 heriots were paid and 240 fines made in court during 1348–9, one might admit that each man or woman taking up land would represent two other adult relatives *not tenants* of the lord. This very low estimate (purposely low because there is no record of the deaths of landless women and children) would give a population of from 600 to 700 adults for Bishop's Waltham—a very large manor. Over eighty different surnames occur in the lists of heriots and in the later Court Rolls. Yet in 1376–7 only 37 customers are mentioned as owing most of the surviving services. These, however, were all below the status of a virgater. It is thus impossible to ascertain the total number even of tenants at Waltham, and quite impossible to discover whether the 240 deaths represent one-third, one-fourth, or any other fraction of the whole population. But grouping roughly thus :

240 deaths of tenants
240 incoming tenants
240 surviving dependants of tenants,

it is obvious that a loss of one-third of the population is an over-pessimistic estimate. If it is true that children and old men suffered less than men in the prime of life, the proportion would be very considerably reduced.

[1] Something must be allowed for the marriages which are included under Fines in the table on p. 78 ; these were perhaps unusually frequent during the plague years. Something must also be allowed on many manors for fines paid on sales or leasing of land among the villeins, which continued unchecked by the ravages of the plague.

[2] In some cases, of course, the same tenement changed hands more than once in the year, and thus the tenants surviving would be less in number than the tenants making fine, but the qualification does not appear to make any serious difference in the figures. The fines for 1349–50 are probably a safer guide than those for 1348–9, as the new tenants for the second year are more likely to have survived. (But cf. p. 217. Addenda.)

The following very tentative table gives first the *ascertain-able* number of unfree tenants on a group of manors in Somerset; secondly the number of heriots paid, and thirdly, an estimate of the adult population based *entirely* on the supposition that each tenant owing works represented a group of three adults. If, as has been shown, each heriot commonly represented a different tenant, it will be clear that the adult population must have been much larger than the number of tenants mentioned as owing works.

On this estimate from two-fifths to one-half of the adult population must have perished, but the mortality is very irregularly distributed.

If it may be assumed that children formed one-third of the total population, as in modern census returns for England, and that children suffered little from the plague, the proportion of deaths sinks to about 33 per cent. These calculations, however, involve a considerable amount of supposition, and are highly unsatisfactory. All the figures used are somewhat suspicious, and they hardly seem to tally with the results shown by the Accounts of Works.[1] Moreover, extremely little is gained by making out an *average* death-rate. The mortality varied widely, not only from manor to manor, but from tithing to tithing, and in discussing the changes in the manorial economy, it must be remembered that immobility of labour, though beginning to break up, is still a very weighty reality.

The general impression gained from an attempt to make any such calculations is that they are singularly useless.

	A. Number of tenants mentioned as owing works.	B. Number of Heriots.	C. Adult population (?) A × 3.	D. Total population (?) A × 5.	E. Population in 1801.
Nailesbourne	81	c. 81	243	405	
Holway	127	175	381	635	
Poundisford	124	179	272	620	
Staplegrove	75	135	225	375	319
Hull	74	66	212	370	683
Rimpton	37 ?	19	111	185	193
Orchard	38	—	114	190	131
	556	655	1558	2780	

[1] Cf. p. 89.

The question of vacant tenements is, however, much easier to solve; the evidence of the tables on pp. 78–9 is quite clear and unmistakable.

Of 18 manors examined 5 had absolutely no vacant tenements in September 1349, 2 had none in September 1350, 4 had none in 1351, while in 1354 4 had none, and 2 had only one still vacant. Taking the 18 manors together, if the 1,340 heriots paid in 1348–9 represent 1,340 holdings, one finds that 1,058 [1] fines were made within the year, while in the following year 128 tenements were thrown on the lord's hands, and 705 [1] fines were made. Thus after making due allowance for the marriages and leases which are included among the fines, it is evident that a very large proportion of the tenements must have been occupied again by 1351. By 1354 only 233 holdings remained vacant, while the heriots during the five years 1349–54 amounted to nearly 1,800. The average number of vacant holdings per manor is thus about 13, but it would be extremely misleading to take this as representing the general state of affairs; the average number on the Hampshire and Berkshire manors was 9, while taking the 6 least affected manors the average is one each.

The number of tenements vacant seems much larger than the loss in rent would lead us to expect. There are two main reasons for this. First, the vacant tenements on the Taunton group are very small holdings. The ordinary villein on these manors held only a ferling-land (10 acres), but it is not these which are vacant,[2] but rather the dwelling-houses, the cottages, crofts and tofts, and odd pieces of land worth small sums of 1d. or 2d. to 1s. In Hampshire the holdings were generally larger, and the empty holdings include a fair number of virgates, though the majority of 'defects' are for smaller plots. Secondly, it is generally possible to divide the lands on which the lord was able to raise the rent on the produce from those which lay derelict. The table is not quite accurate

---

[1] This figure is subject to two qualifications : (a) it includes a certain number of marriages ; (b) it contains a small proportion of cases of sales, sub-letting, or exchange.

[2] I believe it is safe to say that not a single virgate lay unclaimed on the Taunton manors, and very few ferling-lands.

on this point, as the account for some manors is confused. Taking it as it stands, however, only 29 tenements are a dead loss to the bishop by 1354, that is to say, an average of between one and two holdings on each manor made no return whatever. A considerably larger number paid part only of their rent from the produce, but on the great majority the whole rent was raised, and on very many small sums *ultra redditum* are commonly noticed.[1]

A new entry makes its appearance in the accounts, *Exitus terrarum in manus domini per pestilentiam*, which must be balanced against the *Defectus redditus per pestilentiam*.[2] Generally the balance is in favour of the bishop, though the gain is not large. It must be noticed, however, that if the lord could make an actual profit over and above the rents by cultivating the vacant tenements, or by letting them on new terms, he lost the labour services, the heavy occasional fines, the heriots, and the dues of the Court, so far as these holdings were concerned. The net result, therefore, might easily be a loss. What is very noticeable, however, is that in no single case in any year here examined is the loss absolute. The bishop might make a lower rate of net profits; he never failed to find a profit on every manor.

It is not very clear how the vacant tenements were cultivated, nor what class of produce was sold to meet the rent. The standing corn belonged to the chattels of the dead man, and although it might conceivably be sold to provide a heriot,[3] it would not fall to the lord unless the holding came to him as an escheat. In the fairly frequent cases where a widow or next heir refused to make fine for the land on account of poverty or impotence, the lord must probably have lost the

---

[1] It has already been noticed (p. 77) that in some cases the rents may have been raised or even exceeded by letting the vacant holdings at a yearly rent, to tenants who would not make fine and take up the ordinary position of a villein. But as a rule this is not clearly stated. Cf. Adderbury, 1376 (?) : ' Exitus Manerii. Et de vs. de Rogero Daw pro 1 cotland quondam Alicie Aylon ultra certum redditum quousque aliquis advenerit ad finiendum pro eodem.' Similar entries occur at Droxford, and at Cheriton.

[2] Wargrave, 1351-2, *Defectus* : ' De redditu vi*d*. pro uno mesuagio et dimidia virgata terre native que fuerunt Alicie Colt nichil in defectu quia levitur de exitibus et de residuo reddit infra in exitu manerii.'

[3] Cf. p. 55. Cf. Digby, History of the Law of Real Property, p. 213.

rent until he could find a new tenant or until next year's produce could be gathered in. In subsequent years there is little or nothing to show whether the holdings in the lord's hand were cultivated, or used as pasture. Probably if the rough pasture on compact holdings had been sold, the rent might have been raised, and it would certainly be convenient for the lord to retain some extra pasture, for the use of the numerous heriots. It is hard to see, however, that anything could be done with a strip-holding save to cultivate it in the usual rotation. Until extensive enclosure, demanding a plentiful supply of labour, could be carried out, most of the vacant villein tenements could hardly be turned to account for sheep-farming, although, no doubt, they might set free part of the demesne for grazing purposes.[1]

It is interesting to notice how the tenements which were taken up were filled. In reading down a list of fines, one sees that a large number of tenants succeeded in the ordinary way, to their fathers or brothers or husbands.[2] The number of widows retaining land is large, but not specially remarkable; when a daughter succeeded to her father's land—and according to Collinson in the Taunton manors the youngest daughter succeeded to the whole tenement (see p. 50)—her fine on entry is almost invariably followed by a slightly higher fine, paid by her husband 'for her and her land'. Heiresses commonly married within a year of entering upon their inheritance.

When no direct heir by blood was immediately forthcoming, proclamation was made in court, according to the custom

---

[1] A separate entry occurs on some manors of the *Defectus per secundam pestilentiam*, i. e. the visitation of 1361. Such manors often show a larger loss for the second than for the first pestilence, but the entries are a trifle suspicious. *Defectus post pestilentiam* would in some cases be a more accurate heading. For instance, at Bishop's Sutton the defects in 1355 are 3s.; in 1377 there are no defects *per primam pestilentiam*; in 1386 there is a deficit of 1s. 2d. and by 1455 it has increased to 12s. The fact is that the heading may be convenient to cover desertions for which the bailiff would otherwise be responsible.

[2] Of 82 fines at Poundisford in 1348–9, 43 were for land descending from relatives, 17 from land which had escheated to the lord, 14 for sale or sub-letting of land, 6 for marriages, and 2 doubtful. The same tenement is sometimes involved more than once.

of the manor, for several successive law-days. If none of the kindred appeared, the lord looked favourably upon other applicants, who would be willing to take the land on the old terms. In many cases men who were already tenants of the manor would be glad to take up an additional holding; sometimes the tenement or tenements would be split up among a number of applicants. In one case 26 tenants were held responsible jointly for the works of one virgate.[1] In other cases a son or a brother of a tenant would become an independent holder instead of a mere supernumerary. The practice already noticed at Taunton of paying fine for one acre in order to attract to one's self the residue of the tenement seems to point to some competition in securing land. On the other hand, especially on the Hampshire manors, there are signs that some pressure was needed. Many of the entries of fines end with the words *compulsus est*—he was compelled to take up a holding.[2] Who compelled him is not quite clear; probably the bailiff in conjunction with the whole body of customary tenants, for there are other entries stating that a certain man had been chosen or elected by the homage *per totum homagium electus est*.[3] This entry is not common enough to have much significance as to the filling up of vacant tenements, but it is obvious that the homage acted as a body in supplementing the persuasion or coercion of the bailiff, and that they were afraid of being burdened, in their communal capacity, with the obligations of an unoccupied holding.

During the years 1349–50 the normal successor frequently died before he could come and pay his fine; his death is commonly recorded in the entry of the fine which was eventually paid. Occasionally a tenant, generally a woman, is allowed to refuse the tenement on the ground that he or she

---

[1] Meon, 1348–9, Sale of Works. Each of the 26 tenants paid 1*d*. in place of the works due from the vacant virgate. This arrangement dates back before the pestilence.

[2] Nailesbourne, 1350–1, *Defectus per pestilenciam*: ' Robertus le Somenour compulsus finivit et clam recessit et ea tenere recusavit.' Compulsion was evidently not a wholly successful method of dealing with the difficulty.

[3] Cf. p. 51. Cf. Twyford, 1353–4, Fines.

was too poor or too impotent to pay the fine or fulfil the obligations ; in other cases the next of kin might come into court and solemnly renounce his right in full court, whereupon the land was considered to have escheated to the lord.[1]

The taking up of an escheated tenement was apparently the most favourable opportunity of commuting services. ' So-and-so holds such land for rent, because no one would hold it for works ' is a fairly frequent entry both before and after 1349 ; *extenduntur in denarios quamdiu domino placuerit* is another common way of expressing commutation of labour services.

By one or other of these means the vacant tenements were filled up so completely that the manorial organization was maintained almost without alteration ; among the Bishop of Winchester's manors there is not one which suffered any important change of system before 1355. It is useless to deny that the population was greatly decreased ; it seems equally useless to deny that the surplus and surviving population was able to meet the new demands made upon it, and to fill, to a very large extent, the gaps left in its ranks.

This conclusion leads on to the question of commutation, and the results of the Black Death in hastening or retarding its progress. Two or three facts stand out very clearly in the history of labour services on the episcopal manors. The change had already begun in 1208, but it was not yet complete in 1455. It had made very considerable progress by 1349, but was everywhere partial and variable. No single manor in the Account Rolls had entirely commuted its labour services.[2]

---

[1] Twyford, 1353–4, Fines : ' Et de vi*s*. viii*d*. de Adam Gyke pro 1 croft continente xii acras terre purpresture in Suthtwyford que fuit Isabellae Godde et que devenit in manus domini tanquam escaeta, eo quod dicta Isabella demens est per quod redditus et servicia a retro sunt per biennium et de quibus Henricus Gaterigge qui fuit propinquior de sanguine ad finiendum pro eisdem secundum consuetudinem in plena curia ius suum remisit habenda.'

[2] Pillingsbere (Billingsbear) might seem to be an exception, but I am by no means sure that Pillingsbere was ever accounted a manor ; it seems to have had no court, and possibly no demesne. Certain services are done at Pillingsbere by neighbouring manors, e. g. Culham. The Hundred Rolls note that Pillingsbere was a great *purprestura* in the Forest of Windsor, annexed by Adomar, Bishop-elect of Winchester, and enlarged by his successors, and enclosed with a strong fence hedge.

The wages paid in 1348, when compared with the amount of produce raised, would in themselves suffice to show that the main part of the work of the manor was provided by villein services.

In 1376–7 the Account Rolls contain an exact account of the 'Works' of almost each manor;[1] it is therefore clear that labour services still survived and were as widely distributed in 1377 as in 1348. This reduces the problem to more manageable proportions, but even here subdivision is again necessary. First one needs to know what changes took place during the thirty years under consideration ; secondly one needs to know whether these changes were the result of the Black Death itself, or merely the effect of normal economic causes, working out with little or no stimulus from the decrease in population.

Unfortunately the evidence is adequate only on one group of manors—the Taunton group. For the Hampshire manors the evidence of 1377 generally stands alone and must be carried backwards, with some suspicion, to 1348, and supplemented with incidental notices of services elsewhere in the Rolls.

The accounts for the Taunton group are, however, very satisfactory. The entries of services owed, performed, and sold are complete during the whole period under review.[2] It is therefore possible to ascertain (1) whether the supply of labour services was greatly lessened by the Black Death ; (2) whether the practice of commutation made exceptionally rapid progress during this period ; (3) whether, on the contrary, commutation was retarded by the shortage of hired labour ; (4) the disposition of labour services, and the types which tended to survive.

The following tables will make these points clearer than any commentary can do.

It is evident that on the six manors examined all the main types of services still existed—ploughing and harrowing,

---

[1] Cf. p. 62.
[2] I believe they are entered for every year from 1347 to 1377. Later on they are omitted.

harvesting, and week-work are all accounted for. There are no special carrying services, but the lists of the 'manual works' performed shows that the latter could be utilized for all kinds of carting and carrying. Possibly the demesne provided the horses and carts necessary ; carts were certainly made by the villeins as part of their 'manual works'. Moreover, none of this group (except Rimpton) was as far as ten miles from Taunton : the carrying services, therefore, could not have been very burdensome.

It is important to notice how variable the commutation was. Certain services seem to have been uniformly required on the demesne, but others were treated differently from year to year. Some of the ploughing services were performed on all the manors in 1348, and only on one (Poundisford) was the whole of the ploughing commuted by 1377. The same is true of the harrowing services. The harvest services survive everywhere, as one might expect, and are absolutely unchanged in amount by 1377. In the 'manual works' the bishop had a reservoir of undefined and unallotted labour, which could be disposed of as seemed most necessary at the time. The large surplus already mentioned (p. 65) which was normally sold could be drawn upon to make up any deficiencies in the specific services owed by certain tenants. Hence the sums entered under 'Sale of Works' show a marked decrease during the years 1349–52, but the decrease does not denote that commuted services were reimposed, nor does an increase of money gained by such sale imply that more hired labour was required to replace the works sold. The surplus was large enough to cover the 'defects' caused by the pestilence. All the necessary work of the demesne was performed as usual (with the assistance of a few wage-paid servants), and there were still 'works' left over which might be sold. In proof of this statement there are first the condensed entries given in the table on p. 180, and secondly there are the full accounts of the disposition of the manual works, of which a few specimens are transcribed here.

NAILESBOURNE, 1348–9.

Total number of *Opera Manualia* owing	4755

In acquittance to 1 reeve and 1 beadle . . .	98	
,, ,, 1 ploughman	122	
,, ,, 9 *operarii* for festivals . . .	45	
Total number of *Opera* acquitted . . . . —		265
Reaping and harvesting &c. by 62 customers . .	248	
Mowing, and haymaking, 12 acres	96	
Mattocking demesne for winter sowing . . .	15	
Sowing	4	
Harrowing	104	
Making ' grips ' [1] or trenches	17	
Mattocking demesne for Lent sowing	15	
Sowing	4	
Making ' grips '	2	
Hoeing corn	64	
For 1 rook-herd	10	
Repairing bridge	2	
Total number of *Opera* performed		581
,, ,, ,, sold		3863
,, ,, ,, sold (after account was made up) .		61
		4770 [2]

NAILESBOURNE, 1349–50.

Total number of *Opera Manualia* owing	4755

Defects, owing to death of 19 customers . . .	931	
,, ,, ,, 12 ,,	1188	
Total number of defects . . . . . —		2119
Acquittances to the reeve, &c.	220	
,, for festivals	54	
Total number of *Opera* acquitted . . . . —		274
Harvesting the bishop's corn	248	
Haymaking (12 acres)	96	
Mattocking demesne for winter sowing . . .	18	
Sowing	4	
Harrowing	40	
Enclosing the fields known as Ruggewey and La Mersh,		
and mending hedges round meadow . . .	20	
Hoeing	50	
Enclosing	10	
Miscellaneous	102	
Total number of *Opera* performed		588
,, ,, ,, sold		1532
,, ,, ,, ,, (late)		242
		4755

[1] This entry ' *in eisdem terris grapiendis* ' was rather puzzling, but the word appears occasionally in other contexts which suggest that the reason of the process was better drainage. The word ' grip ' is still common in Sussex (and elsewhere) for a shallow trench or open drain. See Murray, Oxford English Dictionary. This entry thus confirms Norden's testimony as to the excellent system of trenching and mattocking common in the Vale of Taunton. Cf. p. 63 note.

[2] This slight inaccuracy appears to be in the original account.

Holway, 1348–9.

Total number of *Opera Manualia* owing   8462

,,   ,,   defects (from 4 tenants)   .   .   308
Acquittances to the reeve, three ploughmen, two
    beadles, one *Messor*, one smith, and two woodwards 1117
Acquittances for festivals   63
    Total number of acquittances   .   .   . ——   1180
Mowing demesne meadow   44
Harvesting bishop's corn   .   .   . 388
For one rook-herd 15
Spreading manure 7
Mattocking land for winter sowing   .   . 89
Harrowing 8
Making ' grips '   26
Mattocking land for Lent sowing   .   . 120
Harrowing 50
Making ' grips '   16
Reaping 609
Mending fences round corn   .   .   . 17
Miscellaneous 157
    Total number of *Opera* performed .   .   .   1546
    ,,   ,,   ,,   sold   5426
                                                8460

Holway, 1349–50.

Total number of *Opera Manualia* owing   8462

,,   ,,   defects (5 tenants)   .   .   .   587
Acquittances as in previous year   .   . 1117
    ,,   for festivals   .   .   . 78
    Total number of acquittances   .   .   . ——   1195
Mowing demesne meadow   44
Harvesting 388
For one rook-herd 15
At the barn 14
Spreading manure 10
Mattocking demesne for winter sowing   .   . 174
Boy leading harrow   18
Making ' grips '   48
Mattocking demesne for Lent sowing   .   . 140
Harrowing 60
Reaping 386
Mending hedges round corn   .   .   . 18
In bladis domini pikkandis   .   .   . 4
Removing rotten hay   20
Enclosing Haydewode   .   .   . 10
Miscellaneous 66
    Total number of *Opera* performed   1415
    ,,   ,,   ,,   sold   5123
    ,,   ,,   ,,   ,,   (late)   142
                                                8462

POUNDISFORD, 1348–9.

Total number of *Opera Manualia* owing	7002
„ „ defects	None ?
Acquittances to reeve, two beadles, and one ploughman	269
Acquittances for festivals 30	
Total number of acquittances	299
Mowing 24	
Haymaking (on 9 acres newly enclosed) . . . 36	
Harvesting (102 customers) 408	
„ (6 *operarii*) 120	
„ (3 *coterelli* and 1 *operarius*) . . . 44	
„ (8 *operarii*) 70	
For one rook-herd 10	
Mattocking for winter sowing 37	
Sowing 4	
Making ' grips ' 5	
Spreading manure 7	
Mending fences 6	
Washing and shearing 159 sheep 16	
Rolling up fleeces 2	
Making hedges 82	
Beating game in park 26	
Total number of *Opera* performed	897
„ „ „ sold	5585
„ „ „ „ (late)	91
	6872

POUNDISFORD, 1349–50.

Total number of *Opera Manualia* owing	7002
„ „ defects	595
Acquittances to reeve, two beadles, and two ploughmen	278
Acquittances for festivals 36	
Total number of *Opera* acquitted	314
Mowing 24	
Haymaking 36	
Harvesting (102 customers) 408	
„ (6 *operarii*) 120	
„ (3 *coterelli*) 44	
„ (8 *operarii*) 70	
For one rook-herd 10	
Mattocking for winter sowing 58	
Sowing 4	
Making ' grips ' 8	
Spreading manure 22	
Mending enclosure 9	
Mattocking demesne for Lent sowing . . . 28	
Sowing 4	
Reaping 24	
Mending hedges 22	
Total number of *Opera* performed	891
„ „ „ sold	5202
	7002

STAPLEGROVE, 1348–9.

Total number of *Opera Manualia* owing	4341
„ „ defects	None
Acquittances to reeve, beadle, and 2 ploughmen . 212	
„ for festivals . . . . . None	
Total number of *Opera* acquitted . . . . ——	212
Mattocking for winter sowing 41	
Making ' grips ' 11	
Making hedges round corn 6	
Mattocking for Lent sowing 16	
Sowing 4	
Spreading manure 4	
Carting manure from *pund-fald* 11	
Haymaking in Castlemead 48	
Mowing and haymaking in Doddehullemede . . 18	
Reaping 90	
Harvesting (47 customers) 188	
At the barn 12	
Collecting rods and making two carts . . . 2	
For one rook-herd 10	
Total number of *Opera* performed	461
„ „ „ sold	3668
	4341

STAPLEGROVE, 1349–50.

Total number of *Opera Manualia* owing	4341
„ „ defects	None
Acquittances to reeve, beadle, and 2 ploughmen . 212	
„ for festivals . . . . . None	
Total number of *Opera* acquitted . . . . ——	212
Mattocking for winter sowing 33	
Making ' grips ' 20	
Mattocking for Lent sowing 20	
Harrowing 20	
Carting manure 6	
Spreading „ 13	
Ditching 12	
Haymaking in Castelmede 48	
„ Dodhullemede 18	
Reaping 100	
Harvesting (47 customers) 188	
One rook-herd 10	
Removing straw 12	
Stacking „ 21	
Mending enclosure round barn and pound . . 8	
Total number of *Opera* performed	529
„ „ „ sold	3581
„ „ „ „ (late)	19
	4341

HULL, 1348–9.

Total number of *Opera Manualia* owing		4993
,, ,, defects		None ?
Acquittances to reeve, beadle, and 3 ploughmen .	432	
,, for festivals	30	
Total number of *Opera* acquitted	——	462
Haymaking (12 customers)	24	
Harvesting (63 ,,)	252	
,, (7 *operarii*)	80	
,, (6 ,,)	120	
Haymaking	14	
One rook-herd	12	
Mattocking demesne for winter sowing . . .	52	
Sowing	4	
Harrowing	124	
Making ' grips '	10	
Spreading manure	6	
Mattocking for Lent sowing	25	
Sowing	4	
Harrowing	17	
Mending hedge round corn	6	
,, road	2	
Hedging, &c.	65	
Hoeing lord's corn	336	
Supplying lord's kitchen	4	
Total number of *Opera* performed		1157
,, ,, ,, sold		3173
		4792

HULL, 1349–50.

Total number of *Opera Manualia* owing		4993
,, ,, defects (9 messuages, 2½ virgates) . .		790
Acquittances to reeve, beadle, and 3 ploughmen .	432	
Acquittances for festivals	36	
Total number of *Opera* acquitted	——	468
Haymaking (as in previous year)	24	
Harvesting ,, ,, . . .	252	
,, ,, ,, . . .	80	
,, ,, ,, . . .	120	
Haymaking	14	
Rook-herd	12	
Mattocking for winter sowing	52	
Sowing	4	
Harrowing	128	
Making ' grips '	8	
Mending hedges	6	
Mattocking for Lent sowing	50	
Sowing	4	
Harrowing	40	
Ditching, &c.	57	
Hoeing lord's corn	290	
Total number of *Opera* performed		1141
,, ,, ,, sold		2448
,, ,, ,, ,, (late)		146
		4993

RIMPTON, 1348–9.

Number of *Opera Manualia* owing	5100
,, defects	None ?
Acquittances to reeve and 3 ploughmen . . . 816	
,, for festivals 335	
,, ,, law-days 42	
Total number of *Opera* acquitted . . . . ——	1193
Threshing and winnowing 84	
,, ... 38	
,, ... 52½	
Ploughing (Lent sowing and on fallow) . . . 16	
Harrowing (1 day with horse=4 works) . . . 70	
Sowing peas 56	
Spreading manure 20	
Making 'grips' 24	
Reaping 200	
Mowing stubble for thatching 68	
Carrying hay, &c. 50	
Harvesting (225½ acres) 451	
Total number of *Opera* performed	1129½
,, ,, ,, sold	2449½
	4772

RIMPTON, 1349–50.

Total number of *Opera Manualia* owing	5100
,, ,, defects	None ?
Acquittances to reeve and 3 ploughmen . . . 816	
,, for festivals 462	
,, ,, law-days 42	
Total number of *Opera* acquitted . . . . ——	1320
Threshing and winnowing 421	
,, ... 77	
,, ... 56	
Ploughing 15	
Harrowing 70	
Sowing beans 52	
Spreading manure 42	
Making 'grips' 20	
Hoeing corn, 'because of the multitude of thistles ' . 315	
Mowing stubble 81	
Carrying litter to Taunton and Knoyle . . . 12	
Haymaking, &c. 266	
Harvesting (203 acres) 406	
Total number of *Opera* performed	1833
,, ,, ,, sold	1880
,, ,, ,, ,, (late)	77
	5110[1]

[1] It will be noticed that several of these totals are slightly inaccurate. I think the fault lies with the original account, because the 1349 lists are more inaccurate than those for 1350, where the 'Defects' are carefully recorded.

The one Hampshire manor (Meon) which has similar accounts arranges them differently ; only carting services, Manual Works, Harvest Works, and Manual Harvest Works are accounted for. The carting services, however, seem to include ploughing, and some of the *Opera Manualia* were utilized for ploughing (Landright). Judging from this list it would seem that almost the whole of the harvesting at Meon was done by hired labour. Moreover, all these services were owed by *operarii* (43 operarii or 15 ?) and none by ordinary customary tenants or virgaters. Commutation here seems to have affected certain classes uniformly. A considerable proportion, too, of the works of the *operarii* were sold. In 1348 the services were sold at the usual 1*d*. or ½*d*. each, but the rates had evidently not become stereotyped, as in 1376 we find the following prices : Carting services 3*d*. each ; Harvest works 2*d*. each ; Manual works 1*d*. each.

MEON MANERIUM, 1348-9.

Opera Carectaria.

748 Owed.

----

 51 Allowed for 3 weeks of Christmas, Easter, and Whitsuntide.
 18 *In consuetudine de Landryght.*
 41 Lacking from the land held by William le Fisshere.
332 Carrying manure.
306 Sold.

----

748 Total.

Opera Manualia.

308 Owed by 7 *operarii*.

----

 21 allowed for 3 festivals.
 10 *In consuetudine de Landryght.*
142 Collecting and spreading manure.
135 Sold.

308

Opera Autumpnalia.

870 Owed by 15 *operarii* (reaping or carting, 2 men with 1 cart) working
     every day from St. Peter ad Vincula to Michaelmas.

----

300 Allowed for Sundays, Saturdays and festivals.
 39 Lacking from land of William Fisshere.
 70 Reaping and binding lord's corn.
470 Sold.

----

879 Total.

[Inaccuracy is in original account.]

Opera Autumpnalia [ad manus].

464 Owed by 8 *operarii* working every day.

160 Allowed for Sundays, Saturdays and festivals.
 82 Reaping and binding.
 20 Spreading manure.
202 Sold.
———
464 Total.

MEON MANERIUM, 1349–50.

Opera Carectaria.

748 Owed.

 51 Allowed for 3 holiday weeks.
 18 Landright.
 41 Lacking from land of William le Fishere.
168 Lacking from lands of 3 tenants.
329 Carting manure.
141 Sold.
———
748 Total.

Opera Manualia.

308 Owed by 7 *operarii*.

 21 Allowed for 3 festivals.
 10 Landright.
204 Collecting and spreading manure.
 73 Sold.
———
308 Total.

Opera Autumpnalia.

870 Owed by 15 *operarii*.

345 Allowed for Sundays, Saturdays and festivals.
 39 Lacking from land of William Fisshere.
105 Lacking from lands of 3 tenants.
381 Sold.
———
870 Total.

Opera Autumpnalia ad manus.

464 Owed by 8 *operarii*.

184 Allowed for Sundays, &c.
 24 Collecting and spreading manure.
256 Sold.
———
464 Total.

A very fragmentary account from Sutton may be added
to the evidence from Meon. [It is evident, however, from
the account given in 1376–7, that only one group of services
is included here.[1]] In 1349–50 seven *operarii* owed 826 works

[1] Cf. p. 110.

(undefined) at Sutton (*ad curiam de Sutton*) ; that is, two days a week from Michaelmas to August 1 except the three holiday weeks, and every working day (excluding Saturdays, Sundays, and festivals) from August 1 to Michaelmas.

Of these 826 the works of one man (118) had been commuted ; 472 were lacking, because the land was in the lord's hand ; 236 were sold at 1½d. each.[1]

In 1353-4 the total owed was 840; of these 320 are definitely stated to have been ' relaxed '—evidently the vacant tenements had been taken up on different terms ; 520 were ' sold ' as before.

So far as this information covers the ground (i. e. on seven manors), it seems clear that labour services were not seriously affected by the Black Death, even in the actual years of the plague, because the surplus of labour generally sold was so large. Hence one may argue that real commutation, apart from 'sale of works', was hardly affected; the methods of agriculture and the organization of the manor were not disturbed, though it is undeniable that the demand for labour was stimulated, and stimulated very unevenly owing to its immobility.

This conclusion may be checked by a consideration of the changes and development of wages.

The only wages really worth considering are the day-wages of occasional hired workmen. It has already been shown that the ½d. or 1d. per day paid for the *Arrura de prece* or the *Messio de prece* is a traditional payment for boon-works, and not of the nature of wages proper. Again the 2s., 5s., or 6s. 8d. per annum earned by dairywomen, reeves, and ploughmen was so small a part of their wages and remained fixed for so long a period that it hardly enters into the question. On the other hand, the wages paid to extra men at harvest, beyond the customers, to occasional workmen such as carpenters, thatchers, masons, and especially to women, as well as the wages paid for piece-work, are very instructive. Much of this occasional work is, however, done

---

[1] In 1348-9 the number of works sold was 649 ; in 1341-2 they were valued at 1d. In 1438 they were still sold at 1½d. to the number of 410

RATES OF WAGES. HAMPSHIRE AND BERKSHIRE.

	1346–7	1347–8	1348–9	1349–50	1350–1	1353–4	1376–7
Thatcher and thatcher's boy	{ 3½d. p. d., 1/9 per week 4½d. p. d.	3d. p. d.	—	—	5d. p. d.	3d. p. d. 4½d. p. d.	4d. p. d. 3d. p. d.
Threshing wheat	3d. per 10 bus.	4d. p. d.	—	—	4½d. p. d.	6d. per qr.	
Threshing, mixed		—	—	—	2d. per qr.	2d. per qr.	
Winnowing		2d. per qr.	—	—	1½d. per qr.	1d. per qr.	
Mowing	4d. p. a. (peas) 5d. p. a. 6½d. p. a. 8d. p. a.	6d. p. a.		3d. p. a. or 6½d. p. a.	6d. p. a.	3d. p. d. 6d. p. a. 8d. p. a.	7½d. p. a.
Reaping, &c.	7d. p. a. 6½d. p. a. 6d. p. a. 3d. per field acre	6d. p. a.		6½d. p. a. 4½d. p. a. 3d. p. d. with meals	8d. p. a. 6½d. p. a.	8d. p. a. 6d. p. a.	8d. p. a.
Carpenter	10d. per week 1/6 „ „ 1/3 „ „ 3½d. per day 2½d. „ „ 3d. „ „	3d. p. d. 2½d. p. d. 4d. p. d.			3d. p. d.	c. 2½d. p. d. 3d. p. d. 3d. p. d.	4d. p. d.
Washing and shearing sheep		—	—	—	—	—	
Repereve	3d. p. d.						
Park-keeper	2d. p. d.				1½d. p. d.	1½d. p. d.	
Hedging	2/6 per furlong.	1½d. per perch					
Ditching		1d. p. d.					
Cutting brushwood		1d. p. d.					
Women collecting straw							
Warrener	1d. p. d.						(?) 3/4 per score (or for 220)
Plumbator	1/- p. d. 7d. p. d.					8d. p. d.	
His boy	2d. p. d.					10d. p. d. (?)	
Janitor	3d. p. d. 1½d. p. d.						

RATES OF WAGES. SOMERSET.

	1346–7	1347–8	1348–9	1349–50	1350–1	1353–4	1376–7
Thatcher and thatcher's	—	3½d. p. d.		—	3½d. p. d.	3d. p. d.	3d. p. d.
boy		2d. p. d.			4d. p. d.		
Threshing wheat	(Valued at 4d. per qr.)	1½d. p. d.	4d. p. qr.	—	1¼d. p. q. oats	—	2½d. p. q.
Threshing, mixed	—	2d. per qr.		—	2d., 2½d. p. qr.	2d. p. qr.	4d. p. d.
Mason	—			—	3d. p. d.		
Mowing	—			—	2½d. p. a. (?)		
Reaping	—						
Carpenter	—	3d. p. d. (valued)		—	3d. p. d.	—	4d. p. d.
Tiler	—	3d. p. d.		—	3d. p. d,	—	3d. p. d.
Ploughing (Saturdays)	—	3d. p. d.					
Ploughing, mattocking, and harrowing	—	1½d. p. d.	6½d. p. a. / 9d. p. a. } valued.				
Ploughing			10d. p. a.				
Park-keeper	—	10½d. p. week	5d. p. a.				

H 2

' *ad tascham* '—at a lump sum for the piece, or by a special bargain or ' convention '. In these cases it is impossible to discover whether the rate has risen or fallen. This system would form an easy means of evading the Statutes of Labourers.

Comparing the rates given above, it is clear that in some cases a rise of 25 per cent. to 33 per cent. seems to have taken place after 1349, but it is difficult to ascertain how large a part was played by such work in the total expenses of a manor. Taking the figures given as expenses in the tables on pp. 162–177, it is remarkable how small is the rise after 1349 ; indeed in several cases there is a fall. Where the rise is at all serious, it may almost always be found to be due to extra and unusual expenditure, e. g. on building, or on buying stock and corn. Thus, though the rise per cent. in wages may be considerable, this rise bears a very small proportion to the usual balance-sheet of the manor. The workmen no doubt profited greatly ; the lord cannot be shown to have incurred serious loss.

These tables are obviously very incomplete, partly, as has been shown, because the bishop appears to have avoided paying day-wages when possible ; partly because the circumstances of the work vary so much that many of the figures in the accounts are useless for purposes of comparison. The Somerset table is specially slight because so little wage-paid labour was needed in the Taunton district. Many more examples could be given, but these represent most of the different rates I have noticed. As a matter of fact, piece-work wages are almost useless, then as now, for exact comparison. An acre of mowing in one meadow may be nearly double the work of an acre in another, while reaping also must have varied very considerably from year to year.

It is remarkable that only one post-pestilence figure in these tables (8*d.* per acre, reaping) cannot be paralleled in 1346 and 1347. The wages of craftsmen[1] are surprisingly high, both before and after 1349 ; the plumber who was so

[1] The entries at Farnham, Winchester, Waltham, and others of the bishop's residences are a mine of information as to the payment of arts and crafts and their development, but a detailed examination of this valuable material would be irrelevant here.

much in request for work on the roofs was paid as much as
10*d.* or 1*s.* per day ; the tiler received 5*d.* a day ; the carpenter
was paid 2*d.* a day for mending carts, 3¼*d.* a day for making
window-frames, or 4*d.* a day for felling trees ; the highly
paid glaziers generally supplied their own materials. No
attempt has been made to distinguish the wages paid on
individual manors, because the figures are so few, and the
work varies from year to year in character. Harvesting, for
example, may include reaping, binding, shocking, carrying
and stacking corn, or only one or two of these processes.
Women's wages are very rarely mentioned ; they are paid
sometimes 2*d.*, sometimes 1*d.* a day ; for unskilled labour of
the same class men were paid at the same rate. However,
in spite of the incompleteness of the figures quoted here, they
are sufficient to show how impossible it is to state, with
Thorold Rogers, that the rise in wages was exactly 48 per
cent., was sudden, and was permanent.

It is useful to compare the rates actually paid with those
payable by the Statute of Labourers (1351).

The regular servants of the manor, ploughmen, shepherds,
and others, were to work as before for a yearly wage and
allowances, at the rate that had been paid in 1347 and four
years previously. On the Winchester manors there was no
attempt whatever to transgress this provision.

Harvesting and haymaking were to be paid at 1*d.* a day ;
mowers at 5*d.* per acre or 5*d.* per day ; reapers at 2*d.* a day
for the first week in August and 3*d.* a day for subsequent
weeks. These rates are evidently lower than those current
on the bishop's estates, with the one exception of the 5*d.*
a day for mowing, which was evidently unnecessarily high.
The rates allowed for threshing (wheat, 2½*d.* per qr., other
grain 1½*d.* per qr.) correspond roughly with those common in
Hampshire and in Somerset.

Artisans' wages, however, are fixed distinctly lower than
those prevalent on the Winchester manors. A master carpenter could evidently earn more than 3*d.* a day before 1349,
while an ordinary carpenter commonly earned 3*d.* rather than
2*d.* ; a ' *mestre mason de franche peer* ' might earn 4*d.* a day

according to the Statute, but this figure sounds very low in comparison with the rates paid to the plumber.

It is interesting also to compare the wages actually paid by the bishop with those complained of by the justices elsewhere. Miss Putnam [1] quotes the following cases, among others:

Reapers . . .	5d.–6d. per day	in Essex.
Mowing . . .	9d. per acre	„ „
„ . . .	10d.–14d. per acre	„ Wilts.
Hoeing (women) .	2d. per day	„ „
Threshing wheat .	3d. per qr.	„ Derby.
„ barley .	2d. „ „	„ Wilts.
Plastering (daubing) .	3d. per day and food	„ „
Sawyer . . .	5d. per day	„ „

These cases certainly sound more like a general rise of 48 per cent., indeed they must often have meant a rise of 100 per cent.; one or two of the figures do not seem to be abnormal, but on the whole, as Miss Putnam remarks, they lend considerable colour to the chroniclers' complaints of the ' malice of servants '. It must be acknowledged, how-ever, that they represent the extreme demands which the Statute of Labourers aimed at suppressing. The Winchester estates gave no parallel reason for intervention, although the wages paid were habitually above those fixed by Statute.

The following lists of the total wages paid on several manors (in Somerset, Hampshire, and Berkshire) in 1376–7 should be compared with the total receipts and expenses for this year (v. pp. 162–77) and also with the accounts of the customary services actually performed between 1376 and 1381. The wages have certainly increased both in total and in rate since 1346, but the figures point to an orderly development rather than to a cataclysmic upheaval ; there are no traces of a great ' social revolution '. The men who could afford to pay £5 or £10 as an entry fine were not as a class swept off their feet by being paid 2d. instead of 1d. a day, and a skilled craftsman only improved without revolutionizing his position when his wages rose from 3d. to 4d. per day. The lord, on the other hand, could well face a rise of 50 per cent. in the total wages when his wages bill amounted to only £8 or £12.

[1] v. B. H. Putnam, The Enforcement of the Statutes of Labourers. New York, 1908.

The analysis of expenses on six manors, which is also
added, should be compared with a similar table for 1346–8
(p. 59).   On five out of the six manors, the expenses are
higher than in the two preceding years, but the amount can
generally be paralleled in quite recent years.   Where the
increase is very large, as at Cheriton, it is evidently accounted
for by extensive purchases of corn and stock, and by building
expense, as well as by the extra labour required in attending
to the ' infirmities ' of the sheep.

WAGES AT SUTTON, 1376–7.

£	s.	d.	
	4	0	1 *fugator*.
	8	0	2 carters.
	4	0	1 shepherd.
	3	6	1 dairymaid.
	2	4	Thatching (4*d.* p. d.)
	1	9	Thatcher's assistant (3*d.* p. d.)
		8	Thatching.
		4	,,
	9	10	Miscellaneous.
	1	0	Carpenter (4*d.* p. d.)
	1	6	Mending walls—*ad tascham*.
	3	8	Thatching.
	3	8	,,
	12	5½	Making and mending hedges.
3	0	10	Park-keeper.
	8	4	Weeding.
	10	0	Mowing.
	4	0	Haymaking.
1	2	10½	Threshing.
1	14	8¾	Harvest works (provisions, &c.).
2	15	3	Bailiff's wages.
12	12	8¾	

WAGES AT TWYFORD, 1376–7.

£	s.	d.	
1	8	0	Smith ?+iron.
	1	6	For *Precariae*, ploughing.
	12	0	Three ploughmen (yearly).
	8	0	Two carters ,,
	3	0	Supervising shearing.
	16	0	Four shepherds (yearly).
	2	0	Dairymaid ,,
	3	6	Thatching (c. 4*d.* p. d.)
	4	0	Swineherd (yearly).
	10	0	Mowing 16 acres.
3	3	10¼	Harvest works (provisions).
1	6	0	Wages of bailiff.
8	17	10¼	

Wages paid at Nailesbourne, 1376–7.

£	s.	d.	
	2	4	To customers ploughing.
	1	4	Customary food provided.
	2	6	*Fugator.*
		8	Carpenter (4d. p. d.).
	1	9	Thatching (3d. p. d.).
	6	0	Shepherd and cowherd.
	13	11	Threshing.
	3	0	Mowing and harvest works.
1	11	6 *	

Wages paid at Harwell, 1376–7.

£	s.	d.	
	6	0	Smith.
		8	Thatcher (4d. p. d.).
		4	Two men carrying wood to Witney.
	9	4	Thatching (4d. p. d.).
	3	8	„ (assistant, 2d. p. d.).
	2	0	„ „
	3	4	Washing and shearing 220 sheep.
	6	0	Shepherd.
2	1	1¼	Threshing.
	7	6	Mowing and hoeing.
1	17	9	Harvest works (about half for provisions)
5	17	8¼	

Wages paid at Stoke, 1376–7.

£	s.	d.	
	1	3	To customers ploughing (*Precariae*).
	4	0	1 *fugator.*
	4	0	1 carter.
		8	Thatching (4d. p. d.).
		4	Carpenter (4d. p. d.).
	(?)4	0	1 shepherd.
	2	0	1 dairymaid.
	10	5	Park-keeper.
1	10	0	„
	6	2	Mowing (customary payments).
	12	11½	Harvest works.
3	15	9½	

Wages at Wargrave, 1376–7.

£	s.	d.	
	3	0	Smith.
1	0	0	Four ploughmen (*in defectu cust'*).
	6	0	Carter.
	5	0	Washing and shearing sheep.
	10	0	Two shepherds.
	5	0	Cowherd.
	8	0	Dairymaid and swineherd (4s. each).
2	14	11½	Threshing.
2	4	1	Harvest works (wages, not provisions).
6	15	0	Serjeant and warrener.
14	11	0½	

* Notice the very small sum spent on wages on the manors where ' *Opera Manualia* ' were superabundant.

EXPENSES, 1349–50.

	Stoke.	*Waltham.*	*Droxford.*	*Cheriton.*	*Sutton.*	*Crawley.*
	£ s. d.	£ s. d.	£ s. d.	£ s. d.	£ s. d.	£ s. d.
Ploughs . . .	illegible	2 10 9½	1 6 0	1 1 10	1 16 1	1 16 7
Carts . . .	1 2 3	2 2 1½	1 0 4	19 1	2 0 8	10 9
Corn bought . .	2 9 9	11 6 7½	—	10 16 6½	7 6 2½	
Stock bought . .	4 17 0	3 14 0	3 12 0¾	7 3 8	6 17 0	10 0
Dairy and	—	16 2½	9 9	—	—	8 0
sheepfold . .	14 11	2 17 2	1 7 10	2 18 6½*	2 0 10½	6 5 2
Household . .	2 5½	3 9 3½	6 7			
			Threshing			
		5 11 1½	1 5 4	3 2 3	8 8 3	19 10
					Hoeing	
Park . . .	1 11 11	3 14 2	—	—	7 6	
		Threshing			Threshing	
Meadows . .	6 2	{1 9 0½	—	—	1 0 10½	2 9 6¾
				Vadimonium	Park	
		3 1 8½	—	5 0 0	12 8	
		Mill		Expenses		
Autumn works . .	1 0 3 }	3 2 5	—	6 11½		
	1 10¾ }	6 17 4½	5 18 4	3 1 2	2 3 8¾	4 12 9
	16 8 7¼ †	58 10 1¼	17 18 2¾	35 0 0½	33 17 1½	21 3 5½

* 'Because of the great infirmity of the sheep.'

† These totals are copied from the roll, and for various reasons do not quite tally with the sum of the items given here. A few of the entries are illegible.

A further examination of the cost of the harvest works over a period of five or six years is also useful corroborative evidence. Only the Hampshire manors and two in Berkshire are given, as the Taunton manors show very small fixed payments, from 2s. to 4s. 2d., which hardly varied between 1284 and 1376, and were probably early commutations of the meals generally provided. Evidently no hired labour was required. On the Hampshire manors the expenses of the harvest fall under three main heads : (a) the cost of bread, beer, and herrings or some other *companagium* for the harvesters ; (b) the cost of hired labour over and above the work of the customers ; (c) the wages of the overseer, *repereve*, hayward, and stacker—generally for the time of harvest only, though the 6s. 8d. of the hayward is a fixed payment per annum ; (d) occasional payments for carts, small payments made for ' *Messio de prece* ' or in commutation of allowances in kind, and a few pence for candles for the watchmen who guarded the corn at night. Most of the accounts show that extra wages had to be paid in 1349 and 1350, but they do not show a steady rise ; the year 1350–1 was a disastrously wet season, and expenses are correspondingly high, but after this year there is generally a drop—sometimes a drop which continues down to 1376. The decrease may be due to decreased expenditure for food for the customers, or to a decrease in the area under cultivation as demesne ; it is not very clear which. It is quite clear, however, that the variations in the cost of getting in the harvest were not very great from year to year, and that the state of the weather and of the crops had at least as much influence as the decrease in the number of the customers. It should be noticed that although the number of customary tenants for whom food was provided is generally given, the figures are misleading ; the number of men working and the number of days worked have often been multiplied together, since in order to calculate provisions, the distinction is immaterial.

There remains one vexed question on which not much light is forthcoming. Did the shortage of labour tend to delay the process of commutation ? A few incidental notices would

COST OF HARVEST WORKS.

	1347–8	1348–9	1349–50	1350–1	1351–2	1353–4	1376–7
	£ s. d.	£ s. d.	£ s. d.	£ s. d.	£ s. d.	£ s. d.	£ s. d.
Downton . . .	1 0 11	17 4	2 5 2	2 1 1½	?	illegible	?
Brightwell . . .	1 4 3	1 4 0	2 10 7½	1 17 6	?	1 4 3	?
Harwell . . .	3 0 6½	3 0 7	2 15 6	2 15 0	?	2 18 10	1 17 9
Crawley . . .	1 14 0½	4 17 6	4 12 9	5 3 8¾	4 9 9	4 18 9½	*3 13 7¾
Bishop's Waltham .	4 15 0(?)	6 16 0½	6 7 4½	5 13 10½	5 7 10	4 18 10½	*3 11 8
Droxford . . .	5 11 10	6 4 10¼	5 18 4	5 8 10	5 13 4	5 16 8	4 8 6½
Beauworth . .	?	1 18 7¾	18 6	15 3¼	?	1 0 2½	19 4
Cheriton . . .	2 17 9½	3 15 7¼	3 1 2	2 12 0¾	3 0 6½	3 8 0	2 11 7
Sutton . . .	2 6 4½	4 2 10	2 3 8¾	2 12 4¾	2 7 0½	2 6 3½	1 14 8¾
Stoke . . .	2 10 4½	2 4 8	1 0 3	1 3 7	1 6 1	1 6 8	12 11¾
Marwell . . .	?	2 0 0	19 2	1 2 8¾	?	1 6 2½	?
Twyford . . .	5 4 5	3 5 4	4 8 2	4 14 11½	4 11 4	4 19 5½	3 3 10¼

lead one to suppose that certain commutations usually made were refused during the first shock of the pestilence.

Occasionally one finds such entries as these : ' Nothing from the men of Netley because they worked this year.' [1] ' Nothing from Alice Quirteslond because she worked with the other workmen.' [2] ' Nothing because 5 ploughmen and 2 oxherds did their works this year.' [3]

At Wargrave works which had been regularly commuted into a fixed rent are demanded again, because the works are worth more.[4]

At Brightwell (1349–50), however, the cost of the harvest works is said to be so high, (a) because the works of three customers who used to work were sold ; (b) because the works of three half-virgaters were relaxed, on account of their poverty; (c) because harvesters were scarce and dear (*messores fuerunt rari et cari*).

Brightwell had apparently just been visited by the bishop's auditors, for one finds in the same year the note ' *compertum est per examinationem auditorum* ' that the rest of the threshing should be done by the customers.[5]

At Droxford a special note is made of the dearness (*caristia*) of workmen ; at Cheriton certain tenants who failed to come were fined 4d. per day each. At Poundisford in 1350–1 the *auditores* found by examination of the Pipe that the tenants ought to plough as much of the demesne for seed as used to be ploughed when there were two ploughs there.

The evidence, however, as to a check in the process of commutation is not clear. As there are no means of calculating the rate of commutation before 1349, so it seems impossible to ascertain whether it went on more rapidly afterwards. Certainly by 1376 the area of land and the

---

[1] Brightwell, 1348–9, *Venditio Operum*.

[2] Meon, *Venditio Operum*.

[3] Twyford, 1349–50, *Venditio Operum*.

[4] Wargrave, 1348–9, *Defectus* : ' In defectu redditus terre Willelmi Herbard tracte in dominicum per annum iii s. qui prius solebat respondere in redditu assise pro operibus et quia opera plus valent, modo operatur.' (The words ' tracte in dominicum ' seem to make nonsense of the above entry. Possibly it is a case of a familiar formula misplaced.)

[5] Brightwell, 1349–50, *Custus Autumpni*.

number of tenants affected by commutation were both much larger, but the commutation was nowhere complete.

It will be convenient at this point to examine in detail the Account of Works mentioned before which was evidently demanded by the bishop in the years 1375-6-7 and irregularly till 1381. In one year or another almost every manor has its account of works. That these accounts were also separately enrolled and preserved appears from a note given under Wargrave in 1377-8 : *Opera custumaria patent in Pipe precedente et in rotulo compoti.* This note also appears under Harwell, 1380-1.

It is unfortunate that there is no direct material for studying the progress of commutation at an earlier date ; these returns show very clearly the position just before the Peasants' Revolt, but they do not permit a close comparison with conditions before the Black Death. The Taunton manors are, however, again an exception, as their records of works are continuous.

The Hampshire returns make several points very certain. Labour services were by no means disused ; still less were the obligations allowed to drop. The numbers of services performed has evidently declined considerably, although one cannot tell from what period the obligations date.

A few examples of the Accounts of Works, in a condensed form, are given below. Others will be found with the Taunton accounts on pp. 89-96.

SUTTON, 1376-7.

	Works due.	Owed by.	Acquittances.	Defects.	Performed.	Sold.	Performed in 1380-1.
Ploughing	280 acres Pd. 2d.	20 virgaters* / 25 half-virgaters / 16 half-virgaters / 3 virgaters	68 acres (mostly relaxed)	164 [many ∴ they have no ploughs]	48 acres	—	24
Harrowing	210 acres	23 virgaters / 25 half-virgaters / 10 cotsetli / 16 half-virgaters / 26 cotsetli / 4 „ / 6 half-cotsetli	42	40	128 acres	—	128
Shearing sheep	220		42	20	136	—	144
Brewing	158		132	26	None eo quod non valent reprisam.	—	None.
Carrying bushes	384		78	84	210	(?)	178
Averagia	128		46	22	60	—	44
Mowing	64		19	11	34	—	31
Loading hay	440		84	84	272	—	268
Tass' Bladi	40			—	40	—	40
Carrying hay	64		15	11	38	—	32
Carrying corn	400		84	76	196	(?)	316
Harvest works (Precariae)	531		105	105	321	—	124
Messio de Gavel	210		60	20	126	—	
Opera Autumpnalia	336		35	42	—	259	(240 sold.)
Opera Manualia	656			82	—	574	(482 sold.)

* Some of the customers plough 2 acres at each sowing; others 6 at each. It is worth notice that there were evidently 110 customary holdings at Sutton, while the fines paid in the two years of the plague amount to 44 and 45, though no tenements were left permanently vacant.

WARGRAVE, 1376-7.

	Works due.	By whom owed.	Acquittances.	Defects.	Performed 1376-7.	Performed 1377-8.	Sold 1376-7.
Ploughing, sowing and harrowing	168	57 tenants	—	90	66	?	4
Threshing	88½	59 „	—	88½	—	—	—
Shearing	64	31 „	2	28	34	34	—
Making hurdles	87	43½ „	—	58	—	—	29
Mowing	69	—	—	24	45	51	—
Turning hay	251	—	3	130	118	148 ?	—
Carrying hay	251	—	3	130	118	118 ?	—
Garrying hay	72	—	—	45	27	42	—
Stacking hay	75	—	3	39	33	33	—
Claustura de Pillingbere	150	—	2	88	—	—	60
Hoeing corn	91	—	1	44	46	56	—
Harvest Precariae	445	—	3	220	216	282	43¾
Messio þ Halnyng [Rypcol]	34 acres	—	—	21	12⅜	—	—
Harvest works	1719	*47 virgates and half-virgates of work-land.	49	1610	40	—	18
Carrying corn	70½	—	—	43½	27		
Stacking corn	83	—	3	39	41		
Superintending	13	—	—	3	10		
Precariae de Culham	73	—	1	43	39 (sic)		
Winter and summer works	†5453	—	131	5322	—		
Works done in common	Carrying timber and corn.						

* 'Et sciendum quod dum predicte xxxii virgate fuerunt omnes in tenura viii virgate operare solebant successive de anno in annum quequidem (sic) opera vocantur opera rotunda. Et modo ii virgate relaxate, xx virgate sunt in manu domini et x solvunt pro eorum opera.'

† 'Et sciendum est de eisdem virgatis viii operantur successive de anno in annum et residuum solvunt per eorum opera prout inferius patebit quequidem (sic) opera vocantur opera rotunda.' This arrangement is also found at West Wycombe.

TWYFORD, 1376–7.

	Works due.	Owed by.	Acquittances.	Defects.	Performed.	Sold.	Performed in 1380–7.
Threshing and winnowing	46 qrs.	3 virgaters, 25 half-virgaters, 4 customers, 18 half-virgaters, 5 ferling men, 2 customers, 30 cottars	12½	12¾	20 qrs. 5½ bus.	—	16 qrs. 3½ bus.
Ploughing	90 acres	—	39*	51	18 acres (*sic*).	—	
Harrowing	32 acres	—	7	4	21	—	23
Carrying brushwood to Wolvesey	62 opera	—	20	16	26	—	23 (sold).
Shearing sheep	306	—	63	72	171	—	156
Mowing meadow at Wolvesey	35	—	13	12	10	—	4
Carrying hay at Wolvesey	10	—	—	—	10		
Carrying and stacking hay	35	—	13	12	10		

* It will be noticed that the occasional sale of surplus works hardly appears in these tables, except in the case of some of the harvest works. It is generally possible to ascertain the amount of genuine and permanent commutation, from the details given as to acquittances and defects, but the entries are so irregularly distributed that I have not noted them. In general, commutation does not account for more than perhaps half of the obsolete services. Others have simply dropped off, for various reasons (see p. 157).

STOKE, 1376–7.

	Works due.	Owed by.	Acquittances.	Defects.	Performed.	Sold.	Sold in 1377–8.
Ploughing	32 acres *	13 customary tenants	—	17½ (7 customers have no ploughs)	15		15
Carrying brushwood to Wolvesey	18 carts 15 men and horses	18 customers 15 ,,	1	—	17+15	—	15+15
Shearing sheep	139	69 customers 1 ferling man.	12	—	127	—	(129 performed).
Mowing	352	114 customers	47	—	305		
Spreading hay (?)	60	—	12	—	48		
Nedrip (or *Messio per acram*)	57 acres	45 customers	4½	—	53		
Harvest *Precariae*	361	—	112	—	249	—	(30 not asked for).
Opera Autumpnalia	3475	—	1044	—	80	2401	2544
Carting and *Opera Manualia.*	6184	—	970	—	2780	2507 (*sic*)	(239 performed). 25

* The acres accounted for are acres *sicut iacent*; that is, four customary acres make one measured acre : the acreage actually sown in 1376–7 amounts to 72 customary acres.

I

HARWELL, 1376–7.

	Works owed.	Owed by.	Acquittances.	Defects.	Performed.	Sold.
Ploughing (Graserth on November 11)	24 acres	32 virgaters	3 roods	3 roods	22½	
Opera Manualia	230 works*	46 virgaters and half-virgaters	31	5	195	
Mowing	47	ditto + 1 customer	6	1	40	
Spreading hay	50	{ 32 virgaters, 15 half-virgaters, 3 cottars }	6	1	43	
Carrying hay	12½	{ 25 virgaters, 20 half-virgaters, 19 cottars }	½	—	12	
Stacking hay	39		6	—	33	
Hoeing corn	150	{ 32 virgaters, 15 half-virgaters, 3 cottars }	18 (21½ not required).	3	107¾	
Opera Autumpnalia (with 2 meals a day)	327	32 virgaters, 15 half-virgaters, 3 cottars; 2 customers; 16 cottars	35 to find one man. { to come themselves, with all their families except the mother and the shepherd. } to find one man.	7	169	(118 not asked for).

Works done in common = Carrying letters, corn, wood, &c. to London, Winchester, Wallingford, or Oxford. Driving sheep.

* An *opus* in this case meant the work of one man till the third hour for the five days immediately after the *quindenam Michaelis*; this heavy service was expended in threshing, sowing, spreading manure, leading the plough, scouring ditches, &c.

DOWNTON, 1375-6.

	Works due.	By whom owed.	Acquittances.	Defects.	Performed.	Sold.	Sold in 1376-7.
Arrura de Grashurch	151 acres	73 virgaters and half-virgaters.	7	26	—	117½	128
Arrura de Prece	274 acres	*	28	{ 66 † / 86 ‡	—	94	4 (79 performed).
Harrowing	205 acres		8	35½	162		
Brewing	94 works		—	—	Not required this year.		
Opera Manualia	2940		882	1764	—	266	(1409 performed).
Carting manure	1624		—	—	1302	?	
Spreading manure	725		—	—	500	?	
Making hurdles	139		—	—	the whole.		
Washing and shearing sheep	332		—	—	220		
Repairs, &c.	136		—	—	98		
Enclosure round barn	167 perches		—	—	107		
Haymaking	1197 works		—	—	825	108	None because no one would buy. 67 not asked for.
Hoeing	156 ,,		—	—	124		
Opera Messionis	1818 ,,		—	—	404 (=202 acres)	613	119 837 not asked for.
Messio per acram	7½ acres		—	—	5½		
Precariae	205 works		—	—	149		(157 performed).
Carrying corn	57 ,,		—	—	55	—	(55 ,,).
Stacking corn	16 ,,		—	—	14	—	(16 ,,).

12

* The *Arrura de Prece* was owed by many different classes of tenants, including the rector and a knight.
† In the lord's hand.
‡ Because they have no ploughs.

CHERITON, 1376-7.

	Works due.	Provenance.	Acquittances.	Defects.	Performed.	Sold.
Ploughing ·	221 acres	38 virgaters / 22 half-virgaters / 25 tenants of the Prior of St. Swithin's.	18 / 4	157	42	
Harrowing ·	249	38 virgaters / 22 half-virgaters. / 20 cotsetlers. / 5 half-cotsetlers. / 4 cottars.	30	178	41	
Harrowing *ad avena-gium*	146* works	38 virgaters / 22 half-virgaters.	14	54	124	
Hoeing and weeding ·	85	[as before]	11	38	36½	
Shearing sheep, &c. · ·	[? 429] 329	Virgaters and cotsetlers find two men per day; half-virgaters and half-cotsetlers find one man per day until it is finished.	54	177	125	73 not asked for.
Loading and carrying hay	320	From the virgaters and half-virgaters.	36	96	140	
Carrying brushwood to Wolvesey	120	From virgaters and half-virgaters.	12	44	64	

* If the lord required more work, he could demand it; if less, the tenants were quit.

CHERITON, 1376–7—(contd.)

	Works due.	Provenance.	Acquittances.	Defects.	Performed.	Sold.
Carrying services .	60	38 virgaters, 22 half-virgaters.	6	22	32	
Brewing . .	49 quarters	38 virgaters, 22 half-virgaters.	2 qrs. 4 bus.	13 qrs. 4 bus.	?	(29 qrs. 4 bus. not asked for).
Harvesting per acre .	1125 works *	20 cotsetlers, 5 half-cotsetlers.	164	800	111	50
Precariae Autumpni .	1095 (30 more than usually required)	38 virgaters, 22 half-virgaters. 4 cottagers. 25 tenants of Ovynton.	110	293	591 †	?
Opera Manualia .	1640	20 cotsetlers	—	1394	240¼	

Works done in common { Carrying timber, &c., for enclosures, building, &c.; finding men for building; mowing meadow at Wolvesey; maintaining palings round park at Waltham; carrying writs or letters } Not accounted for.

* A work = reaping ¼ acre of wheat or barley, or 1 acre of oats, taking one sheaf per acre as perquisite.

† This calculation is obviously incorrect; the number of works performed does not agree with the details given, but the method of calculation is unusually involved.

A separate Compotus Roll for the Year 1400–1 gives an account of the Opera, and shows that very nearly as many services were performed in that year as in 1376. Cf. Eccles. Com. Various, Bdle. 66.

A drastic condensation of the above lists gives the following results :

Manor.	Kinds of Services mentioned.	Kinds of Services performed wholly or in part.
Cheriton	8	6
Sutton	15	12
Wargrave	19	15
Twyford	8	8
Bishop's Waltham . .	14	14
Downton	16	13
Stoke	9	9
Harwell	9	9

The proportion of the works performed to the amount owed is often very small, but remarkably few had died out altogether on any one manor. Thirty-two different classes of services are mentioned for these eight manors. Some ploughing, though often very little, survived on them all ; the other services varied from manor to manor. *Opera Manualia* seem to have had a different meaning in Hampshire and in Somerset, for the Hampshire class was evidently rapidly disappearing. At Harwell a definition is given which perhaps explains the difference. An *Opus Manuale* meant one man working for five days immediately after the fortnight of Michaelmas, every day to the third hour. Such a heavy and rigid service would be less desirable than the very elastic arrangements of the Taunton manors.

Summarizing again, the following table aims at showing which classes of services survived, and which died out entirely ; no attempt is made to show what fraction of the service due was actually performed, as the details are all given in the preceding tables.

	Cheriton.	Sutton.	Twyford.	Waltham.	Stoke.	Wargrave.	Harwell.	Downton.	Downton.*
Ploughing . . .	P	P	P	P	P	P	P	O	P
Harrowing . .	P	P	P	—	—	P	—	P	P
Shearing . . .	P	P	P	P	P	P	—	P	P
Hoeing . . .	P	—	—	P	—	P	P	P	P
Precariae Autumpni	P	P	—	P	P	P	—	P	W
Opera Autumpnalia	P	O	—	P	P	P	P		
Carrying corn .	P	P	—	—	—	P	—	P	W
Carrying services .	P	P							
Brewing . . .	O	O	—	—	—	—	—	—	O
Carrying brushwood	P	P	P	P	P				
Mowing . . .	—	P	P	P	P	P	P		
Turning hay . .	—	P	—	—	P	P	P	P	P
Stacking corn . .	—	W	—	W	—	P	—	P	W
Carrying hay . .	P	P	P	P	—	P	P		
{ *Messio de Gavel*									
{ *M. per acram* .	P	P	—	—	P				
Opera Manualia .	—	O	—	—	P	—	P	O	G
Carting manure, &c.	—	—	—	—	—	—	—	P	P
Threshing . . .	—	—	P	—	—	O			
Making hurdles .	—	—	—	P	—	O	—	P	O
Stacking hay . .	—	—	P	W	—	P	P		
Claustura . . .	—	—	—	—	—	O	—	P	P
								{ P	P
Messio per Halnyng (?)	—	—	—	—	P	—	{ P	P
								{ P	P
Superintendence .	—	—	—	—	—	P			
Opera yemalia et estivalia . .	—	—	—	—	—	O			

P=performed in part.   O=not performed at all.   W=the whole performed.
* Partly paid *de prece*.

The Taunton accounts show much the same state of affairs (cf. p. 88); the classes of work are far fewer, but hardly any of these classes have been entirely and permanently commuted on any of the manors.

Manor.	Classes of Work mentioned.	Classes of Work performed.
Holway	8	5
Nailesbourne . . .	7	5
Poundisford . . .	8	4
Staplegrove . . .	9	5
Hull	7	5
Rimpton	2	2

It is interesting to notice the sharp contrast between the highly specialized services of the Hampshire manors, and the broad classification and elastic arrangements of the Taunton group ; the latter appears to be the more progressive system from an agricultural point of view. If, however, the traditional test of villeinage—not to know at night what one was to do in the morning—carries any weight, the tenants of the Taunton manors, in spite of their material prosperity, must have been far less free than those in Hampshire. This is quite in harmony with the normal contrast between western and eastern or central England. In this connexion it is remarkable that some services (e. g. threshing) on the Somerset manors were valued for commutation at a rate above what was actually paid in wages ; threshing wheat was valued at 4d., and generally performed for 2½d. or 3d.

With regard to the specially vexed question of the commutation of ploughing services, yet another table may be useful. It has already been shown that some ploughing services were still exacted on all the manors in 1348 ; this list gives the exact amount performed in 1376-7. It is remarkable that complete commutation should have taken place on so few manors.

PLOUGHING SERVICES PERFORMED IN 1376.

Manor.	Due.		Performed.
Bishopston . . .	{ 92 acres		None. Not required.
	41 „ de prece	,,	,, ,,
Knoyle	49		None.
Fonthill	36		,,
Brightwell . . .	{ 25		,,
	40		2
Harwell	24		22½
Adderbury . . .	156		105
Wargrave	168		66
West Wycombe . .	108		76¼
Ivingho	571½		88½ *
Waltham St. Laurence .	84		38
Culham	54		9
Morton	13½		13½
Bentley	43		38¼
Highclere	103		15 †

* This very large number is probably an old calculation, as only 366 acres are accounted for here. Ivingho had adopted sheep farming since the early part of the thirteenth century.

† At Highclere ploughing was owed by the cotsetlers, a very unusual arrangement.

Manor.				Due.	Performed.
Overton	.	.	.	468¼	9½
Itchingswell	.	.	.	147	42
Woodhay	.	.	.	120	33
Burghclere	.	.	.	207 *	54
North Waltham	.	.	273	18
Ashmansworth	.	.	.	75	12
Sutton	.	.	.	280	48
Alresford	.	.	.	98	14
Cheriton	.	.	.	221	42
Wield	.	.	.	32	10
Beauworth	.	.	.	40	6
Meon	.	.	.	216	? †
Hambledon	.	.	.	No entry.	
Meon *Ecclesia*	.	.	.	18	18
Hambledon *Ecclesia*	.	.	152	? ‡
Fareham	.	.	.	202	9
Bitterne	.	.	.	None due.	
Twyford	.	.	.	90	18
Stoke	.	.	.	32	15
Marwell	.	.	.	278	42
Mardon	.	.	.	537	111
Crawley	.	.	.	25	8

* The ploughing due at Burghclere must have sufficed for the whole demesne, as 204 acres were actually sown.

† At Meon 64 acres of ploughing were excused *quia non fecerunt huiusmodi arrura causa reprisae.*

‡ A similar note occurs at Hambledon (*Ecclesia*) and at Fareham with the further information that ploughing was there performed *ad cibum domini*. At Overton 4 virgates were excused their ploughing *quia reprisa excedit valorem*. Cf. p. 157.

Another group of questions concerns the effect of the Black Death on the position of the lords of manors, and on the growth of the system of 'farms' and leases.

As regards the actual profits of the Bishop of Winchester, he would seem to have gained rather than lost during the two years of the pestilence. A glance at the balance-sheets on pp. 162–77 will show how his gains arose. The only two items which show a large and consistent increase are the heriots and the fines. In some cases the heriots had been commuted, and the increase stands out clearly in the account; in others the heriots, being paid in kind, can only be found in detail in the Stock Account, with no attempt at valuation—their presence, however, is betrayed by the rise in the item 'Sale of Stock' for the next year or two.

As to the fines, their amount is increased enormously;

some idea of the number of fines is given on pp. 78–9, but their total monetary value shows an increase of from 3 to 25 times as much as in normal years (in Hampshire), or in Somerset from 1½ to 10 times as much. The average increase would be from 4 to 6 times as much as usual. It is very largely from these immense lists of fines that so much information as to tenements can be gathered.

As has already been shown, it is impossible to tell, except in a very few cases, whether fines were raised or lowered on account of the Black Death, because the pre-pestilence fines were so disproportionate. Probably a few remissions were made, but no serious change followed.

The total amounts paid in fines seem to have decreased after the Black Death, but no one reason accounts for this. The number of tenements thrown on the lord's hands is partly responsible; the practice of sales and sub-letting among the tenants may have declined; the fines on unusual occasions may have been hard to exact; the practice of leasing for lives still further reduced the numbers; there may well have been a movement against the arbitrary amounts of the fines;[1] the gradual leakage from the manors during the later fourteenth and early fifteenth centuries must have played its part.[2]

For the time being, however, the increased receipts from the fines and heriots gave the bishop a large surplus of ready money. It is a curious commentary on the alleged ruin of

[1] The 'Terrarium Domerhamense domini Ricardi Beere, abbatis Glaston.' for 1518 (see p. 20) gives some interesting examples of fixed fines, with the corresponding rents, and notes as to whether one heriot, several heriots, or no heriot was to be paid. There is no relationship whatever between the Rent and the Fine ; though the rents were obviously customary and not economic, ranging from 3d. to 5d. an acre. Thus rents of 7s. 4d., 30s., 43s. are all combined with a fine of 3s. 4d., payable by ' Tenants by the custom of the Manor'. The *Nativi* paid fines which were sometimes equal to a year's rent, sometimes to half, a third, three-quarters, one-fifth, one-thirteenth, four-fifths or any other fraction of a year's rent ; in two cases only the fine exceeds one year's rent. Among the free tenants the fines are generally lower, representing $\frac{1}{7}$ to $\frac{1}{20}$ of a year's rent, though in one case the fine (of £5) represents the rent for about a year and a half. The number of heriots payable by each free tenant is noted *ut patet per copiam* ; in one or two cases capons are paid as a fine.

[2] Cf. Davenport, Economic Development of a Norfolk Manor.

the country-side, and the impossibility of obtaining labour, to find that he was able by 1354 to spend £145 in building operations at Marwell, and £119 at Sutton. Wherever the expenses appear to have increased enormously during the years immediately following 1349, it is always wise to look for the expenditure on buildings and repairs, or on the purchase of stock. The receipts of the year 1350–1 should, in like manner, be carefully scrutinized. It was a year of disastrous floods and tempests, which swept away houses and mills as they stood, and most of the hay crop. Had it not been that the corn of the previous year had been to a large extent left on the lord's hand, famine must have been added to the ravages of pestilence. As it was, wheat rose to 10s. per quarter in 1351, and to 14s. in 1352. This year was the low-water mark in the manorial receipts; afterwards they climb steadily up again, either to the average of the pre-pestilence period, or to a higher figure. Of the ten Hampshire manors examined, by 1353–4 seven show an increase in the receipts above the average for the years 1346–7 and 1347–8, while of the other three, two had shown an increase in earlier years, and all had increased their profits considerably by 1376–7. On the Somerset manors, on the contrary, a slight decrease is general, but the inflation of receipts in 1349 and 1350 had been much greater.

If, then, the bishop made any changes in the organization and management of his estates, it was not because of pecuniary pressure, but because the whole fourteenth century is a period of change, and the increased use of money as a means of exchange acted as a powerful economic solvent. Two main changes might have been made : the demesne might have been leased out or farmed, either as a whole or in small parcels, or it might have been turned down for pasture and used for sheep-farming. The change might have been even more drastic if the whole manor had been farmed.

Something has already been said of sub-letting and of 'farms' before 1349; it is necessary to go back a little to see what changes are made at a later date.

Early in the thirteenth century a few of the more remote

manors (e.g. Fonthill, Bishopston, Fawley, Rimpton) had been farmed; possibly the perquisites of the court were sometimes included in the farm. But the practice does not seem to have been very general. The only manor I have found which appears to have been farmed more or less consistently is that of the hamlet of Otterford, which probably had no separate court, but owed suit of court at Holway.

In 1284 it was farmed for £11; the bishop retained the 'issues' of the manor, which in this case consisted of pannage, hundredpenny, brewing, and tithing penny, amounting to 11s. 6d.

In 1346–7 it was farmed by Christina de Shordych for £16. The bishop reserved the *Consuetudines* (13s.) (i.e. pannage, hundredpenny at Martinmas, and hockdaieswite); the 'issues' of the manor, 4s. (i.e. the perquisites of St. Leonard's Fair); and the proceeds of the court (i.e. fines of land, marriages, heriots, *Perquisita Curiae*, stallage, hundredpenny, hochedaieswyte, pannage, and *forisfactura*. The first four of these items were due at Holway).

Early in 1349 Christina de Shordych died; no one else would take the manor at farm, and the account for 1348–9 thus consists partly of the farm, partly of the actual receipts.

In 1349–50 and 1350–1 it was still unfarmed, and the total receipts were £15 13s. 3½d. and £16 3s. 3¼d. The sale and commutation of works had evidently made considerable progress in this hamlet; nearly £2 of the total £16 are accounted for by 'works'.

In 1351–2 Otterford was farmed for a term of years for £5 5s. 6½d. for the first year, and afterwards for £7 5s. 6½d. for a term of ten years. The farm, however, could only have included the demesne, the mill, and certain specified services.[1]

In 1376–7 the hamlet was farmed and had been farmed

---

[1] Otriford 1351–2, *Firma.* 'Et de cvs. vid. ob. de firma manerii de Otriford cum molendino per annum hoc anno et abhinc per terminum x annorum proxime sequencium annuatim viili. vs. vid. ob. exceptis & salvis domino toto redditu Assise dicti manerii, finibus terrarum, maritagiis, heriettis, perquisitis curiae, stallagiis, hundredpeny, Hokhedaieswite, pannagiis porcorum, et forisfacturis. Ita tamen quod dicti firmarii habeant avericia bladorum et herbagii suorum [cum ?] omnibus averagiis (?) provenientis de extraura durante firma predicta.'

for nine years to Adam atte More, for a term of thirteen years. The £8 0s. 4½d. which he paid included the manor and the mill, but excluded as before the assized rents, fines, marriages, heriots, perquisites, hundredpeny, hokedaieswite, pannage, forisfactura, pundfald, stallage, and strays. The farmer undertakes to maintain the house and buildings in good condition. The whole entry ends *Et hec faciet fideliter.* The only other ' farm ' which I can find recorded before 1349 is that of Ashford (? a hamlet of Meon), which paid £10 a year. A third part of the ' farm ' was held by John Blackman, whose son John Blackman paid a fine of £2 in order to succeed to it.[1]

The sales between villein tenants with reservation of a rent-charge are interesting when given in full, because they throw some light on the motives for sale, and show, too, how the fourteenth-century sales and sub-letting are closely connected with the older ' farms ' of provisions and necessaries. The following example will illustrate this.

Poundisford, 1347-8, Fines and Marriages :

' Et de vi*li*. xiii*s*. iiii*d*. de Roberto Burgeys pro uno mesuagio dimidia virgata terre native et i roda terre de Overland in decenna de Southtrendle ex redditione Nicholai le Whyte habendis et eciam ut possit retinere ii acras dimidiam terre native in decenna de Trendle sine calumpnia domini quas prius tenuit, et concedit dictus Robertus dicto Nicholao et Agneti uxori eius ad terminum vite eorumdem iiii quarteria dimidium frumenti, i quarterium fabarum, iiii bussellos siliginis, iiii bussellos pilcorn, et i porcum precia ii*s*., et ipsi Nicholao quolibet anno dum vixerit i parem sotularium et unum garniamentum album, et predicte Agneti annuatim unum parem sotularium et quolibet altero anno i garnia-mentum de colore et quando contigerit unum eorum decedere medietas predicte pensionis cessabit.'

It is sometimes difficult to distinguish between a sale reserving a rent-charge and a lease, as both involved a sur-

---

[1] This same John Blackman, who appears to have been a villein, must have paid fines to the amount of £18 13s. 4d. for his father's holdings : v. Meon, 1347-8, Fines and Marriages.

render, and the terms are not always explicitly given. In several cases a lease seems to be indicated rather than a sale.

Such leases occur from time to time both before and after 1349, but as a rule the terms are not given. At Droxford (1350–1) a cottage and curtillage with one acre of villein land were surrendered, with rent-charge, for term of life, of 2 quarters 5 bushels of barley and one piece of linen cloth per annum.

The following sales or leases appear at Meon in 1353–4:

(*a*) A virgate of land for 1 quarter of wheat four times a year, for term of life.

(*b*) A cottage and one rood of land at an annual rent of 4*d*.

(*c*) A messuage and a virgate of land for the following rent:
½ bushel good wheat per week;
6 yards (virg') russet cloth at All Saints';
2 pieces of linen and two pairs of boots on the feasts of All Saints' and St. John the Baptist;
4 pairs of shoes of the value of 1*s*. per pair, at the four quarters;
1 cow pasturing with the cows of the tenant.

(*d*) A messuage, a virgate and 4 acres of wood for:
1 bushel of corn (wheat and barley) per week.
7*s*. sterling at the Purification of the B.V.M. and the Nativity of St. John the Baptist;
2 carts of brushwood annually;
1 hall with room, garden, croft quit of all services;
1 horse or cow bought with the beasts of the tenant.
The bailiff was to arbitrate in case of disturbance.

A similar entry is noted at Staplegrove 1350–1, among the fines. 'Et de xv*s*. Stephano Wadyn pro i messuagio i ferlingo terre native in decenna de Holeford ex redditione Ade Pitte-path. Ita quod idem Stephanus inveniet eidem Ade annuatim duo quarteria et unum busellum frumenti, unum quarterium et unum busellum siliginis et unum busellum pilcorn, novem virgas panni grisi et unam parvam donam dum vixerit habenda.'

These sales and leases among tenants seem to have two main motives, either the more convenient rearrangement of land, or the more comfortable and less responsible provision for old age. Hence they were nearly always renewable from year to year or for term of life. A tenant *ad voluntatem* would be ill-advised to grant leases for term of years.[1] Hence such few leases as one finds for fixed terms are leases from the bishop.

But such leases are very rare on the Winchester estates. A few had evidently been granted *per cartam*, generally for term of life, before the Black Death. A few are found for term of life direct from the bishop, between 1349 and 1359; still fewer for term of years. As a rule only small plots are thus leased, and there are no signs whatever that the whole demesne was leased, or the whole manor farmed, as a result of the shortage of labour or the increase of sheep-farming.

The leases for nine years, common in Berkshire during this decade, which were generally allowed to fall in at the end of the nine years,[2] were almost unknown on the Winchester estates. I have only found one stock and land lease definitely so-called, which occurs at Morton (Berks.) in 1351–2 by indenture. The first entry merely relates the fact of the lease;[3] in subsequent years a catalogue is given of the land sown, of the corn in hand, and of the live and dead stock on the manor. Most of the items are valued in money, and the bishop might choose, at the end of the lease, in what form they should be returned to him.

A lease on very favourable terms, directly due to the Black Death and to the deserted condition of the tenement, occurs at Downton in 1349–50. A certain toft and a plot

---

[1] Several leases for short terms of years are entered in 1284, e. g. at Poundisford and Holway, but such leases seem to have dropped off by 1348, or possibly the terms are not entered among the fines.

[2] v. Miss E. C. Lodge, in Victoria County History, Berkshire, vol. ii, Social and Economic History.

[3] Morton 1351–2: 'Compotus eiusdem a festo sancti Michaelis anno domini Willelmi Episcopi vi^{to} usque ultimam diem Aprilis proxime sequentis per xxx septimanas et ii dies anno consecrationis dicti Episcopi vii^{mo}. Et tunc consentitio (?) fuit per dominum quod dictum manerium dimitteretur ad firmam per x annos subsequentes dicto domino Episcopo existente superstite quod quidem manerium ab Gula Augusti extunc proxime sequente dimittetur Iohanni atte Berghe ad terminum supradictum cum bladis crescentibus et stauris in eodem [anno ?] sub communi forma in quadam indentura inde confecta et in Thesauro dicti domini Episcopi remanente.'

for a fulling-mill (ruined), together with three pieces of meadow, 10 acres of land belonging to the mill, one croft containing 36 acres, 6 crofts of the waste, enclosed with hedges and ditches, and 19 acres of *terra borda* were taken over by the son of the miller for a fine of 1s., on condition that he should rebuild the mill with his own materials, except the timber, which was provided by the lord. All arrears of rent were to be excused to him, and he was to pay a rent of 20s. a year for term of life.

These few specimens of leases and ' farms ' direct from the lord are not, however, merely examples of a common item in the accounts ; they are all that I can find before the year 1355. On the Taunton manors, where the *Firme* are already entered separately, there is little or no change in the entries between 1345 and 1355, though there is a tendency for the ' farms ' to disappear—sometimes reappearing again as the more precarious Sale of Pasture.

By 1376–7, however, the section *Firme* yields more information and shows the direction of development. The ' Sale of Pasture ' entry grows longer and is more scrupulous in recording the sale of tiny plots or strips of grass-land. The *Firme* have also largely increased in number and in value ; the holdings ' farmed ' now include pasture, meadow-land, fishponds, cottages, mills, arable land, plots enclosed on both sides, woods, and pasture in woods, and road-side pasture.

At Holway the crofts of arable land, and small plots of the demesne (*c.* 4 acres) were let for terms of twenty years unless the lord could let them better (*carius*) within that time. Seventy acres of reedy meadow around the *vivarium* were let on the same terms for the high rent of £17 6s. 8d. (nearly 5s. per acre). Arable land varied from 1s. 1½d. to 8d. per acre. At Rimpton arable land was leased at 6d. per acre, and meadow-land apparently at nearly 4s.

At Downton a large slice of the demesne (88 acres) was farmed to seven of the customary tenants, apparently at about 8d. per acre, while a croft of pasture was farmed in order that it might be enclosed.

The entry *Firme* also occurs on one or two other manors, e.g. at Adderbury 15 acres of demesne, i.e. all that *cultura* known as Goldwell furlong, with another small *cultura*, were let for 16s. for as long as the lord shall please. Five acrelands or cotlands among the tenements vacant *per pestilenciam* were let *ad firmam*, but the fact is easily overlooked, as the entry is made among the *Exitus manerii.*

A few specimens of the Somerset 'farms' and sales of pasture are given below:

HOLWAY, 1376–7.

Sale of Pasture.

£	s.	d.	
	6	8	for winter pasture.
	1	6	,, winter and summer pasture.
	3	0	,, winter pasture.
	2	8	,, for winter and summer pasture.
	6	8	,, winter pasture.
	2	0	,, ,, ,,
	1	6	,, pasture *circa firm'* (sic).
	2	0	,, winter pasture.
		6	,, pasture around the oats.
	18	0	,, winter and summer pasture.
		6	,, pasture around wheat.
	11	0	,, ,, (*terra frisca*).
		6	,, ,,
	1	6	,, ,, on road from Taunton to Shordych.
		6	,, ,, ,, Holway.
	1	6	,, ,, *infra Berton.*
	6	0	,, ,, on 7 plots of Haydon.
	6	8	,, winter and summer pasture in Hampwode.
	7	10	,, pasture in 8 plots.
		6	,, ,,
	10	0	,, 10 of the lord's oxen from August 1st to Martinmas.
1	4	0	,, *retropastura* [1] in Wydemede.
1	0	0	,, newly enclosed pasture in Corfe.
	1	10	,, pasture on *terra frisca.*

£6 17 2

For 3 plots sometimes pasture nothing because sown.
,, 1 plot ,, ,, ,, *quia supra ad firmam.*
,, 1 ,, ,, ,,. ,, for lack of buyers.

Firme.

s.	d.	
9	0	for 2 acres 1 rood meadow.
6	0	,, 1 fish-pond.
	8	,, 1 cottage belonging to the said fish-pond.
9	4	,, 13 acres arable land and 1 acre of land *undique inclusa* of the demesne, let for term of 20 years (this year the 9th) *nisi infra tempus predictum carius possit dimittere.*

[1] i.e. pasture after mowing (?).

£ s. d.
   4   6   for 4 acres arable land of demesne (lease as above).
   4   6   ,, ,,   ,,   ,,   ,,   ,,
   5   8   ,, 8 ,,   ,,   ,,   ,,
17 6 8   *De firma LXX acrarum arundinarum prati et pasture circa*
              vivarium de dominica domini sic dimissarum Willelmi Portman
              et . . . (7 other tenants) *ad terminum XX annorum hoc anno*
              IX° nisi infra tempus predictum carius possit dimittere.

N.B. These leases appear to date from the first year of William of Wykeham's episcopate. Cf. p. 159.

Thus it may be fairly clearly shown that the Bishop of Winchester did not resort to the leasing of land immediately after the Black Death, that the prevalence of leases had made some but not very much progress by 1376–7, and that the practice of leasing the whole demesne or the whole manor was almost unknown on his estates. The stock and land lease hardly figures in the accounts, and both the smaller and the larger plots of leased land were frequently granted to men of villein status, while leases to groups of villeins were fairly common.

It remains to be seen whether any marked movement towards sheep-farming can be detected. There is certainly a close connexion between long leases and enclosures; only a lease for years or for term of life would make the tenant willing to bear the expense of hedging and ditching. The land 'farmed' would generally seem to have been small plots or closes of arable land, or compact pieces of the demesne, or crofts and larger stretches of pasture land. On the downs it would seem that there was no hard and fast line between arable and pasture; a 'farmer' might use his plots and crofts of land for sheep or for corn as he pleased, or interchangeably.[1] The increase in the number of sheep owned by the tenants may therefore have been very considerable, without exciting notice in the accounts.

For the demesne there are exact figures for the sheep kept by the lord for a period of over 200 years. The subjoined table will show a very large increase between 1208 and 1376, but the increase would seem to have been gradual. No marked rise occurs between the years 1345 and 1355. Occasionally one seems to trace the change in the accounts. In 1381–2

---

[1] Cf. Taunton group under 'Sale of Pasture', and Surveys, Earl of Pembroke (Roxburghe Club), for Wiltshire.

Henlee (Henley-on-Thames) appears probably for the first time, and seems to have been starting as a sheep-farm. Two acres of the demesne were let out for sowing at 4*d.* per acre ; pasture to the extent of 46*s.* 8*d.* was leased from the Prioress of Kingston ; most of the expenses consisted of the purchase of stock ; a large proportion of the receipt was *forensic* (i.e. sent from other manors for a special purpose), and most of it was expended. This, however, is only an isolated instance, not borne out on other manors.

NUMBER OF SHEEP (ALL CLASSES) BETWEEN 1208 AND 1455.

	1208–9	1347–8	1353–4	1376–7	1455
Bishop's Waltham .	920	572 (?)	556	588	1071 (?)
Clere . .	1164	{ Highclere 412 Burghclere 427 }	403	433	
			529	763	
Woodhay .	383	319	317	508	
Itchingswell .	253	408	637	637	
Brightwell .	200	{ Apparently none	None [110 during year]	280	
Harwell .	305	{ Apparently none	306	179	
Witney .	683	646	861	1240	
Downton .	1764	1179	1220	1212	
Overton .	775	1146	1120	1118	
Fareham .	283	370	400	427	
Wargrave .	190	185	230	454	
Bitterne .	90	242	161	369	
Wycombe .	212	323	590	1093	321 (to farmer)
Mardon .	581	513	791	1232	
Farnham .	498	225	199	467	
Sutton .	495	733	649	909	451
West Meon .	1276	1225	1562	1503	
Hambledon .	533	669	937	1145	
Crawley .	1063	1088 (?)	1000	1020	1897
Twyford .	1627	1555	1281	1283	951 (farmer)
Stoke . .	None	186	209	201	
Cheriton .	591	716	967	817	549 (farmer)
Beauworth .	132	316	456	420	266
Wield . .	331	388	410	460	
Rimpton .	None	None	None	None	
					1380–1
Knoyle .	1048	1307	1495	1597	1727
Ivingho .	—	568	488	588	734

The comparatively slow growth of sheep-farming may be checked by the careful accounts kept of the acreage sown; the following table shows how slight were the variations, and how impossible it is that serious changes should have been made as an immediate consequence of the Black Death.

It is true that four out of the seven Somerset manors and three out of the six Hampshire manors examined show a clear decrease in the amount of arable land by 1354, and the decrease is generally equally visible in 1376. But only in one case does the decrease reach nearly 50 per cent. (Marwell), while on some manors it sinks to about $2\frac{1}{2}$–3 per cent. (cf. Rimpton, Crawley, and Bishop's Waltham), and the average loss is not much above 15 per cent. This is partly balanced by an actual gain of about 30 per cent. at Hull in 1353–4.

The further drop in the figures by 1376 may be accounted for by the practice of leasing out part of the demesne, and does not necessarily imply a smaller area under cultivation. Downton, for example, which apparently shows a decrease of 108 acres of arable, had, as is seen elsewhere, leased out 88 acres of the demesne to one group of tenants.

The acreage sown varies irregularly in normal years, and the rotation of crops is irregular, but on the whole the evidence points to a three-course system, modified by a considerable use of beans, peas, and vetch; about equal quantities of barley and oats were grown on most manors, and these together generally equal the acreage under wheat. The yield of wheat seems to have been about 1 quarter to 10 bushels per customary acre, the amount sown varies from $1\frac{1}{2}$ to $2\frac{1}{2}$ bushels per acre.

In Somerset $1\frac{1}{2}$ bushels sown apparently gives as good a yield as $2\frac{1}{2}$ bushels in Hampshire, but comparison is not easy, owing to the variations in the use of the word acre.[1]

(Somerset and Wilts.)	ACREAGE SOWN.					
	1347–8	1348–9	1349–50	1350–1	1353–4	1376–7
Hull	197	105(?)	203	174	257	201
Nailesbourne . .	81	80	75	52	52	88
Poundisford . .	132	89	93	88	109	90
Holway . . .	240	231	$243\frac{1}{2}$	239	illegible	191
Staplegrove . .	159	172	169	143	159	165
Rimpton . . .	220	218	203	$203\frac{1}{2}$	215	$147\frac{1}{2}$
Downton . . .	295	259	271	$286\frac{3}{4}$	256	187

[1] Cf. p. 50.

(*Hants*)	1347–8	1348–9	1349–50	1350–1	1353–4	1376–7
Stoke	84	69	81½	70½	81½	72¾
Marwell . . .	146	85½	50	81	77	78
Twyford . . .	255	208	212½	223	232½	242
Bishop's Waltham	172	210½	140	167	164	165
Crawley . . .	245	219	219	251	237	200½
Sutton . . .	163½	153	134	142	157	161

The increased area of enclosed land is difficult to estimate, because the notices of it are so very indirect, but steady progress seems to have been made in this direction all through the fourteenth century and particularly during the latter part of it.

The wages paid for hedging and ditching would alone show this. At Bishop's Waltham in 1347–8 about £10 was spent in planting hedges; similar work was undertaken at Droxford; at Twyford in the same year £4 13s. 9d. was spent on enclosing, and £3 12s. in 1348–9 on new ditches and on enclosing the warren. Repeated notices show the cost of reclaiming and hedging crofts and 'purprestures' for the demesne, sometimes for arable purposes. The numerous exchanges between the tenants were probably followed by enclosure, but of this there is no record. However, by 1376 it becomes increasingly common to find a villein's holding reckoned in 'closes', or to hear that such and such plots are enclosed on both sides. The uniformity of the virgates is breaking down fast; by 1376 it has become necessary to enumerate all the separate acres and all the crofts of a tenement and to explain in which *cultura* the acres lie.

Moreover, the three or four great fields, with their general names, Northfield, Middlefurlong, Medfurlong, and the like, begin to break up into smaller units, and one hears of a *cultura* called Nyenacres, or Tenacres, or Goldwellfurlong, which is divided between two or three tenants. The later Court Rolls and the fines in the Account Rolls show more frequent entries of large and quite irregular holdings, of which almost each acre is named or described. Bishop's Waltham, for example, between 1390 and 1400 contained holdings of about 22 acres (falling into seven different categories); of 48 acres in many small purprestures; of about 15 acres in 14 different plots; of 50 acres (of five kinds); of eight plots amounting to 17 acres; of 51 acres in eleven separately mentioned plots. The fines payable for such holdings vary from 6s. 8d. to £10 and £16. At Holway in 1387 a fine of £20 was paid for a holding of between 40 and 50 acres. The chief point to notice is that all these holdings are defined in detail; it is no longer sufficient to say ' one virgate and 6 acres of purpresture '; the regular rotation of strips has entirely gone, or is no longer a safe guide. This, however, is going far beyond the immediate effects of the Black Death.

The last problem which naturally occurs to one's mind, the connexion between the Black Death and the Peasants' Revolt, finds no solution in the documents on which this study is based. It has been shown that there is absolutely no sound evidence for retrogression or greater severity in exacting services after 1349 on the Winchester estates. Certainly the bishop's manors were considerably more conservative than the rather miscellaneous groups examined by Mr. Page in the ' End of Villeinage in England ', but it is impossible to show that this conservatism (reflected in the returns of works in 1376) owes its origin or its strength to the devastations of the Black Death. Thus there is no apparent ground for dissatisfaction on the bishop's manors; his tenants were without doubt prosperous and were increasing in wealth and importance towards the critical years 1377–82. The hand of the bishop, though heavy, was firm and consistent, and his demands were probably being spread over an increasing population. He was an absentee landlord, and, as such, probably gave more scope to the communal action of the tenants than the man on the spot would be likely to allow. Above all, on so well-organized an estate there was little or no room for arbitrary action.[1] Hence, so far as I can see, there was no real discontent. Men were allowed to remain away from the ' lands of St. Swithin ' or to settle upon them for very small annual payments, hardly more galling than

[1] Elsewhere the fines are spoken of as ' arbitrary '; it is perhaps rather the proportion of fine to area which was arbitrary. There is no evidence that the fines for different tenements were not fixed, with variations for different circumstances.

the red rose of the freeholder. Only 4s. 6d. was paid at
Wargrave for permission to leave the manor altogether.
In the rolls for 1380-1 and 1381-2 there are no traces of
participation in the Peasants' Revolt, save at Southwark and
Winchester. Here and there the lord takes the chattels of
a felon, or the chattels of a fugitive villein, but such cases
are few and far between. There is a certain leakage from the
manors all through this period; villeins were apt ' to go
away secretly ' and to be no more found. There is nothing,
however, to show that the bishop had any real trouble with
his tenants. The Winchester and Southwark entries are
interesting, but fall outside the scope of this inquiry.

So far certain definite questions have been proposed, and
their answers sought. In corroboration of the conclusions
suggested, it may be useful to go systematically through the
Account Roll, showing what kind of differences are produced
by the Black Death. The material for this inquiry is contained in the tables on pp. 162-77; all that need be attempted
here is a brief commentary.

As has already been shown, the reeve continued during
the years of pestilence to render his accounts precisely as
before; the arrears from the previous year were punctually
paid, although it is noticeable that rather large sums were
left at Michaelmas 1349 to be entered as arrears for the
year 1349-50. On one group of smaller and poorer manors [1]
(in North Hampshire and Berkshire) the arrears were not
paid quite punctually; a year or two's grace was allowed,
or some special arrangement was made, and the bishop let
off the tithing-penny and small sums for the king's fifteenth.

The rents of assize are entered without change, but
a special entry of *Defectus per pestilentiam* is inserted, in
addition to the ordinary defects and acquittances. The net
rent, therefore, is the significant figure. On many manors
these ' defects ' had entirely disappeared by 1354; on others

[1] i. e. Bentley, Ashmansworth, Burghclere, North Waltham, and others.
See table on p. 179. Cf. Cobbett, Rural Rides (1885), vol. i, pp. 43 and 70, for
an estimate of the poverty of the soil in this district; at Highclere and
Burghclere, he says, they have enclosed commons, worth, as tillage land,
not one single farthing an acre.

a small sum is still entered in 1376, and on some there are
two entries, the *Defectus per primam pestilentiam* and the
Defectus per secundam pestilentiam (i.e. the plague of 1361).
In no case, however, is the loss above £6 per annum and it
is frequently quite small sums of less than £1. The two
manors which lost most severely in rents show a ' defect '
of about 20–25 per cent., and this figure is only maintained
for about two years. The amount of loss must be compared
carefully with the long lists of vacant tenements on some
manors ; it is not nearly so large as the numbers would lead
one to expect (cf. p. 82). The manors which were visited
by the second pestilence are almost the only ones which still
show the loss in 1376. The ' acquittances ' were generally
somewhat less, because the regular servants of the manor
died during the year and were not immediately replaced by
tenants on the same terms. This method of payment, however, shows neither extension nor abandonment during this
period.

The issues of the manors commonly show a marked decline.
The produce could not be sold, because there were no buyers.
The extra supplies of forage, of hay and straw, of pasture
and dairy produce were not bought, because of the uncertainty
of life ; the regular dues, such as pannage and tithing-penny,
necessarily decreased, while in the cases where the *Opera
Vendita* were included among the issues of the manors, there
was a further source of decrease. Some of the produce,
notably the hay, could be kept over to the next year, and
consequently in the ' excessively ungenial ' season 1350–1
there were considerable stores of old hay to be used or sold.
The decrease in the amount of the *Exitus Manerii* is found
on all the manors here examined ; the recovery generally
takes several years. It is rather difficult, however, to ascertain
the average value of the produce, because occasional items
occur which raise the amounts to a quite abnormal figure.
Wood, for example, might be cut every nine or ten years,
or only when required : £24 of the issues at Sutton in 1354
was due to the sale of wood. The sales of pasture declined
very considerably during the two plague years, but generally

recovered again in a year or two or were balanced by an increase under *Firme*. On a few manors the lord would seem to have retained more pasture in his own hands (cf. p. 73). The question of leases has already been considered; the figures in the table under *Firme* do not throw much light on the question. The sale of stock was immediately influenced by the heavy mortality among the villeins; the large number of heriots (generally horses, oxen, and cows) has been mentioned; as a rule they were not long retained by the lord, but were sold. Many of the *Venditio Stauri* entries show considerable inflation for two or three years. The year 1350–1, however, was a year of great mortality among the beasts and especially among the sheep. The sale of corn at first falls off for lack of demand, but the corn was stored, and large sums were made in the following years by the sale of old corn. It is curious to notice that on the Somerset manors the demesne corn which was grown by the labours of the customary tenants was afterwards to a considerable extent sold to those same customers—a strong proof both of the prosperity of the tenants and of the force of custom. The prices of corn quoted in the rolls follow fairly closely the calculations of Thorold Rogers, but are rather lower in 1350 and the early part of 1351.

The 'sale of works' has been dealt with at sufficient length; here it may suffice to say that it generally declined during the year 1349–50, as the surplus which could be sold was much smaller, but it never disappeared entirely, and it had gone up again to a normal or greater amount in a very few years.

The most significant entry in the account is the fines and marriages. Dr. Jessopp [1] has remarked that the landlords must have emerged much richer than before from the visitation of the plague, and he speaks particularly of the extraordinary amount received from heriots and fees. But he gives no details, and this particular point does not seem to have attracted the notice of economic historians. Certainly it has never been shown that the entry fines meant exactly the

[1] v. Jessopp, The Coming of the Friars and other historic essays.

difference between large losses and large profits to the lord. When an item in the receipts which stands normally at about £40 rises in one year to £191, or a normal entry of £16 rises to £109, it is obvious that the balance sheet will be largely affected by this change.

The evidence of the fines as to population and the number of deaths has already been discussed, and the unusually high fines of the bishop's manors have been noticed. It is evident from these entries that all the ordinary business transactions went on as before during the two years into which the plague falls. Men succeeded to the holdings of their fathers or brothers, and were able to find large sums of ready money— £3 or £5 or £10—even in the period of acutest distress. Leases were granted and taken up, sales and exchanges were made between the villeins—perhaps not as frequently as before, but still frequently enough to show that the panic was not universal. Marriages were frequent, not only of widows and heiresses, but also of the landless daughters, married both within and without the manor. If the Court Rolls for these years had survived, they must have shown a large increase in the total receipts, though the purely judicial fees, the perquisites of the court, certainly dropped off. The proceeds of the court were, however, decreasing for a variety of reasons, and where the entry fines are accounted for separately, the decline was visible long before 1349. With better organization many of the petty agricultural offences, such as breach of pasture or of wood, must have disappeared. The entry of heriots has also been discussed; it is valuable direct testimony to the number of deaths, but otherwise not much is to be learned from it. In very few, if any cases, was the bishop compassionate enough to forgo his heriot, but once or twice nothing could be found to seize—neither beasts nor money nor produce of any kind.

On a normal manor these are the chief sources of revenue; on some, extra items appear. *Recognitions* decline rapidly, generally because the absent villein was dead; the *Consuetudines* also go down, though they recover again in a few years. The *Dona*, which are found on some of the Thames valley manors, also mark the decreased numbers. The *Firma Molendinae* often showed a heavy loss and the mill was sometimes allowed to get out of repair. This is especially true of the fulling-mills of Wiltshire. All these, however, are comparatively small sums. The outstanding fact is that the increased gains from fines and heriots were able to outset the loss on every other count. Thus the lord had a lump sum of additional capital in his hands, with which to meet the strain of the next few years, while readjustment was taking place.

Turning to the second schedule, the expenses, one finds that the first effect of the Black Death was increased economy. So far as the expenses consisted in buying materials, utensils, and the like, a considerable saving is effected for a year or two, while the customary payments in money or in kind for *precariae* grew less, and the harvest meals and the annual feasts cost less. Sometimes the total cost of the ploughs was more, sometimes less than before; generally it is more, because a little extra labour had to be hired. The same is true of the carting expenses. It is curious to find that the purchase of corn and stock goes on in spite of the plague, with no very consistent variations.

The expenses of the dairy and the sheepfolds are generally higher; women's wages had gone up, and the sheep needed extra care during these two critical years. The cost of the household and of necessaries is commonly cut down; improvements, building operations, repairs, the purchase of tools, &c., were certainly checked, though, as has been shown, building went on again with great vigour in a year or two's time. The cost of mowing, hoeing, threshing, and other occasional services reflects the influence of the sharpened demand for labour, but this item, together with the autumn works, has been already treated in connexion with wages.

A close examination of the expenses, however, merely serves to show that they were by no means uniformly increased, and that where they were increased, the loss was small, compared with the gain on receipts. The Appendix C, which gives the actual balance for four years on all the bishop's manors not specially examined in this study, will corroborate this statement, although the profits in some districts are much smaller than in the Winchester and Taunton groups.

The third part of the account, the stock and corn schedule, contains only one or two features which bear on this inquiry, and these have been treated elsewhere. The heriots which were still paid in kind occur here, and the area under cultivation is ascertained from the bailiff's corn account.

The 'account of works' has also been sufficiently discussed.

This examination of the account in its systematic order merely serves to confirm the conclusion that the attack of the pestilence was sharp and widespread, though irregularly distributed, but that its effects were short-lived. The actual figures speak for themselves far more lucidly than any commentary.

ADDENDUM

As has been already pointed out, there are many Court Rolls for the latter years of the fourteenth century for most of the Winchester manors; as a rule, however, they yield little new information.

The Bishop's Waltham and Bitterne Rolls, for example, are very numerous for the episcopate of William of Wykeham. From them one may gather various disconnected pieces of information. In 1389–90 over eighty-five different surnames appear in the Waltham Court Rolls for one purpose or another; leases for seven, five, and three years are noted; a fine of £16 is paid for a mixed holding, of which the largest unit was one ferling-land; five shillings was claimed for the 'farm' of one cow during two years, the defence being that the cow was useless during that time.

Various scraps of parchment, tied up with the rolls, contain lists of sheep and corn, the names of reeves, or notes of the expenses of the lord's visits. On one of these visits 'good and able' cider ought to have been provided, whereas what was provided was neither 'full nor able'.

About 1380 the *enrolling* of title begins to be mentioned,

after a surrender had been made in full court; a woman recovers the land of a cousin after search made in the records of the Pipe at Wolvesey; three tenants do not come into court to make fine, and are amerced 1s. 6d.; heriots appear to rise with fines, as one sow and 5s. is paid in one case. At Bitterne it is clear that fines were sometimes paid for crofts˜ on the sea-shore (see p. 45) and for marsh holdings, though such fines are small. In one case a day is appointed to Walter Assheldon because he had alienated *per scriptum suum v acras de tenura sua finabili*—an interesting example of the common desire to evade the obligations of villeinage.

The Pipe Roll for 1381–2, for which there seem to be no corresponding Court Rolls, has a striking example of *Deodand*; £5 is paid for a cart and five horses forfeited for having caused the death of Chrispina (?) Wyntere. This salutary custom must have greatly increased the safety of the high roads! The Court Rolls contain some evidence of desertions of villeins, but these are not so frequent as they appear to be elsewhere.

On the whole, then, the Pipe Rolls furnish much the best material for inquiry, though occasional details may be added from the Court Rolls. The latter are, however, only useful for discussing conditions twenty or thirty years after the pestilence, as no contemporary rolls have been preserved.

CHAPTER III

SOME GENERAL CONCLUSIONS

THE first question which naturally arises after an examination such as is contained in the two previous chapters is this—How far does it advance our knowledge of the results and importance of the great pestilence ? This is, professedly, only an attempt to study certain local effects of the Black Death. The one fact which seems to stand out with real certainty is the partial and irregular character of the visitation. Therefore any conclusions drawn exclusively from the manors contained in the Winchester Pipe Roll may justly be confronted with dissimilar evidence drawn from other groups of manors or from other districts. Yet the mere bulk of material contained in the Winchester Rolls and its continuity are exceptional. Hence a few general conclusions seem to possess a considerable degree of probability.

These conclusions may be summed up in the following way. The estates of the Bishop of Winchester during the fourteenth century show no revolution either in agriculture or in tenure, but changes are effected by a continuous economic evolution ; no period of anarchy follows upon the appearance of the Black Death, but there is evidence of severe evanescent effects and temporary changes, with a rapid return to the *status quo* of 1348 ; the period of greatest change in the matter of commutation of services begins after 1360, possibly after 1370, and the rapidity of the change is evidently not immediately due to the Black Death.

Each of these statements has been supported by statistics, which, although on no point exhaustive of the material supplied by the Winchester Pipe Rolls, are, it is hoped, representative. It remains to be seen how far such assertions are in harmony with the opinions of recent writers on the history of mediaeval agriculture.

It is unnecessary to go back to Thorold Rogers and the idea of a complete revolution in the methods of agriculture and in the system of tenure.[1] Every subsequent investigation has tended to discredit the cataclysmic view of economic history.

It is generally admitted that ' the Black Death can no longer be elevated to the position of a constant economic force '.[2] Yet traces of the older view are still evident in every general work on mediaeval economic history ; the old stock phrases die hard, even though the conclusions may have been modified. Thus Archdeacon Cunningham makes use of Maitland's work on the ' History of a Cambridgeshire Manor ' to show how the process of commutation may have been affected by the plague, and goes on to pronounce that ' it seemed as if the agriculture of the country was completely ruined '.[3] Yet if Maitland's essay proves anything, it proves that the theory of revolution is untenable. Moreover, the ' complete ruin ' of the agriculture of a whole district or country is an improbable supposition.

Again, in the ' Historical Outline of Land Ownership in England ', which is prefixed to the ' Report of the Land Inquiry Committee, 1913 ', vol. i, Dr. Slater writes, ' The resident body of workers in villages was so reduced that cultivation could not be efficiently carried on under the old system ' ; and again, ' it was equally impossible for them [the landlords] to cultivate their demesne lands profitably either with forced or with hired labour '. The problem was solved, he asserts, by the increase of sheep-farming and by the adoption of the stock and land lease, whereby ' the demesne lands were allotted to the poorest of the peasantry '.

The briefest examination of the Winchester Pipe Roll shows how entirely inapplicable these statements are to a large number of manors in south-western England.

Other writers speak of the period of anarchy, the unparalleled losses and disasters, the wholesale devastation of the Black Death. Such language is generally an echo of the

---

[1] Seebohm's controversy with Thorold Rogers (Fortnightly Review, vols. ii and iii) is mainly concerned with questions of population, and Seebohm's opinion as to the economic revolution did not substantially differ from that of Rogers.

[2] Vinogradoff, English Hist. Rev., xv. 775.

[3] Cunningham, Growth of English Industry and Commerce, fifth edition, vol. i, p. 332.

chroniclers, or of Thorold Rogers, and is seldom based on any very thorough examination of first-hand evidence.[1] The constant difficulty is to get any exact information showing that changes which followed the Black Death were in any real sense due to it. Probably the most valuable work on the whole subject, since Thorold Rogers, is the collection of material in ' Le Soulèvement des Travailleurs d'Angleterre ' by André Réville, published with an historical introduction by Ch. Petit-Dutaillis. The strong emphasis there laid on continuity and gradual development has influenced all subsequent writers on economic history, and has practically killed the revolution theory, save in casual phrases in text-books. M. Petit-Dutaillis in his essay on the causes of the rising of 1381[2] has recently reviewed the literature on fourteenth-century manorial history which has appeared since 1898, and most of it seems to corroborate his views.[3]

Miss Davenport's ' Economic Development of a Norfolk Manor ' is valuable in its method and general suggestions, but Forncett, the subject of her study, is geographically too widely separated from the Winchester manors to afford a basis for close comparison. Similarly, Miss Putnam's ' Enforcement of the Statutes of Labourers during the first decade after the Black Death ' has been useful in studying the rise in wages, but there seems to be little or no evidence in the Pipe Rolls that might illustrate the working of the statutes on the Bishop of Winchester's manors.[4]

Other work on the economic development of the fourteenth century has appeared in the form of scattered articles in various publications and periodicals. The most useful of

---

[1] Even Mr. Tawney, after some cautious remarks on the probable effects of the Black Death, decides that its result was ' enormously to accelerate tendencies already at work '. Tawney, Agrarian Problem in Sixteenth Century, p. 90.

[2] Studies Supplementary to Stubbs's Constitutional History, vol. ii, Manchester, 1914.

[3] He does not, however, discuss in any detail Mr. T. W. Page's ' Disappearance of Villeinage in England ', which ought perhaps to rank as the most serious contribution to his subject since Réville's work.

[4] See chap. ii, pp. 100-2. It is possible that the frequent contracts with craftsmen, who were paid lump sums for definite pieces of work, were due to the desire to evade the statutes.

these are the articles on Social and Economic History in the 'Victoria County History', which give opportunity for a reconsideration of the question county by county.

The evidence of these articles is probably the most valuable test of my conclusions, as the writers generally draw upon sources other than the Pipe Rolls in treating of those districts which are covered by them. The severity of the plague, the general economic conditions, and the importance of its results might reasonably be expected to be similar within the bounds of one county, though local conditions must still be taken into account. The writer of the Berkshire article on Social and Economic History[1] particularly emphasizes the transient character of the results of the Black Death, which she describes as having been severe but not lasting in this county. All the changes which are commonly ascribed to the pestilence had begun to appear in normal Berkshire manors before 1349, and the process of change continued long after 1381. The writer finds little evidence of reaction in the matter of commutation, due to the decreased population, but there are many signs of temporary derangement of the normal system, with subsequent reversion to the *status quo* of 1348. Thus the number of leases increased rapidly during the first year or two after the visitation of the plague, but the leases were commonly for a period of nine years, and at the end of the term they were not renewed. Roughly speaking, a period of ten years shows an almost complete recovery in Berkshire. If the two striking cases of Harwell and Brightwell be added, the effects of the Black Death might be minimized still further.

For Oxfordshire[2] the material is rather scanty, and the writer finds some traces of reaction, and notes the heavy valuations at which services were commuted. She sums up,

[1] V. C. H. Berkshire, vol. ii, Miss E. C. Lodge, Social and Economic History.
[2] V. C. H. Oxon., vol. ii, Miss B. A. Lees, Social and Economic History. If the Winchester Pipe Roll entries for Witney and Adderbury and Culham had been used for the article, more evidence would have been available for Oxfordshire, and the general impression that it suffered rather severely from the plague would have been confirmed.

however, by concluding that in the majority of cases the old services were continued without further commutation.

The author of the corresponding article for Somerset[1] believes that the material effects of the Black Death were comparatively evanescent, and she analyses the rapid and almost complete recovery of the manor of Wellow, as shown in its ministers' accounts. The dislocation of the ordinary system seems, however, to have left a ' legacy of discontent '.

The Winchester Pipe Roll has been used to some extent for the article on Hampshire,[2] but by a rather unfortunate chance the manors selected for special examination appear to have been exceptionally hard hit by the plague. Burgh-clere in the north-west has been taken as typical, whereas good reason may be shown for regarding this part of the county as somewhat exceptional (cf. p. 135). The manors round Winchester have been more hastily treated, and indeed the writer has sought rather for evidence of the ravages of the Black Death than for an estimate of its permanent effects. Cheriton, for which several striking figures are quoted, suffered far more severely than its immediate neighbours, both in 1349 and in 1361. The author, however, although she emphasizes the results of the pestilence, is very ready to admit that such results were local and curiously uneven. She suggests that Fareham in the south and most of the manors in the north-east corner show comparatively few traces of the plague. Nevertheless, Fareham supplies a striking instance of the rapid growth of commutation between 1346 and 1352, and of a corresponding rise in the working expenses of the manor. The inconsistency suggests once more to the reader that changes which accompanied the Black Death were often due to very different causes.[3]

[1] V. C. H. Somerset, vol ii, Miss G. Bradford.
[2] V. C. H. Hampshire, vol. v, Miss Violet M. Shillington.
[3] I cannot follow the writer of this article in her statement that ' for many years after the Black Death a carefully compiled list of the numbers and kind of the labour-services due from the tenants . . . formed an important item in the accounts of the manors ' [of the Bishopric]. From a careful examination (confirmed by two independent searchers) of almost every Roll between 1346 and 1376, it appears to me certain that no additional accounts of services were inserted in the Pipe Roll during this period.

The whole article seems to show that commutation had advanced far more rapidly on the lay manors of the country than on the episcopal estates.

Of the many short articles in periodicals, modelled to some extent on Maitland's ' History of a Cambridgeshire Manor ', few, if any, demand notice here. As a rule, they treat of districts or of periods outside the limits of this study. Two, however, deal directly with the question of the Black Death and commutation of services. Mr. K. G. Feiling's notes on ' An Essex Manor in the Fourteenth Century ',[1] and Mr. H. L. Gray's article on ' The Commutation of Villein Services in England before the Black Death ',[2] have been referred to elsewhere in connexion with certain points raised in them. Both articles, however, are to some extent criticisms of a more important work. · Mr. T. W. Page, in his ' Disappearance of Villeinage in England ',[3] has made a serious attempt to reach a sound general conclusion as to the Black Death based on a study of ministers' accounts. As such, his work has been my constant standard of comparison, and it will be useful to set the conclusions drawn from a single group of manors side by side with Mr. Page's assertions, based on a less detailed survey of a large number of manors of many types.

Mr. Page makes several very definite statements about the conditions of labour and of the manorial economy in the fourteenth century. His study deals with material very similar to that of the Winchester Pipe Roll, but representing many different estates and different methods. Broadly speaking, his contention is that little commutation had taken place before 1349, and that it took place very rapidly afterwards, and had become general and far-reaching by 1381. There is little doubt that he is right in claiming that great changes

Minute accounts appear for certain Somerset manors (v. p. 62), but these were normal long before the Black Death. Similar accounts for other manors appear for a few years after 1375, but these are apparently due to a change of policy (under William of Wykeham) and not in any sense to the Black Death (see p. 159).

[1] English Hist. Rev., April 1911.   [2] English Hist. Rev., October 1914.
[3] Originally published, in slightly different form, as ' Die Umwandlung der Frohndienste in Geldrenten . . . Englands.' Baltimore, U.S.A., 1897. Republished in English, New York, 1900.

took place between 1348 and 1381, but thirty years might well suffice for a period of rapid transition, even without a catastrophe to mark its beginning. To prove that the Black Death was really responsible, it must be shown that the change was particularly marked between 1350 and 1360, and that the process continues along the same line until 1380. This Mr. Page's evidence does not show with any precision. His methods have been criticized more than once, but it is necessary to repeat some of the criticisms in order to show whether any useful purpose can be served by comparing his results with those drawn from the Winchester accounts.[1] The sharp distinction which he has drawn between the *Spanndienste* and the *Handdienste*, the team-work and the hand-work, has been objected to as far too definite and clear-cut. Both types of labour-services were commonly used in 1348; indeed on some manors even the works known as *Opera Manualia* were frequently employed in team-work. The broad classification of services as *Opera Hiemalia, Estivalia*, and *Autumpnalia*, and *Precariae* is unsatisfactory when compared with the very varied classifications found on the Winchester manors. As has been shown above (pp. 39 and 118), this is no mere question of nomenclature. The classification of services had a considerable influence upon their survival.

The geographical distribution of Mr. Page's manors has also been criticized; his evidence is drawn almost exclusively from the south-east of England. This, however, is a defect only when a universal conclusion is sought or a comparison of his results with the evidence drawn from different local groups is desired. Again, Mr. Page has been criticized for the exclusively ecclesiastical character of his material. Obviously the available material is on the whole predominantly ecclesiastical. It would perhaps be more fair to criticize him for not having grouped his evidence more strictly, so that it might have been possible to distinguish certain differences between lay and ecclesiastical estates, or again between monastic and episcopal estates.

[1] Cf. Vinogradoff, E. H. R. xv. 775; Feiling (K. G.), E. H. R., April 1911; and Gray (H. L.), E. H. R., Oct. 1914.

The most valid criticism of the work, however, is that Mr. Page gives far too little opportunity of judging of the value of his assertions. He has examined a very large number of ministers' accounts and set down certain conclusions drawn from them. But he quotes so little from the actual documents that there is no opportunity of testing his results. He asserts that half, or the whole, or a very few of the services had been commuted, but the statement has to be taken on faith. An examination of the Winchester ministers' accounts shows that it is extremely easy to overlook indispensable evidence, if one is not familiar with the account-keeping of a particular group of manors. It is impossible to accuse Mr. Page of having overlooked such evidence, but it is equally impossible to accept his results without further examination.[1] A much closer study of what might be termed the ' diplomatic ' of manorial accounts seems to be needed if our knowledge of the subject is to be seriously advanced.

The more important of Mr. Page's conclusions, however, demand careful examination and form a most useful standard of comparison. It may be useful to summarize them very briefly, in order to show how far they hold good for the Winchester manors.

Mr. Page asserts (a) that more hand-work than ploughing or team-work was performed by the villeins just before 1349 ; (b) that very little hand-work was commuted by 1350 ; (c) that during the plague agricultural affairs were in a condition of anarchy, while bailiffs' accounts frequently show a break ; (d) that servile burdens were often slipped by the villeins in collusion with stewards and reeves ; (e) that the Black Death caused no increase of burdens of those villeins who remained ; (f) that the tenants frequently paid fines for non-performance of services, and that desertion was very frequent ; (g) that the landlord could very seldom let the land of dead tenants to new ones on the old conditions ; (h) that the Black Death

---

[1] Mr. Page's classification of the manor of Hutton, Essex, as one on which the services were ' about half performed ' at three different dates, is definitely disproved by K. G. Feiling, English Hist. Rev., April 1911, ' An Essex Manor in the Fourteenth Century '.

gave an impetus to the system of leases ; (*i*) that the Black Death caused a considerable diminution of cultivated land ; (*j*) that commutation of services to a money-rent was very frequent by 1380, though often only temporary ; (*k*) that villein status remained unchanged after the Black Death ; (*l*) that a general leakage from the manor is observable after 1400.

It will readily be seen that some of Mr. Page's conclusions are borne out by the evidence of the Winchester estates, while others are directly controverted.

To recapitulate the points of difference or agreement :

It is probably true that more hand-work than team-work was performed by 1349, and yet ploughing services survived on at least thirty-four of the Winchester manors as late as 1376, and can be traced on almost all of them in 1349 ; they cannot therefore be ignored. Even where the actual ploughings were commuted, the lord frequently made a bargain with the villeins that ploughmen should be supplied by them in rotation, and thus commutation did not imply wage-paid labour. Again it is true of the Winchester manors that comparatively little hand-work had been commuted by 1350, yet two necessary modifications must be added. The *Opera Vendita* must be excluded from consideration as not implying true commutation, but merely sale of surplus labour. It is not clear that Mr. Page anywhere makes this distinction ; he certainly mentions the sale of surplus labour at Warboys in 1380, but in writing of commutation generally he does not distinguish different kinds. Secondly, it must be admitted that although commutation of hand-work had not gone far on any of the episcopal manors regarded as a whole, yet it is fairly usual to find that an individual villein had had the whole of his services commuted, either permanently or at the lord's pleasure. Thus, though the demesne was still cultivated by villein labour, there were many individual villeins who did not work on the demesne.

The condition of anarchy said to have been usual during the plague years is absolutely unparalleled on the Winchester estates, while only one or two cases of dishonesty on the part

of the reeves, in returning too many ' Defects of Rent ',
appear to have been detected. No evidence is forthcoming
that they were suspected of dishonesty in dealing with
services.

On the other hand, the Winchester Rolls confirm the statement that the Black Death caused no increase of the burdens
of those villeins who remained—so far as it refers to burdens
definitely imposed or increased by the lord. But all services
which were done in common, for an unspecified length of
time (such as sheep-washing, carrying brushwood, building,
carrying letters); would be made heavier by the loss of
population ; the man who held two virgates would find his
burden materially heavier if two of his sons died, while the
offices which were filled in rotation from among the villeins
would tend to press more severely. Moreover, in one or two
cases, at least, there was definite reaction. ' The services are
performed now, because the work is worth more than the
money ' (cf. p. 108).

As to the great difficulty of finding new tenants who would
take up the vacant holdings on the old conditions, one can
only say this is very unlike the experience of the Bishop of
Winchester and his bailiffs. The immense sums paid in fines
show how willing the survivors were to take up the vacant
holdings on the old conditions. On a very few manors
a considerable number of virgates remained vacant for some
years, but the reason would seem to be decrease of population,
or some special local circumstance, rather than dislike of the
old conditions. It has been shown already that the Black
Death gave no impetus whatever to the system of leases on
the Winchester estates between the years 1350 and 1360, and
although leases were more common by 1376, even then no
very important extension of the practice had taken place.
The area of cultivated land apparently decreased, if the
figures given above (p. 132) may be regarded as typical, but
on the manors thus quoted the average loss is not as much
as 20 per cent., and it is difficult to say how far this is permanent, or how far it was compensated by the leasing of
small parcels of the demesne. The decrease in the area

cultivated by the villeins would seem to be negligible, with one or two striking exceptions, while the growth of small enclosures by the villeins themselves probably increased production.

Mr. Page's conclusion that commutation of services to money-rent was very frequent by 1380, although it was often only temporary, corresponds roughly with the evidence of the Winchester Pipe Roll; but one cannot assume that all the services which were not performed had necessarily been commuted. The customal included in the Pipe Roll for 1376–7 shows that very many of the services had simply dropped out, either because they were not demanded, or because the holdings were now held on other terms, or remained vacant. A clear distinction is drawn in the accounts of some manors between works which had been definitely 'relaxed', and those which were 'defects'. The 'defects' are generally not balanced by any increase of the rents of assize, nor, in many cases, of the leases; they speak rather of a gradual process of rural depopulation, which generally does not date back as far as 1349. Villein status certainly remained unchanged on the Winchester manors, although various circumstances were combining to make the seigneurial court less and less important, and thus the practical enfranchisement of the villein tended to precede any change of theory. With regard to the alleged general leakage from the manors observable after 1400, the date lies outside the scope of this inquiry, but the gradual leakage is clearly marked on the Winchester manors before 1381, though the number of fugitives was probably not very great. The clause which Mr. Page quotes as frequently inserted in the agreements to let derelict lands for money-rents 'until another shall come to take the land on the old terms' is fairly common in the Winchester accounts, but seems to be rather formal than significant. The tenant holding under such a clause probably had as much security of tenure as he was likely to want.

Thus the inevitable conclusion is that the Winchester Pipe Rolls abundantly confirm some of Mr. Page's assertions, and definitely contradict others, while in a few cases the evidence cannot be tested clearly enough to make any comparison. Mr. Page has examined a minimum of about 88 manors ; the Winchester Rolls contain about 60. Whence comes it that such complete contradiction is possible ?

It is partly a matter of geography ; partly a question of method ; partly a question of different systems of estate management. Two or three counsels of perfection in considering the evidence seem to demand attention. Geographical limitations should be very closely defined, and physical conformation and grouping should be allowed due weight. Division by counties is sometimes useful, but it is of more value to distinguish clearly such districts as the valley of the Itchen, with its fringe of down-land ; the North Hants and Berkshire downs ; the manors on the indented coastline of Hampshire ; the Thames Valley ; the former forest-lands of North Oxfordshire ; the famous low-lying arable and meadow land of Taunton Dean, again with a fringe of downs. Such grouping will throw a flood of light on the peculiarities of manorial custom, or the eccentricities of manorial history.

Different groups of estates should be treated separately. If it were possible to investigate the accounts of a great monastic house in the fourteenth century as fully as those of the Bishop of Winchester may be examined, another type of management would probably stand out. What uniformity of method there had been in the twelfth and thirteenth centuries breaks down before the new needs of the fourteenth century. The changes in the value of money, the growing prosperity of the villein, the sudden shock of the Black Death, the gathering cloud of discontent—all these were met and dealt with by different expedients. The ways and means of an Oxford college may have been very different from those of the Bishop of Winchester, the Abbot of Battle, or the canons of St. Paul's. Even within the boundaries of one county, one group of manors may have commonly accepted the innovation of the stock and land lease, while the next had seen no reason to depart from the traditional methods of villein tenure.

If the policy of several great institutions, collegiate,

monastic, and episcopal, during the fifteenth century, could be studied in detail, and compared with the policy of other great landlords, much light might be thrown on the enclosure movements of the fifteenth and sixteenth centuries.[1]

Side by side with a stricter definition of geographical districts, and a sharper classification of estates and systems of estate-management, it seems desirable to demand a more precise treatment of the materials for manorial history. It has already been suggested that, for the solution of such a problem as the results of the Black Death, ministers' accounts supply the most reliable evidence. The vast mass of such material will never be published *in extenso*. The task of examining it is very lengthy and not lightly to be under-taken twice. It is therefore much to be desired that con-clusions drawn from it should be justified as far as possible by direct quotation, and some statistics. If this were more generally done, it would be possible to compare the results attained by different writers, and to check the broad dog-matizing of text-books.

Finally, one very pertinent inquiry may be made in criticism of the modern estimate of the results of the pestilence. If the rapid change in the social and economic position of the peasants and small holders of England be not due to the Black Death, to what cause or causes may it more justly be assigned ?

The question needs an answer. Perhaps it is drawing too sharp a line to ask when and why the nature-economy was transformed into a money-economy. There never was a period in the known history of England when a manor was carried on by a pure nature-economy, without the intervention of money. There has never yet been a period when a pure money-economy has abolished the nature-economy in English agriculture. The system of payment in kind is convenient, sometimes even convenient to both parties in the transaction,

---

[1] The result of the policy of great monastic houses has been shown by Dr. Savine, in Oxford Studies in Social and Legal History, vol. i, English Monasteries on the Eve of Dissolution; the origin of this policy might be traced in the early fifteenth century.

and not even twentieth-century supplies of coinage have sufficed to put an end to it. It is wise, therefore, to seek a diversity of causes for the change, and to allow to each some weight.

One of the great reasons for change is undue conservatism. The rigidness and inadaptability of labour-services and payments in kind led, almost as soon as they were established, to a kind of ' optional commutation ', or rough valuation in money, of which sometimes the lord, sometimes the tenant might take advantage.

The increased demand for money has been ascribed to many causes, notably to the Crusades and to the general increase of trade. The truth seems to be that when once a nature-economy or system of services is changed at one point, the whole structure begins to totter. The king had long been substituting money payments for military services ; the change spread downwards. The use of money and the amount in circulation in England increased rapidly during the thirteenth century ; the accumulations of the Templars, the activity of Italian merchants and bankers, and Edward I's reform of the coinage are but a few among the many proofs which might be cited. By 1346 the French wars had created a new need for coin, and Edward III made many attempts to meet the demand—notably by the introduction of a gold coinage and by laws requiring the import of bullion in payment for wool. The ruin which he brought upon the great banking-house of the Bardi shows the extent of his borrowing.

The fact that the Italian bankers were from this time largely replaced by native financiers proves that the currency in England must have been more adequate in amount, and more readily exchangeable than it had been fifty or a hundred years before.[1]

With changes in the circulation came changes in the value

[1] It is interesting to notice that Winchester must have been admirably situated with regard to the circulation of coin. The great fair, the proximity of Southampton, the residence of the Bishop, the frequent visits of the King and Court, the passage of armies on their way to France, the Pilgrims' Way, which passes through or near several of the Bishop's manors, would lead one to expect early commutation, such as in Kent is often ascribed to special economic conditions. Yet one actually finds great conservatism.

of money. The labourer who in the fourteenth century paid
½d. instead of doing a day's work paid at this rate, nct
because he was singularly lazy or unskilled, but because the
old valuations were out of date. A fall in the value of money
always presses hard upon the recipients of fixed incomes or
traditional fees. The labourer who commuted his services on
an old valuation enjoyed an unearned increment as certainly
as did the copyholder of the end of the sixteenth century.[1]

It is true that the fall in the value of money, while it
would greatly enhance the charm of commutation to the
villein, would render it less and less acceptable to the lord.
The ½d. paid by the villein would not buy a day's work in
1348 (even apart from the question of food allowances),
and only the crying need for greater flexibility, for greater
' mobility of income ' could reconcile the lord to commutation
on this traditional valuation. Yet the reconciliation was
effected. The villein whose dues were fixed by custom
enjoyed the benefit of the change in value, while his standards
of living and his need for expenditure of money hardly
altered. Hence he was able to accumulate a considerable
stock of capital, in money, in cattle, and in household goods ;
the fact is attested by the large sums paid in fines and by the
valuation of a villein's confiscated chattels at £5 or £6. It
might indeed be asserted, with much probability, that the
accumulation of capital during the Middle Ages, which laid
the foundations of English industrial development, was in
great measure the work of the villein, of the small capitalist,
sheltered by custom until his little hoard became the instru-
ment of his enfranchisement.

In yet another way, the result of the change is seen. As
the value of money fell, prices rose, and it seems safe to
assume, with modern economists, that wages tended to rise
less rapidly than prices.[2] This, at least, is the conclusion

---

[1] Cf. Maitland, History of a Cambridgeshire Manor.

[2] Cf. also the elaborate valuation of services in the *Cartularium Mona-
sterii S. Petri Gloucestriae* (Rolls Series), vol. iii ; the Extents dated 1265
contain numerous notes that a certain service *valet ultra cibum* 1d (or 2d.
or ½d.). The Metebedripe, worth ½d. *ultra cibum*, left a very narrow margin
for a rise in prices.

forced upon one by the frequent complaint that the customary meals supplied by the lord cost more than the labour was worth. This complaint was made on many manors belonging to the Bishop of Winchester, in spite of the fact that if one may judge from the cost of the ' Autumn Works ' the meals provided were not very lavish, the average cost being 1*d.* or 1¼*d.* per head for each *Precaria.* Many of the works were performed without food or drink, and in some cases the meals seem in turn to have been commuted for small customary payments to the villeins. But the complaint that the system was working at a loss comes also from Brightwaltham (Berkshire),[1] Hutton (Essex),[2] and from Banstead (Surrey),[3] as early as 1325, and is reflected in contemporary literature.[4] 'The work is not worth the breakfast' (or the *reprisa*) occurs several times in the Winchester Pipe Rolls, and obviously forms a very strong reason for the tacit dropping of labour-services. By 1376 the entry is considerably more frequent, and applies to ploughing as well as to harvest-work (see p. 121). On the Battle Abbey estates a tenant might bring to the harvest *Precariae* as many helpers as he pleased, who must all be allowed to join in the harvest supper. It is easy to see how the lord might suffer from ' assistance ' of this kind.

As has been suggested above, on many manors the majority of the services owed were simply dropped, neither sold nor commuted. They were evidently in many cases inefficient, expensive, and inelastic ;[5] the supply of hired labour increased with every change that broke down the traditional immobility of the labourer. Certain specified services tended to become useless. Thus many of the more personal services owed to the bishop were likely to become obsolete, or to be commuted

---

[1] See Camden Society, Battle Abbey Custumals.

[2] English Hist. Rev., April 1911, ' An Essex Manor in the Fourteenth Century '.

[3] English Hist. Rev., July 1913, p. 623.

[4] Cf. Langland, Piers Plowman, B. Passus vi, 309–14. ' The labourers that have no land to live on but their hands ', says Langland, ' will not be content with penny-ale and bacon, but demand fresh flesh or fish fried or baked, and that chaude or plus chaud.'

[5] If the lord could save 1¼*d.* on the food provided, and obtain 1*d.* or ½*d.* as commutation, he could evidently hire men at 2*d.* or 3*d.* per day, and might well obtain more efficient labour.

during the fairly frequent vacancies, when the temporalties
of the see were in the king's hand.

A combination of such natural causes led to the entire
disuse of labour services.[1] The chief offices of the manor were
sometimes filled in rotation by the villeins, and in some cases
the lord would probably seek to retain a permanent shepherd
or stockman by making the position more attractive; in one
case towards the end of the century a man *gave up* his land to
become the lord's shepherd;[2] the *Opera rotunda* of Wargrave
and Wycombe and Waltham St. Lawrence show another form
of rotation. The growth of enclosure, the increase of pasture-
farming, the leasing of the demesne, all tended to lessen the
need for labour-services, although perhaps only to a slight
extent. With the partial enclosure and consolidation of the
villein holdings, the virgate tends to be obscured, and the
virgate was the unit of assessment of villein services. Some
of the tenants cease to have ploughs or plough-beasts, and
are perforce allowed to substitute ' hand-work ' for ' team-
work '. Others again prospered and accumulated holdings
until they could send their own sub-tenants or hired men to
the lord's demesne work. Every change of this kind made the
system harder to work. Assart land had always paid regular
money-rents; a few derelict lands taken up on new terms
after the Black Death had been granted at money-rents; the
lands of deserters were frequently let at a rent, yearly or on
lease, ' because no one would hold them for works '; the
letting of small parcels of the demesne still further extends the
rent-system. With so many examples of a money-economy
all around them it is small wonder that the virgaters and
semi-virgaters became dissatisfied. The Black Death had
given a momentary shock to agriculture, and the chief result
of that shock had been a slow-growing conviction that times
were changing, and that agriculture might well change too.

[1] It should be noted, however, that the practical disuse was very gradual,
extending all through the fifteenth and sixteenth centuries; while even
as late as 1707 the neighbouring manor of Crondal was leased with all the
works not heretofore arrented into money. (Hampshire Record Society,
Crondal Records, 1890.)

[2] Wycombe, 1376–7.

The immobility of labour had received a rude blow—all the more effective because the plague had visited village after village with strange irregularity and partiality. The Black Death did not, in any strictly economic sense, cause the Peasants' Revolt or the breakdown of villeinage, but it gave birth, in many cases, to a smouldering feeling of discontent, an inarticulate desire for change, which found its outlet in the rising of 1381. As to the abolition of villeinage, the process was clearly not complete in the sixteenth century.

The Winchester estates were affected by these natural causes in common with all southern England. They preserved a more conservative system than secular estates, as a rule, and the bishop had perhaps less need of actual money than the military leaders who followed Edward III to France. Moreover, very considerable sums accrued to him even before commutation became general. Is there any point in the history of the bishopric at which the process of commutation might be expected to receive a powerful stimulus?

In 1367 William of Wykeham, the man 'wise of castle-building', was finally invested with the bishopric of Winchester; in 1371 he resigned the Great Seal, and is said to have turned his attention to his episcopal estates, and to building-operations, both on his manor-houses and on the cathedral, though the latter scheme was suspended almost at once; in 1369 he began to buy land for his future college in Oxford; by 1376 he was supporting poor scholars both at Winchester and in Oxford; in 1376 he had seventy poor scholars lodged at his expense in various halls in Oxford; between November 1376 and June 1377 (the period of his brief disgrace) the temporalties of his see were in the king's hand, although the revenues were ultimately restored to him. In 1379 the poor scholars, who had been dispersed in 1376, returned to Oxford; in 1382 Wykeham's College in Winchester received its foundation charter.

Wykeham's New College of Saint Mary of Winchester in Oxford was based upon a system of direct money-allowances; each Fellow had one shilling a week and 'livery' once a year, while the Warden received £40. This system must have imposed an appreciable burden upon the revenues of the bishopric during the early years of the two foundations ; the concurrent policy of buying estates with which to endow the colleges must, however, have created a far sharper demand for ready money.

It is, of course, possible that these dates have no significance in the history of commutation on the episcopal estates—that they merely mark coincidences. Yet the coincidences are unusually striking. From fifteenth-century entries in the Pipe Roll it appears that the year 1367 was regarded as marking an epoch in the process of commutation, though the roll itself records no remarkable change. Perhaps, like ' the time of King Edward ', it had come to mean simply the days before the upheaval. It is certainly remarkable that the founding of New College should exactly coincide with the moment at which the bishop began to make stricter inquisition into the amount and value of the services due to him. (The inquisition is not due to the seizure by the king, as it begins in 1375–6, whereas the seizure only takes place in November 1376.) A motive for commutation is thus clear and pressing. Very little proof, however, is forthcoming. At Harwell, in 1380–1, it is recorded—*De firmis terre et tenementorum que nuper fuerunt Thome Gateway nichil hic quia assignati per dominum ad solvendum apud Oxoniam pro sustentatione pauperum scolarium domini ibidem.* This is the only entry of the kind that I have found, but of course it is equally probable that the allowances were paid out of the bishop's general revenues, and not directly from any single manors.

If this suggestion bears examination, it would prove that the process of commutation on the Winchester estates was more seriously affected by William of Wykeham's magnificent projects than by that traditional parent of all economic development, the Black Death.

APPENDIX

MANOR ACCOUNT ROLLS

A. WINCHESTER GROUP. I. BISHOP'S STOKE.

Reeve	1346–7 Robert Edrad	1347–8 William atte Thorne	1348–9 ?	1349–50 Peter Ailward	1350–1 P. Ailward and John Peyhan	1351–2 John Peyhan	1354–5 John Pehon	1376–7 Peter atte Nashe	1385–6 —	1455 J. Coupere and John Colswayne
Receipt	£ s. d.	£ s. d.	£ s. d.	£ s. d.	£ s. d.	£ s. d.	£ s. d.	£ s. d.	£ s. d.	£ s. d.
Arrears	10 1 5½	3 6 0	2 16 0	25 2 8¼	19 9 3¼	11 9 0¼	25 14 9¾	13 12 6	1 0 0	19 9 5½
Assized rents	19 12 10¾	19 12 10¾	19 12 10¾	19 12 10¾	19 12 10¾	19 12 10¾	19 12 10¾	19 13 1¾	19 13 1	19 19 4¼
Increment										
— Acquittances	11 0	7 0	11 0	12 0	12 0	12 0	12 0	12 0	12 0	7 0
— Defects	1 7 6	1 7 6	1 7 6	1 7 6	1 7 6	1 7 6	1 7 6	1 10 2	1 10 8	1 10 8
— Defects *per pestilentiam*	—	—	? 4 4	2 6	1 6	1 0	None	None	None	
Net rents	17 14 4¾	17 18 4¾	17 9 0¾	17 10 10¾	17 11 10¾	17 12 4¾	17 13 4¾	17 10 11¾ 2 6 4*	17 10 5¾	18 1 10¼
Issues of the manor	26 16 7½	27 5 2¼	14 16 6	18 11 1½	18 18 3	19 18 7½	21 11 5½	13 6 11	13 8 8	5 9 9½ 10 6 4†
Fines and marriages	7 0 4	7 0 2	52 0 6	11 9 6	5 13 8	3 19 8	2 4 2	4 13 4	12 0 0	1 5 4
Heriots										
Perquisites of the court	2 0 9	1 8 9	12 0	1 10 2	1 1 6	14 7	1 2 5 11 6 0‡	1 15 0 13 11§	c.3 0 0	19 8
Sale of stock	3 7 0	5 3 2	5 8 6	5 3 8	2 12 6	6 3 6	15 16 7	17 16 4	13 0 6	} 1 3 4
„ corn	17 7 10	8 12 0	8 0 0	5 6 1	3 9 7	3 8 2¾	8 6 3	15 19 1	13 1 6	}
„ works	—	—	—	—	—	—	—	7 13 6½	6 18 7½	19 8 8
Total Receipts ‖	78 10 7¼	70 6 11¼	104 16 7¼	62 19 2¼	55 17 9¾	60 10 7	110 11 7½	95 12 2¼	84 0 6¾	76 5 7¼
Expenses	18 17 2½	15 9 0	9 19 7	16 8 7¼	28 6 9½	17 5 6½	23 2 10	16 1 2½	18 15 6½	6 4 1
Balance paid	56 7 4¾	51 11 11¼	69 14 4	27 1 3¾	14 12 0	27 10 0¼	72 4 2¼	63 2 11¾	65 5 0½	
„ due	3 6 0	3 6 0¼	25 2 8¼	19 9 3¼	12 1 7½	15 15 0¼	3 18 7¼	16 8 0	(Quit.)	
Total Balance	59 13 4¾	54 17 11½	94 17 0¼	46 10 7	26 13 7½	45 5 0½	76 2 9½	79 10 11¾	65 5 0½	70 1 6¼

* Mill. † Farm of demesne and mill. ‡ Forensic receipts. § Late receipts.

‖ The total receipts given in these accounts generally differ slightly from the sum of the items given above, as I have occasionally omitted

	1346–7			1347–8			1348–9			1349–50			1350–1		
Reeve	Adam le Palmere			Adam le Palmere			Robert Germayn			Adam Skot			Adam Scott		
Receipt	£	s.	d.	£	s.	d.	£	s.	d.	£	s.	d.	£	s.	d.
Arrears . . .	22	11	1½	6	10	0	13	11	8	108	13	5½	34	7	8½
Assized rents .	83	9	10½	83	9	10¼	83	10	3½	83	10	3½	83	10	3½
Increment. . .		—				5		—			—				4
— Acquittances .		16	0		14	0		12	6		14	0		14	0
— Defects . .	1	13	2	1	13	2	1	13	2	1	13	2	1	13	2
— Defects *per pestilentiam*		—			—			5	6	1	7	3		None	
Net rents . . .	81	0	8½	81	3	1½	[80	19	1½]	79	15	10½	81	3	5½
Issues of the manor	26	6	7¼	51	14	11	25	13	11½	17	13	3¼	21	16	8
Fines and marriages	24	14	2	34	8	10	134	15	5	49	7	6½	13	7	2
Heriots		?			—		4	3	0		?			18	0
Perquisites of the court	8	9	3	10	11	2	5	7	8	6	7	6	7	0	0
Sale of stock . .	5	7	10	20	2	10	18	11	2	21	4	11	10	5	4
„ corn . .	16	1	4¼	42	0	10½	18	4	6½	25	19	0½	28	11	3
„ works . .	37	2	10½	37	2	10½	[37	2	10½]**	37	2	10½	37	2	10½
Total receipts .	218	18	3	280	6	4¾	345	15	1¼	245	1	0¾	205	9	7½
Expenses . . .	56	6	7¼	97	14	10¾	55	6	7	58	10	1¼	55	6	4
Balance paid . .	156	1	7¾	168	19	10	181	15	0¾	152	3	3	113	18	2
„ due . .	6	10	0	13	11	8	108	13	5½	34	7	8½	36	5	1
Total Balance .	162	11	7¾	182	11	6	290	8	6¼	186	10	11½	150	3	3

	1351–2			1354–5			1376–7			1385–6			1454–5		
Reeve	Adam Scott			Robert Parry			John Hody			?			John Lekestede, reeve		
Receipt	£	s.	d.	£	s.	d.	£	s.	d.	£	s.	d.	£	s.	d.
Arrears . . .	36	5	1	48	4	3¾	58	14	0½	103	14	3	127	3	2¼
Assized rents .	83	10	7½	83	14	7½	83	17	8½	illegible			84	4	4½
Increment. . .		—			—			—			1	0		16	3½
													8	11	6*
— Acquittances .		14	0		16	0		14	0		14	0		12	0
— Defects . .	1	13	2	1	13	2	1	13	2	1	16	2	4	8	5
— Defects *per pestilentiam*		None			None			None			None			None	
Net rents . . .	81	3	5½	81	5	5½	81	10	6½	81	8	10½	88	11	9
							1	7	11†	1	7	1†		2	6†
Issues of the manor	25	16	8¾	27	8	2½	26	5	4	31	4	8	17	2	9‡
							15	5	4§		—		12	10	8§
Fines and marriages	18	3	2	14	11	0	11	18	4	38	18	0	11	16	1
Heriots		14	0		9	0		11	0		—			13	0
Perquisites of the court	8	1	3	9	12	4	8	1	11	16	11	2	5	17	1
				5	16	11‖	3	6	1¶	9	17	4‖			
Sale of stock . .	17	7	9	12	17	2	17	7	8	14	10	1	1	5	8
„ corn . .	28	8	8½	65	14	8½	21	6	2	15	1	11			
„ works . .	37	2	10½	37	2	10½	37	6	4½	37	3	1½	43	7	2½
Total receipts .	225	10	10¾	260	18	9	283	0	8½	372	14	4	308	13	10¾
Expenses . . .	69	7	5	94	1	5½	35	15	8	51	8	4	15	17	8¼
Balance paid . .	107	19	1¾	138	12	1½	207	7	7	213	3	9			
„ due . .	48	4	4	28	5	2	39	17	5½	107	2	3			
Total Balance .	156	3	5	166	12	3½	247	5	2½	320	6	0	292	16	2½

* New rents of demesne. † Annual recognitions. ¶ Late receipts. ‡ Farms. ** Roll damaged. § Mills. ‖ *Catalla Felonii.*

III. DROXFORD.

	1346–7	1347–8	1348–9	1349–50	1350–1	1351–2	1353–4	1376–7	1385–6	1455
Reeve	Ralph de Gosewelle	Ralph de Gosewelle	John atte Hatche	John atte Hatche	?	John le Shepherd	John le Shepherd	Wm. Orplyngton, John Russell	?	R. Sanne, Reeve; Philip Knight, Farmer
Receipt	£ s. d.	£ s. d.	£ s. d.	£ s. d.	£ s. d.	£ s. d.	£ s. d.	£ s. d.	£ s. d.	£ s. d.
Arrears	6 8 0½	4 13 0¾	10 4 2¼	27 3 8	9 3 9	13 17 0¾	3 18 0	3 0 0	4 0 4	30 14 3½
Assized rents . .	25 3 9½	25 3 9½	25 4 3½	25 4 3½	25 4 3½	25 4 3½	25 4 3½	25 4 5½	25 4 5½	25 4 5½
Increment . . .	—	6								
— Acquittances .	4 0	5 4	3 4½	5 4	5 4	5 4	5 4	5 4	5 4	6 3½
— Defects . . .	10 0	10 0	10 0	10 0	10 0	10 0	10 0	10 0	10 0	1 16 8
— Defects *per pestilentiam*	—	—	? None	16 3	None	None	None			
Net rents . . .	24 9 9½	24 8 10½	24 10 11	23 12 0	24 8 11½	24 8 11½	24 8 11½	24 9 1½	24 9 1½	23 1 6
										1 6
Issues of the manor	6 2 4½	6 15 4¾	5 2 9¼	5 17 1¾	6 4 0½	6 8 1¾	8 0 3¾	8 11 0½	10 3 6½	4 4 10½
										*2 19 8
								1 10 6†	—	‡6 14 1½
Fines and marriages	7 4 2	4 5 8	46 12 6	4 9 4	4 12 8	5 19 8	9 10 4	5 0 0	15 0	14 4
Heriots	—	—	—	—	—	—	—	—	1 0	
Perquisites of the court	1 14 10	2 3 6	14 5	?	15 10	1 1 9	14 0	6 1½	illegible	1 9 8
Sale of stock . .	3 6 8	6 3 7¾	9 17 9	11 18 5	8 4 11½	15 12 7	6 10 5	15 2 7	illegible	7 14 0
„ corn. . .	19 12 11	17 0 6	6 8 9	20 6 7¾	14 13 9¾	22 13 9¾	17 17 3	19 6 7¼	21 2 8	3 8 3¾
„ works . .	9 6 10¼	9 6 10½	9 6 10½	9 6 10½	9 6 10½	9 6 10½	9 6 10¼	9 6 10¼	9 6 10¼	8 16 10¼
Total receipts . .	75 0 6¾	73 10 10¼	107 7 8¾	82 8 2½	73 13 3¾	90 5 3½	69 19 2½	86 13 4¼	95 8 4¼	90 1 9½
Expenses . . .	24 2 2	26 9 9	21 18 4½	17 18 2¾	19 19 5½	19 17 8½	24 16 2	13 1 9½	illegible	11 3 1
Balance paid . .	46 5 4	36 16 11¼	57 12 4½	55 6 2¾	39 16 9½	50 10 6	38 6 10½	67 9 6¾	64 10 8¼	
„ due . .	4 13 3¾	10 4 2	27 17 8	9 3 9	13 17 0¾	19 17 1	6 16 2	6 2 0	1 13 4	
Total Balance . .	50 18 7¾	47 1 1¼	85 10 0½	64 9 11¾	53 13 10¼	70 7 7	45 3 0½	73 11 6¾	66 4 0¼	78 18 8½

Not in the Roll for 1453.

* New rents and services. † Late receipts, &c. ‡ For demesne lands.

Reeve	1346–7 John atte Gate, Michael de Somborne	1347–8 Michael de Somborne (serviens)	1348–9 Michael de Somborne and Wm. Hude	1349–50 William Hude	1350–1 William Ude	1351–2 William Ude	1353–4 William Ude	1376–7 Stephen Syward	1385–6 ?	1454–5 T. Cripps, Farmer; John Martyn, Reeve
Receipt	£ s. d.	£ s. d.	£ s. d.	£ s. d.	£ s. d.	£ s. d.	£ s. d.	£ s. d.	£ s. d.	£ s. d.
Arrears	3 1 6¼	6 8	1 0 0	8 0 0½	1 3 10¼	13 8¼	19 6	2 8 10	2 4	7 0
Rents of assize	5 16 10	5 16 10	5 16 10	5 16 10	5 16 10	5 16 10	5 16 10	5 16 10	5 16 10	5 16 10
Increment										
— Acquittances	6 6	4 0	5 9	5 0	5 0	5 0	5 0	5 0	5 0	5 0
— Defects	2 6	2 6	2 6	2 6	2 6	2 6	2 6	2 6	2 6	1 6 10¾
— *Defectus per pestilentiam*	—	—	18 0	1 9 2	1 4 6	15 1	9			
Net rent	5 7 10	5 10 4	4 10 7	4 0 2	4 4 10	4 14 3	5 8 7	5 9 4	5 9 4	4 4 11¼
Issues of the manor	1 7 1	1 8 ?	18 9½	10 8	7 2½	8 6	18 7½	1 8 9	1 5 10½	{1 4 4¾ / 2 10} 3 0 0*
Fines and marriages	4 0	4 0	5 15 8	1 14 0	12 0	9 0	11 0	1 14 0	1 4 0	4 0
Heriots										
Perquisites of the court	9 8	10 2	3 4	5 9	3 3	10 0	5 2	10	8 7	16 0
Sale of stock	4 11 5	2 12 8	1 5 0	1 5 4	?	1 16 8	4 7 6	7 4 10	3 7 10	1 10 10
,, corn	8 17 1	10 12 0¾	3 5 1	10 10 7	5 2 0	6 7 0	5 7 11½	16 4 9	16 15 11	
,, works	—	—	—	—	—	—	—	—	—	2 2 6
Total receipts	[25 18 7¼]	20 19 7¼	16 10 10¾	19 16 3¾	11 12 0½	14 13 0½	19 9 2	34 13 6	29 8 9	12 17 10
Expenses	13 15 2¾	10 11 9¼	4 13 9¼	11 14 1	9 18 4¼	12 11 4½	12 10 2	9 19 8¼	13 12 3¼	5 2 7
Balance paid	7 7 7	9 7 9½	3 17 1	6 18 4	9 0	1 2 7½	6 19 0	21 4 11¾	15 16 5¾	
,, due	6 8	1 0 0	8 0 0½	1 3 10¼	13 8½	19 0½	—	3 8 10	—	
Total Balance	7 14 3	10 7 9½	11 17 1½	8 2 2¼	1 2 8½	2 1 8	6 19 0	24 13 9¾	15 16 5¾	7 15 3

* Farm.

V. CHERITON.

Reeve	1346–7 John Damene	1347–8 John Damene	1348–9 Richard Basset, John Damene, William Damene	1349–50 Wm. Damene	1350–1 John de Edyntone	1351–2 William Damene	1354–5 William Damene	1376–7 William Damene	1385–6 ?	1454–5 Nicholas Aghneld, Farmer; Thomas Agneld, Reeve
Receipt	£ s. d.	£ s. d.	£ s. d.	£ s. d.	£ s. d.	£ s. d.	£ s. d.	£ s. d.	£ s. d.	£ s. d.
Arrears	4 10 8	None	3 8 3¼	21 13 6	9 14 8¼	12 4 7¾	22 6 5	None	None	14 14 6½
Rents of assize	33 18 8¾	33 18 8¾	33 18 8¾	33 18 8¾	33 18 8¾	33 18 10¾	33 18 10¾	33 19 0¾	33 19 0¾	33 19 0¾
Increment	—	—	—	—	2					
— Acquittances	1 6 6	1 8 6	1 2 0	19 0	17 6	1 0 0	1 0 0	1 9 0	1 11 0	5 0
— Defects	4 19 8	4 19 8	4 19 8	4 19 8	4 19 8	4 19 8	illegible	4 19 8	4 19 8	4 19 8
— *Defectus per pestilentiam*	—	—	5 4 8¼	5 19 10½	3 17 11	2 15 9	illegible	d. p. p. p. 2 6	—	1 6 0
				?	—	—	—	d. p. s. p. —	—	4 15 1
Net rent	27 12 6¾	27 10 6¾	22 12 4½	22 0 2¼	24 3 9¾	25 3 5¾	illegible	27 7 1¾	27 5 0	22 13 3¾
			*2 0					*4 15 4	4 15 4	*1 13 4
Issues of the manor	8 13 0¾	8 12 7	5 18 3½	7 0 11¼	8 5 10½	9 1 6¼	7 16 2½	9 8 1½	10 5 2	2 3 9½
								‡4 16 5½	‡4 14 5½	‡8 5 6
Fines and marriages	5 12 8	6 9 3	16 3 8	19 2 0	2 12 6	2 8 6	1 19 0	2 1 8	3 8 4	2 17 0
Heriots										
Perquisites of the court	2 15 5	2 10 2	1 5 9	2 6 0	3 2 7	1 11 1	2 11 10	1 13 8	3 17 8	1 9 8
Sale of stock	4 11 3	8 0 4	3 15 0	7 3 5	18 18 11	16 17 4	18 8 9	20 12 0	10 0 4	†9 0 0
,, corn	23 11 10½	29 10 7	10 8 3¾	7 17 0	11 17 8	26 18 5½	29 8 8	53 3 6¼	57 12 7	3 14 4
,, works	—	—	—	—	—	—	—	—	—	8 6 6
Total receipts	74 11 6	84 10 2¾	62 7 11¾	84 14 6¾	71 4 11	84 5 7½	88 12 5¼	124 12 7	132 3 8¼	75 5 5
Expenses	19 16 10½	14 0 3½	13 10 0¼	35 0 0½	18 13 1¼	17 6 1¾	36 15 7	18 13 11	22 14 11¾	20 14 5½
Balance paid	54 14 7½	67 1 8	27 4 5½	39 19 10	40 7 2¾	57 16 8¼	46 15 10½	84 15 8	109 8 8½	
,, due	—	3 8 3¼	21 13 6	9 14 8¼	12 4 7¾	9 2 9½	5 0 11¾			

d. p. p. p. — *Defectus per primam pestilentiam.*

Reeve	Thomas Hockeley	John atte Gate	Thomas Hockeley and John atte Gate	Thomas Hockeley	Thomas de Hockeley	?	John Colegrym	John Yatelyng	?	Robert Colegrym, Farmer; John Syward, Reeve
Receipt	£ s. d.	£ s. d.	£ s. d.	£ s. d.	£ s. d.	£ s. d.	£ s. d.	£ s. d.	£ s. d.	£ s. d.
Arrears	1 16 8	None	7 16 4	31 7 4	25 1 11½	11 2 6¾	42 8 2½	9 16 2½	18 9 9¼	63 19 5¼
Rents of assize	51 13 6½	51 13 8	51 13 8	51 13 8½	51 13 8½	51 13 8½	51 13 8½	52 0 2½	52 0 2½	52 0 2½
Increment	[1½]									
— Acquittances	1 0 6	1 3 0	1 8 0	19 0	1 8 0	1 5 0	1 8 0	1 8 0	1 7 0	5 0
— Defects	18 9	18 9	18 9	18 11	18 11	18 11	18 11	4 14 9	4 14 11	4 14 11
— *Defectus per pestilentiam*	—	—	4 10 3½	2 5 6	1 12 0	1 11 2	3 0	D. p. p. p. —	1 2	12 0
								D. p. s. p. 9 6	9 6	3 18 1
Net rents	49 14 1½	49 11 9½	44 16 6	47 10 3½	47 14 9½	47 18 7½	49 3 9½	45 7 9½	45 6 7½	42 10 2½
Issues of the manor	14 5 4½	19 6 3¾	9 7 7½	8 13 3¾	c. 8 1 2	16 7 2	41 5 3	{ 22 3 0½	{ 24 16 9½	{ 2 5 3½
									† 5 12 6	
			*1 7 0	—	*2 15 0	—	—	†3 7 6	† 32 19 4	‡20 7 7½
										3 15 0
Fines and marriages	8 9 6	10 7 (?)	30 7 8	17 16 8	5 10 0	10 12 9	5 2 10	6 6 0	5 5 8	4 4 0
Perquisites of the court	4 8 9	4 17 5	4 16 7	2 5 10	c. 3 5 8	3 15 9	3 7 7	10 11 8	8 9 9	1 17 5
Heriots							§75 14 8			
Sale of stock	5 15 8	11 15 5	7 6 4	8 15 0	4 3 0	9 16 10	29 15 6	24 14 4	12 4 4	5 4 10
,, corn	21 10 1	16 6 1½	15 6 2½	14 11 4¾	13 12 7	20 1 1	12 11 0	19 9 6	None ?	
,, works	—	—	—	—	—	—	—	—	—	15 6 1
Total receipts	105 4 6	114 13 10	114 9 0¼	103 13 2	88 19 11¼	114 5 0½	272 8 9	143 19 5	160 18 6	161 9 5
Expenses	45 1 7¼	30 18 10½	26 18 4¼	33 17 1½	37 19 9½	50 1 9¼	164 8 8	38 8 2¼	46 5 8¾	18 11 7½
Balance paid	60 2 10¾	75 18 8	56 3 4	44 14 1	39 17 7	44 3 10½	39 0 10	69 15 11¼	90 3 11	
,, due	—	7 16 4	31 7 4	25 1 11½	11 10 6¾	19 19 4½	68 19 3	35 15 3½	24 8 10¼	

* Reliefs. † Lands in lord's hand. ‡ Farms, &c. § Forensic receipts.

D. p. p. p. = *Defectus per primam pestilentiam.* D. p. s. p. = *Defectus per secundam pestilentiam.*

VII. CRAWLEY.

	1346–7	1347–8	1348–9	1349–50	1350–1	1351–2	1353–4	1376–7	1385–6	1454–5
Reeve	John atte Hall	?	John atte Hall	John atte Hall	John atte Halle	John atte Hall	John atte Hall	John Trig	Thomas Cuppere	William Sely, Farmer; Thomas Davy, Rent Collector
Receipt	£ s. d.	£ s. d.	£ s. d.	£ s. d.	£ s. d.	£ s. d.	£ s. d.	£ s. d.	£ s. d.	£ s. d.
Arrears	None	None	1 10 0½	4 2 0¾	1 17 8	16 11 0¼	12 3 7¼	10 0	4 6 8	2 0 9
Rents of assize	15 0 11	15 0 6?	15 0 11	15 0 11	15 0 11	15 0 11	15 0 11	15 0 11	15 0 11	15 2 7
Increment										
— Acquittances	2 5 0	2 5 0	1 2 8	1 1 0	15 8	15 8	15 8	1 3 8	1 3 8	1 10 4
— Defects	1 0 4	1 0 4	1 0 4	1 0 4	1 0 4	1 0 4	1 0 4	1 0 4	1 0 4	1 5 8
— *Defectus per pestilentiam*	—	—	—	6 0	9 6	1 4 0	6 0	None	1 1 0	1 2 0
Net rent	11 15 7	11 15 2	12 17 11	12 13 7	12 15 5	12 0 3	12 18 11	12 16 11	11 15 11	11 4 7 4 0
Issues of the manor	9 3 10¾	9 15 8	5 18 0½	10 2 1¾	10 3 1¼	10 6 1	12 13 5	{ 9 12 7¼ { 14 11	11 10 1 9 4	10 15 9 } 1 8 8 } *
Fines and marriages	13 4	16 0	11 14 8	4 1 4	c. 3 10 0	2 6 8	2 12 0	13 4	15 4	1 6 8
Heriots										
Perquisites of the Court	18 8	13 11	8 8	10 9	16 8	18 4	1 13 8	19 1	1 5 8	9 4
Sale of stock	4 0 4	9 2 6	8 16 8	12 2 4	16 9 4	21 6 8	12 4 2	14 1 4	18 2 4	2 8 0
„ corn	32 18 10¾	37 11 5	14 0 8½	27 6 9¾	31 14 8	49 0 4¼	26 19 0½	21 12 0	31 8 6	
„ works	—	—	—	—	—	—	—	1 6 10½	1 5 0	2 6 0
Total receipts	59 19 5	69 19 10	55 0 2¼	68 7 3¾	76 13 5	97 3 7¼	69 8 10½	63 0 5¾	81 1 2	34 9 9
Expenses	22 13 2	15 14 1½	19 2 9½	21 3 5½	28 12 9½	17 18 5¾	22 3 5¾	18 9 0¾	20 8 7¾	10 4 11½
Balance paid	37 6 3	52 14 8	31 15 4	45 6 2½	31 9 7¼	51 11 8	40 15 5¾	41 16 6	60 3 10¼	

	1347–8	1348–9	1349–50	1350–1	1351–2	1354–5	1376–7	1385–6	1454–5
Reeve	?	William atte Thorne	William atte Thorne	William atte Thorne	?	William Herfu ?	William Crowde	?	Andrew Park, Reeve and Farmer, Thomas Coote, Rent-Collector
Receipt	£ s. d.	£ s. d.	£ s. d.	£ s. d.	£ s. d.	£ s. d	£ s. d.	£ s. d.	£ s. d.
Arrears	None	None	2 10 4½	11 14 0½	13 4 4¼	85 12 7	10 10 5	10 0 9½	22 0 0½
Rents of assize . . .	27 19 9¼	27 19 9¼	27 19 9½	27 19 9½	27 19 9½	27 19 9½	27 19 11½	28 0 0	28 0 5½
Increment									
— Acquittances . .	8 0	(?) 8 0	13 0	13 0	13 0	16 0	16 0	18 0	16 0
— Defects	3 12 0	3 12 0	3 12 0	3 12 0	3 12 0	3 12 0	4 7 8	4 7 8	4 7 8
— *Defectus per pestilentiam*	—	2 10 7	2 14 6	3 10 4½	1 7 10	10 10	—	—	1 0 0
Net rents	23 19 9¼	21 9 2½	[21 0 3½]	20 4 5	22 6 11½	23 0 11½	22 16 3½	22 14 7½	21 16 9
									1 0
Issues of the manor .	11 15 9½	{ 6 7 8	7 13 10	7 16 4½	8 3 5½	10 18 11½	{ 15 4 6	21 9 11½	{ 13 6 5
		{ 2 0 10	?	?			{ 12 0		{ 1 10 0
Fines and marriages .	2 16 8	10 10 0	6 19 8	8 4 10	17 4	2 6 4	1 1 8	1 19 4	15 4
							10 0*		
Perquisites of the court	1 13 1	8 1	1 5 2	10 6	16 0	1 4 10	18 2	3 0 6	1 0 0
						† 15 14 7¾	7 ‡		
Heriots									
Sale of stock . . .	1 1 10	{	6 17 6	15 13 8	4 5 7	7 9 0	7 18 8	9 14 0	10 0
,, corn	5 9 8	{ 10 17 2¾	12 18 0	3 6 4	4 16 1½	10 13 2	c. 16 0 0	13 1 3	—
,, works . . .	(?)	1 6 2	2 0 10	2 0 8	2 2 8	2 2 8	4 6 3	2 13 7¼	12 9 8
Total receipts . . .	47 2 5	54 6 5	71 7 11½	(?) 62 11 7½	48 6 11½	186 9 1¾	c. 60 0 7½	87 13 5¾	73 9 3
				[69 10 10¼]					
Expenses	32 14 8¼	17 1 7¼	22 5 0¾	28 0 3½	16 14 2½	§ 159 7 11¼	17 8 9¾	31 10 11½	15 13 11½
Balance paid . . .	8 18 4¾	34 13 4	37 8 2	18 0 9	16 2 0¼	19 2 6	47 11 4¾	?	
,, due . . .	—	2 10 4½	11 14 0¾	16 10 7¼	15 10 8¾	7 18 8½	12 0 5	6 7 1½	

* Relief. † Forensic receipts. ‡ Annual recognition. § Includes about £145 for building.

IX. TWYFORD.

	1346–7 *	1347–8	1348–9	1349–50	1350–1	1351–2	1353–4	1376–7	1385–6	1454–5
Reeve . . .		Richard Coke	William Herfu	Jordan de Custon	Jordan de Custon	?	Adam Wyke	Robert Powrte	?	John Dyper, Farmer, Walter Horsham, Rent Collector.
Receipt	£ s. d.	£ s. d.	£ s. d.	£ s. d.	£ s. d.	£ s. d.	£ s. d.	£ s. d.	£ s. d.	£ s. d.
Arrears . . .	9 6 7½	6 1 0	1 6 10¾	9 15 2	10 12 4	8 18 10¼	25 9 5½	38 17 10	109 15 1½	35 9 8
Rents of assize	54 7 8½	26 7 11	26 7 11	26 7 11	26 7 11	26 7 11	26 7 11	26 10 3	illegible	27 5 5
Increment . .										
— Acquittances	2 0 6	2 4 6	1 13 3	1 9 0 (?)	1 13 6	1 14 3	1 19 3	1 2 0	17 0	1 7 0
— Defects . .	3 17 0	5 0	5 0	5 0	5 0	5 0	5 0	5 0	?	5 0
— *Defectus per pestilentiam*	—	—	6 16 7½	5 17 3	4 17 7	3 12 0	2 8 9	1 10 6	2 2 5	7 18 6
Net rents . .	48 10 2½	23 18 5	17 13 0½	18 16 8	19 11 7	20 16 3	21 4 11	23 12 9	illegible	17 14 11
Issues of the	19 5 4	11 1 2	4 5 8¼	9 0 1½	7 12 8¾	10 4 8	12 0 5	{ 17 0 6½	{ 14 12 9	12 5 5
manor								1 2 0	1 10 8	6 8 0
Fines and marriages	10 19 4	4 10 8	15 0 10	15 7 6	7 1 10	1 14 8	5 0 8	3 6 2	1 10 4	3 13 8
Perquisites of	4 6 6	2 4 8	17 4	1 13 1	1 2 1	1 3 3	1 0 6	1 14 0	3 3 1	1 0 6
the court .							7 4 8 ‡	3 13 6 ‡		
Heriots . .	—	—	—	—	—	§ 4 1 11¾	§ 4 9 7¾	§ 3 6 8½	§ 5 7 2¾	§ 7 1 6¾
Sale of stock .	31 19 7	26 6 0	10 4 6	25 12 5½	18 2 6	13 14 4	30 11 8	42 14 8	44 16 4	16 3 4
,, corn .	25 7 2	18 3 4	damaged	17 18 5½	12 18 4	17 10 8	33 8 11½	22 16 7½	24 15 11	
,, works .	13 13 9	9 18 8	4 19 4	3 11 11 ‖	2 18 6	2 19 6	3 7 6	3 5 2	2 1 8	11 1 10
Total receipts .	161 10 4¾	109 6 10	62 13 4¼	99 2 8¾	74 8 0½	77 13 5¾	120 9 2½	161 12 9¾	243 12 6¼	114 12 0¾
Expenses . .	72 6 5¾	52 13 5½	23 9 1¾	39 1 0¾	54 18 11¼	24 8 5¼	40 14 5	35 8 9¾	42 3 0	17 15 2¾
Balance paid .	83 2 9	54 16 6	29 9 0½	49 9 4	9 15 3	37 4 2¾	65 8 3	62 3 10	72 16 2	
,, due .	6 1 0	1 16 10¾	9 15 2	10 12 4	9 13 10¼	16 0 9¾	7 1 10½	64 0 2	128 13 4¼	

* This entry probably includes Marwell. ‡ Forensic receipts. § Mill.

‖ Eighteen tenements were left in the lord's hands. Labourers were hired for the harvest in default of customers.

Minister	1284–5	1340–7 Richd. Hardyng	1347–8 John Hardyng	1348–9 Ade atte More	1349–50 Ditto	1350–1 Ditto	1351–2 ?	1353–4 Ade More	1376–7 ?
	£ s. d.	£ s. d.	£ s. d.	£ s. d.	£ s. d.	£ s. d.	£ s. d.	£ s. d.	£ s. d.
Arrears	?	24 9 7¾	17 1 7½	26 2 10½	153 15 9	118 9 2	91 10 4¼	49 3 6	14 10 4
Rents of Assize	62 15 7½	73 17 6¾	73 17 10¾	73 17 10¾	73 17 10¾	73 17 10¾	73 17 10¾	73 17 10¾	75 1 3¾
Increment	—	4							
— Acquittances	1 1 0	1 0 0	1 1 0	1 1 0	1 1 0	1 1 0	1 1 0	1 1 0	1 1 0
— Defects	3 2 5	3 18 3	3 18 3	3 18 3	3 18 3	3 18 3	3 18 3	3 18 3	4 14 0
— *Defectus per pestilentiam*	—	—	—	3 15 10½	3 9 11½	1 14 1½	3 14 8	1 3 10	No entry.
Leases	—	3 0 4	3 2 4	1 10 8	2 2 4	2 2 4	2 2 4	2 2 4	19 1 10
Custom	{ 1 lb. cummin { 6 lbs. wax	6 3 2½	5 17 4	*c.* 4 0 3	5 2 3½	5 2 3½	5 11 0	5 8 6½	5 13 9½
Annual recognition	—	11 1½	10 6½	7 7	6 11	4 8	4 5	4 0	6 7
Issues of the manor	23 5 2½	3 3 6	12 18 6	2 8 0	6 1 5	4 15 9	5 0 1	6 6 4	6 9 0
Sale of pasture	—	16 4 6	12 14 2	3 7 8	5 15 10	5 3 4	6 0 11	6 17 6	6 17 2
,, corn	—	56 4 6½	55 11 2½	4 10 5	55 7 1¼	61 10 5	35 15 9	36 18 4½	43 4 6½
,, stock	—	8 8 9	1 5 8	5 8 7	8 5 0	3 0 8	12 6 4	2 9 8	4 17 0
,, works	[4 2 0]	16 16 4¾	18 13 7¼	*c.* 18 5 4½	17 10 8	17 12 7½	18 5 0¼	18 2 2¾	21 18 3½
Fines and marriages	13 7 0	54 19 4	34 11 3	191 2 2½ 1 11 6*	105 17 7	35 14 1	11 14 6	13 13 8	26 13 4
Perquisites of the court	?	9 9 1	7 9 10	4 8 6	6 3 10	8 8 3	5 8 0	29 19 11	8 2 1
Heriots in pence	—	5 0	4 0	2 9 6	16 0	9 6	7 0	2 0	
Miscellaneous	—	1 3 5½	10 6	1 12 4½	2 5 7	7 5 10	2 15 0½	1 4 7½	3 3
Total receipts	103 11 10	269 17 6¼	239 9 2½	333 16 5½	434 19 0	337 3 6	[torn]	240 7 6	227 5 7¾
Expenses	5 3 2	21 6 2¾	32 6 4	13 14 11	15 3 5¼	39 17 7¼	25 19 9¼	12 11 0	13 6 4½
Balance paid	98 8 8	231 9 8	181 0 0	166 5 9½	298 3 0	205 15 6½	140 6 0	189 14 5	199 16 8
Owing	—	17 1 7½	26 2 10½	153 15 9	121 12 6¾	91 10 4¼	97 19 0	38 2 1	12 7 4

* Relief.

II. POUNDISFORD.

Minister	1284–5 ?	1346–7 Richd. Hardyng and Th. Cavisgrave	1347–8 Th. Camisgrave	1348–9 Th. de Camisgrave and Walter de Robert (?)	1349–50 Walter Coulyng	1350–1 Stephen Godard	1351–2 Stephen Godard	1376–7
	£ s. d.	£ s. d.	£ s. d.	£ s. d.	£ s. d.	£ s. d.	£ s. d.	£ s. d.
Arrears	?	1 8 0½	4 16 5¼	6 0 1¾	42 9 1	69 10 5¼	45 13 8	3 0 0
Assized rents	38 8 0¼	42 4 3¾	42 4 9¾	42 5 11¾	42 5 11¾	42 5 11¾	42 5 11¾	42 10 6¼
Increment	—	6	1 2					
— Acquittances	1 7 9¼	1 6 8¼	1 6 8¼	1 6 8¼	1 6 8¼	1 6 8¼	1 6 8¼	1 6 8¼
— Defects	19 3½	1 5 3½	1 5 3¼	1 5 3¼	1 5 3½	1 5 3½	1 5 3½	Torn
— Defects *per pestilentiam*	—	—	—	1 9 4¾	1 13 1	1 0 10¾	16 6¾	None
Leases	—	1 6	1 6	2 0	2 0	2 0	2 0	2 0
Custom	—	5 12 9	5 10 0½	c. 5 6 2½	5 0 4	5 4 6½	5 3 0½	5 13 6
Annual recognition	4½ lbs. wax 1 ploughshare	7 6	7 0	4 9	2 9	1 9	1 6	None
Issues of the manor	18 18 2	2 15 0	7 4 7	3 8 0	7 9 0	6 18 0½	7 13 3	12 5 9
Sale of pasture	—	4 9 7	4 16 9	1 4 5	10 2	3 3	5 6	13 0 (5 6)
,, corn	45 13 8¼	25 0 11¼	23 0 5	6 3 1	7 12 0	13 11 1	12 14 7	15 15 5¾
,, stock	—	1 1 4	9 0 3	5 14 5	14 19 2	7 9 1	8 6 8	13 19 6
,, works	(Included in issues)	15 12 4¼	17 3 10½	17 2 9	15 16 10	14 18 3	15 18 10½	19 4 10¼
Fines and marriages	22 1 6	11 6 4	29 19 4	67 16 0 18 4*	85 9 0	12 4 10	16 17 0	29 12 4
Perquisites of the court	29 13 10	6 12 1	6 12 7	2 19 11	5 2 7	6 10 6	4 0 5	5 7 11
Heriots in pence		6 0	5 6	2 12 0	19 6	6 6	5 6	4 0
Miscellaneous	†12 4	11 1	—	1 5 7½	5 14 10	1 3 10	4 6 8½	1 17 1
Total receipts	130 18 0¾	114 7 4	148 12 3¼	159 2 3	235 5 4¾	183 17 9½	159 16 1¾	147 17 8½
Expenses	12 18 0¾	18 3 3¾	27 2 1½	13 4 4	14 4 11	24 13 0	20 5 2½	23 5 1½
[illegible]	118 0 0¼	91 17 7	115 10 0	103 8 10	151 5 0½	114 3 0	93 6 2	118 6 8

	1284–5	1346–7	1347–8	1348–9	1349–50	1350–1	1351–2	1353–4	1376–7
Minister	—	Roger Pegge	Roger Pegge	Nicholas Kempe	John Crugge	John le Rouk	John le Rouk	John Rouk	Wm. Shaldon
	£ s. d.	£ s. d.	£ s. d.	£ s. d.	£ s. d.	£ s. d.	£ s. d.	£ s. d.	£ s. d.
Arrears	—	9 16 7½	21 7 6½	4 11 4	29 2 4¾	51 18 3¼	37 16 3	20 19 7¼	11 16 8
Assized rents . . .	20 14 10½	26 16 5½	26 16 5½	26 16 5½	26 16 5½	26 16 5½	26 16 5½	26 16 11½	26 17 6½
Increment	—	—	—	—	—	—	6		
— Acquittances . .	9 6	8 3	8 3	8 3	8 3	8 3	8 3	8 3	8 3
— Defects	—	8 0	8 0	8 0	8 0	8 0	8 0	8 0	8 0
Defects *per pestilentiam*	—	—	—	1 7 10¼	1 6 11	12 6	None	8 7	None
Leases	—	12 6	12 6	2 6	2 6	2 6	2 6	2 6	10 6
Custom	—	3 4 9	3 3 10½	3 0 0½	2 14 1½	2 18 3½	2 17 4½	3 9 0	3 5 5½
Annual recognition .	6½ lbs. of wax	3 6½	3 6½	2 9	1 6	1 3	1 0	9	2 0
Issues of the manor .	11 19 5½	2 5 7	2 17 8	3 0	2 4 2	1 3 9	5 9	3 18 0½	3 2 8
Sale of pasture . . .	—	5 5 7	4 11 0	3 6 11	2 3 3	1 13 3	2 9 5	1 14 7	4 11 3
„ corn	—	43 18 11¾	41 4 11	12 10 3	33 2 7	34 5 10½	19 17 7¼	31 10 11¾	37 1 11¼
„ stock . . .	—	4 10 6	13 4	7 10 0	3 0 8	4 7 0	4 14 0	1 15 0	4 15 4
„ works . . .	—	11 9 8½	13 1 3¼	13 0 5¼	c. 10 18 0	11 16 9¼	11 14 5¼	11 13 4¾	14 6 7¾
Fines and marriages .	7 6 8	14 16 6	13 2 8	44 13 10	61 1 2	17 12 2	10 4 4	9 13 8	6 8 8
Perquisites of the court	10 18 10	4 10 1	4 6 6	1 9 6	2 15 8	4 9 10	2 17 8	4 12 6	3 16 0
Heriots in pence . .	—	2 0	5 0	1 14 6	8 0	5 0	3 6 ?	2 6	1 6
Miscellaneous . . .	—	1 11 2	—	1 4 0¾	1 11 11½	5 6 7½	5 14 1½	4 17 0	1 0 1½
Total receipts . . .	43 11 2	128 7 8¾	131 10 0¼	148 1 5¼	174 4 10¾	161 8 3½	124 6 8	120 2 4¼	117 0 0½
Expenses	13 14 6	15 11 6½	22 4 8¼	7 16 3½	10 16 2½	26 11 4¼	Illegible	24 8 5	11 15 3½
Paid over	29 16 8	91 8 8	74 14 0	111 2 9½	111 3 4	97 9 0	71 18 8	67 15 4	94 18 1
Owing	—	21 7 6½	34 11 4	29 2 4¾	52 5 4¼ 7 1 remitted	37 16 3	Illegible	27 18 7	10 6 8

IV. NAILESBOURNE.

	1284–5	1346–7	1347–8	1348–9	1349–50	1350–1	1351–2	1352–3	1376–7
Minister	—	John Cade	John Waterman	Roger de Torre	Roger de Torre	Roger atte Torre, John Waterman		John Waterman	Adam atte Mersch
	£ s. d.	£ s. d.	£ s. d.	£ s. d.	£ s. d.	£ s. d.	£ s. d.	£ s. d.	£ s. d.
Arrears	—	12 16 7	26 9 5¾	2 17 10¼	18 0 0¾	26 10 8¼	—	2 9 7½	None
Assized rents	21 2 6½	26 19 2¼	26 19 5¼	26 19 5¼	26 19 5¼	26 19 5¼	—	26 19 5¼	27 11 6¼
Increment	—	3							
— Acquittances	1 12 0	1 1 0	1 1 0	1 1 0	1 1 0	1 1 0	—	1 1 0	1 1 0
— Defects	7 1½	7 1½	7 1½	7 1½	7 1½	7 1½	—	7 1½	7 1½
— Defects *per pestilentiam*	—	—	—	c. 4 14 9½	3 12 8¾	13 0¼	1 10 3¾	1 1 11¾	None
Leases	—	1 11 4	1 11 4	1 11 4	1 9 8	1 11 4	1 11 4	1 11 4	1 1 4
Custom	—	3 4 6½	3 1 8	2 19 0	2 19 11½	2 18 4	—	2 17 4½	3 8 9½
Annual recognition	2 plough shares 6½ lbs. wax	1 3	9	9	3	4	—	8	3 4
Issues of the manor	9 4 1	2 1 0	2 3 6½	2 10 8½	4 4 4	4 0 9	—	4 18 0	7 9 4
Sale of pasture	—	5 11 0	5 2 9	14 1	c. 1 0 8	1 11 0	—	19 8	3 0
„ corn	28 11 0½	36 0 7¼	21 16 5½	10 4 11	9 5 0	12 7 6	—	9 18 8½	14 4 2½
„ stock	—	1 13 3	1 6 0	1 16 0	3 10 8	6 13 0	—	4 6 6	5 0 0
„ works	[1 18 0]	9 12 11¾	9 12 6¾	9 12 8¼	4 3 9½	6 0 7¾	—	5 14 5¼	9 16 5½
Fines and marriages	3 18 10	7 9 8	4 2 8	16 18 8	10 3 8	14 10 6	—	2 16 8	2 6 4
Perquisites of the court	6 1 10	3 7 0	2 16 2	1 18 7	2 17 8	4 9 11	—	23 0 1	2 13 7
Heriots in pence	—	1 0	4 6	1 5 6	2 6	8 0	—	1 0	1 0
Miscellaneous	—	6 8½	3 5¼	17 9¾	1 1 5	—	—	3 0 3½	18 6
Total receipts	63 0 4½	109 8 2¾	104 2 8	74 4 5	80 14 8	106 0 3½	—	86 3 8¼	74 9 3¼
Expenses	12 7 2½	13 6 10½	8 19 9¾	7 18 7¾	4 18 1¾	17 7 0½	—	10 6 6¾	11 1 5½
Paid over	50 13 2	69 11 10½	92 5 0	48 5 8½	49 5 10	67 11 0	—	54 10 8	59 17 9¾
Owing	[illegible]	[illegible]	[illegible]	[illegible]	[illegible]	[illegible]	—	[illegible]	[illegible]

V. STAPELGROVE.

	1284–	1346–7	1347–8	1348–9	1349–50	1350–1	1351–2	1353–4	1376–7
Minister	—	Rob. Pogenham	Wm. Dawe	Nich. Essisbury	Nich. de Egebury	Nich. de Eggisbury	Ditto	Nich. de Eggisbury	Wm. Dawe
	£ s. d.	£ s. d.	£ s. d.	£ s. d.	£ s. d.	£ s. d.	£ s. d.	£ s. d.	£ s. d.
Arrears	—	2 3	9 0 11½	19 15 8¾	82 14 7½	97 1 4¾	51 19 0	37 10 9¾	10 0 0
Assized rents . . .	30 0 6½	44 5 0½	44 5 0½	44 5 0½	44 5 0½	44 5 0½	44 5 0½	44 5 0½	44 6 11
Increment	1 1								
— Acquittances . .	16 0	16 0	16 0	16 0	16 0	16 0	16 0	16 0	Illegible
— Defects	2 0	6 6	6 6	6 6	6 6	6 6	6 6	6 6	6 6
— Defects *per pestilentiam*	—	—	—	1 2 11¾	1 5 0½	13 11	12 4	7 6	None
Leases									
Custom	—	4 12 5	4 6 2½	4 2 4½	3 14 7½	3 10 11	3 16 0	4 3 1	Illegible
Annual recognition .	8½ lbs. wax	7 10	5 6	5 3	5 3	1 1	Illeg.	1	
Issues of the manor .	8 10 4	2 4 8	1 8 9	10 0	17 2	17 3½	19 6	2 13 2	?
Sale of pasture . . .	—	2 13 3	2 4 9	1 5 6	1 2 0	19 0	1 2 8	1 3 2	?
,, corn . . .	—	33 7 0	24 8 8¼	7 2 4¾	18 0 0½	18 8 0¼	32 19 2¾	20 17 0½	18 4 11½
,, stock . . .	—	4 2 6	1 0 0	5 18 7	4 17 10	4 13 10	6 9 0	4 10 10	3 13 0
,, works . . .	[1 5 9]	11 9 5¾	11 17 9¾	12 1 1¾	11 13 6	11 8 3	11 15 8	11 1 7½	11 11 11
Fines and marriages .	11 7 0	16 15 0	21 14 4	109 9 6	81 1 2	21 5 2	11 1 10	26 7 8	2 0 4
Perquisites of the court	17 9 8	5 5 7	4 0 11	2 8 11	2 18 3	4 4 0	2 19 6	5 17 1	6 5 4
Heriots in pence . .	—	4 6	2 0	1 18 0	6 0	9 6	6 6	4 0	1 0
Miscellaneous . . .	—	1 14 2½	8 2	1 6 9½	2 1 6½	5 2 2	3 4½	15 9	1 3 6
Total receipts . . .	55 4 5½	126 1 2¾	124 0 7½	208 3 9	250 19 5¾	210 9 3	156 2 6¾	157 9 4¼	104 4 9
Expenses	4 12 2	12 5 2¼	24 16 7½	8 0 5½	9 2 0	23 16 11	17 1 10	16 13 2¼	9 3 10½
Paid over	50 12 3½	104 15 1	79 8 3	117 8 7	144 16 1	134 0 0	94 6 8	106 18 0	95 0 10½
Owing	—	9 0 11½	19 15 8¾	84 14 7½	97 1 4¾	52 14 4	54 14 0¾	33 18 2	Quit

VI. RYMPTON.

Minister	1284–5	1346–7 Robt. atte Wood	1347–8 Robert atte Wood	1348–9 Ditto	1349–50 Ditto	1350–1 Ditto	1376–7 John Boye
	£ s. d.	£ s. d.	£ s. d.	£ s. d.	£ s. d.	£ s. d.	£ s. d.
Arrears	—	1 10 11¾	15 8¾	2 2 6	6 4 3	18 13 2	None
Assized rents	4 18 0	5 3 0	5 3 0	5 3 0	5 3 0	5 3 0	5 3 0
Increment							
— Acquittances	2 11 0	2 11 0	2 11 0	2 11 0	2 11 0	2 11 0	2 10 0
— Defects	1 0	1 0	1 0	1 0	1 0	1 0	1 0
— Defects *per pestilentiam*	—	—	—	None	None	None	None
Leases	—	2 8? 0	2 18 0	2 11 10	*4 5 0	*3 18 11¼	2 19 0
Custom	—	15 3	15 6	14 11½	13 11	14 0	14 10½
Annual recognition	—	4 4	4 2	2 4	2 4	1 10	1 9
Issues of the manor	7 17 9	5 16 9	5 11 8	3 3 1	4 11 3	7 7 8	4 18 4
Sale of pasture	(1 6 1*)	4 1 3	3 15 1	3 4 9	2 19 8	3 3 7	5 0 1
,, corn	23 19 1½	30 17 2	45 11 2	3 12 4½	51 2 1½	40 10 2¾	27 8 0¾
,, stock	—	4 14 8	9 15 0	3 13 2	17 2 11	5 11 10	11 0 2
,, works	(No fines entry)	4 16 5½	4 4 2½	5 2 0¾	3 18 4	4 4 8	4 13 6½
Fines and marriages	5 6 6	8 0 0	11 12 8	14 9 4	7 10 0	11 0	3 0
Requisites of the court	—	1 1 0	1 11 10	18 5	1 8 5	17 1	1 13 11
Heriots in pence	—	—	1 6	4 0	None		
Miscellaneous	—	2 0	—	16 0¾	1 6 10½	1 11 6	
Total receipts	40 15 5½	65 17 10½	88 11 9½	41 3 4½	98 1 10	70 3 4	61 4 8¾
Expenses	17 16 0½	17 5 1¾	19 1 7¼	10 8 9½	25 14 1	12 19 11½	5 11 7¼
Paid over	22 19 5	47 17 0	67 7 8¼	24 10 4	53 14 7	41 18 6	54 5 1½
Owing	—	15 8¾	2 2 6	6 4 3	18 13 2	15 4 10½	1 8 0

* Mill.

Minister	1264–5 —	1346–7 Ralph Jones, Geoffrey Hakebond	1347–8 Ralph Jones, Geoffrey Hakebond	1348–9 William Denge	1349–50 William Denge	1350–1 William Denge	1354–5	1376–7
	£ s. d.	£ s. d.	£ s. d.	£ s. d.	£ s. d.	£ s. d.	£ s. d.	£ s. d.
Arrears	—	46 3 11¼	41 16 2¼	75 10 10	71 9 11¼	57 14 0	—	74 5 10½
Assized rents	55 19 0	70 5 7½	70 5 7½	70 5 7½	70 5 7½	70 5 7	—	70 14 6½
Increment	5 5							
— Acquittances	3 11 8	2 3 8	2 0 8	1 4 3	1 7 0	1 5 8	—	1 14 0
— Defects	2 5 1	2 16 7	2 16 7	2 16 7	2 16 7	2 16 1	—	2 15 0
— Defects *per pestilentiam*	—	—	—	6 6 9	10 19 4	2 2 3	1 0 0	1 6 0
Leases	—	3 0 0	3 0 0	3 0 0	3 0 0	3 0 0	—	5 14 6
Custom	1 lb. cummin and 1 lb. chalk?	6	6	6	6	6	—	6
Annual recognition	5 7	14 1	14 7	9 1	c. 8 4	8 4	—	3 9
Issues of the manor	54 2 2½	33 17 4	34 10 6	15 7 8¼	14 10 4½ ¶4 19 0	21 10 8 ¶14 8 6	— ¶10 16 7	29 15 3¾ ¶11 8 4
Sale of pasture	—	7 11 0	7 1 9	3 3 8	5 13 7	6 4 3	—	7 8 1
,, corn	37 12 6	40 4 5	35 15 5¼	10 8 8¼	41 11 7¾	48 12 2	—	24 15 7½
,, stock	*3 9 2	† 45 19 0	† 48 1 0	† 18 2 9¾	† 24 3 9	† 27 14 1	—	† 15 19 0½
	1 19 1	13 1 9	10 11 1	24 5 0	13 16 0	30 16 8	—	21 17 6
,, works	—	—	None	None	—	None	—	5 15 8
Fines and marriages	5 4 10	7 15 0	18 6 4	72 11 4	45 6 6	13 3 4	15 0 0	5 0 8
Perquisites of the court	13 11 9	10 16 6	9 13 6	5 0 8	9 10 7	9 3 5	—	14 6 7
Heriots in pence	[6 5 2]	19 0‡	—	5 0 §	—	1 10 4‡	—	1 14 7
		18 4‖	—	—	—	—	—	—
Miscellaneous	7 1	2 6 6	3 7	3 7 3½	2 17 5½	—		
Total receipts	177 13 3	230 9 4½	235 9 7¼	215 4 9½	220 14 11¼	232 10 2	—	283 4 7¾
Expenses	38 3 9½	46 5 1¼	45 14 8¼	c. 41 15 0	53 4 10¾	46 15 2¼	—	21 18 5
Paid over	139 9 5¼	142 8 1	114 9 0¾	illegible	109 16 0½	100 12 8½	—	148 3 0¾
Owing	—	41 16 2	75 5 10¼	c. 62 0 0	57 14 0	85 2 3¾	—	113 3 2

* Mill, Fishpond. † Mill. ‡ Green wax. § Relief. ‖ Felon's chattels.
¶ Lands in the lord's hand.

C. NET BALANCE OF MANORS NOT EXAMINED IN DETAIL.

Manor.	1347–8	1348–9	1349–50	1351–2
Taunton	768 0 4	681 9 6½	904 7 0	574 0 4¾
Borough of Taunton	c. 45 6 9½	39 15 11	42 16 2½	57 15 11
Otterford	—	11 8 2¼	13 12 2¼	21 10 11
Borough of Downton	9 3 11	7 16 8	8 0 10	10 18 7
Knoyle *	59 6 4¾	29 13 5½	32 3 11½	34 18 11½
Hynedon	8 6 7½	8 4 2½	8 1 8½	8 11 7
Bishopston * . . .	50 8 8½	43 2 10½	†69 11 10¼	78 0 6½
Fonthill *	24 2 11	11 5 8¾	24 8 7¼	28 16 2½
Upton *	9 18 4	1 18 6¼	3 1 4½	12 3 8
Meon (Manor *) . .	206 5 3¾	278 5 5¾	207 3 7	237 10 0¼
Meon (Church *) . .	88 18 3	?50 12 9	89 0 3½	103 16 1¾
Hambledon * . . .	88 18 1	96 4 4	59 8 10½	95 5 3
Hambledon (Church) .	80 1 4¾	?2 7 6½	†69 2 2½	57 14 8½
Fareham	77 12 7¾	87 11 7½	66 17 8½	71 10 8
Brockhampton . .	72 3 7¾	198 11 11	105 6 7	55 6 3½
Alverstoke . . .	57 18 9¼	86 2 4½	c. 59 17 3½	67 19 10½
Gosport	6 9 0½	4 3 7½	4 14 4	4 16 2
Mardon *	77 15 10¼	128 18 3¼	67 4 8¼	33 6 3¼
Bitterne	18 18 2	?	16 18 7¾	?
Alresford (Manor *) .	81 0 6½	52 10 1¾	90 15 8¼	71 9 7
Alresford (Borough) .	19 16 0	17 18 6	18 15 9½	18 ? ?
Wield *	20 3 8¼	7 9 8½	10 4 7½	12 8 2½
Ivyngho	123 16 5¼	111 4 5¼	‡59 6 1¾	66 14 3
West Wycombe * . .	89 18 1½	71 16 7¾	51 10 6	69 17 2½
Morton	34 12 11¼	19 18 2	14 4 10½	21 5 6¾
Wargrave * . . .	61 1 5½	80 18 11½	92 14 7½	65 15 4
	2178 2 8½	2129 8 7	2189 10 2¼	1879 12 3¾

N.B.—Twelve manors out of 26 show an increased balance; 13 manors out of 26 show a decreased balance; 1 is doubtful. Of the 13 showing a decrease, 5 do not include wool, and therefore their accounts are incomplete; while in one or two cases there is a special reason for increased expenditure. Seventeen manors had a decreased balance in 1348–9; 7 manors had an increased balance in 1348–9; 9 manors had an increased balance in 1349–50; 17 manors had a decreased balance in 1349–50. Of 17 manors whose expenses are clearly given, twelve show a decrease, 5 an increase in expenditure. The total result to the Bishop was an average loss of a little over £100 per annum, or about 5 per cent.

* The manors marked thus with an asterisk sent their wool separately to Wolvesey, and it is therefore not included in the cash account. The manors not marked may also have sent wool to Wolvesey, but there is no direct evidence of this. Hence the apparent loss in receipts may not always imply a real loss to the Bishopric.

† The receipts marked thus include considerable sums for old corn, remaining from the previous year, i.e. £18 at Bishopston, and £52 at Hambledon (Church), where large quantities of corn were received as tithe.

‡ This drop is largely due to building operations, and heavy increase of expenses.

D. NORTH HAMPSHIRE AND BERKSHIRE GROUP.

Net Balance.

	1347–8			1348–9			1349–50			1350–1			1351–2		
Bentley	65	3	5¼	*86	17	5¾	38	11	6¼	14	15	5	21	10	4¼
Borough of Overton .	10	11	7½	9	9	0½	10	1	5½		?		6	6	3½
Manor of Overton .	76	12	5¾	34	6	8¾	50	12	8½	75	13	6¾	77	10	1
North Waltham . .	7	17	8	9	17	6¾	16	11	1¾	6	1	10½	9	12	0
Waltham St. Laurence	42	1	1¾	65	18	5¼	55	4	6¼	47	13	1¼	40	8	2¼
Ashmansworth . .	13	5	1¼	*15	1	4¾	20	14	0	1	17	4¼	5	7	7¾
Burghclere . . .	113	0	2	*124	10	7½	93	17	4¼	44	9	9	92	13	11
Highclere	31	0	7	35	12	4½	24	11	10¼	32	16	9½	28	11	11¾
Newtown	7	13	8	7	15	11	7	12	10		?		7	13	10
Woodhay	54	4	6	38	13	8¼	60	6	8	49	7	6½	49	13	1¼
Itchingswell . . .	44	2	4½	35	0	9½	33	9	10	33	15	0¾	27	3	2½ †

* Arrears not fully paid off in following year.

† The average loss on the 4 years 1348–52 amounts to about 17 % ; if the table had been continued for two years the recovery shown would have been more complete.

E. LABOUR SERVICES* DURING THE BLACK DEATH.

NAILESBOURNE.

	Works due.	1346–7	1347–8	1348–9	1349–50	1350–1
		Performed.				
		Partly	Partly	Partly	Partly	Partly
Threshing .	{ 6 qr. 6 bus. 13 qr. 5 bus.	52½ sold	52½ sold	52½ sold	32½ sold	43¾ sold
Ploughing per acre .	54½ acres	All performed	All performed	28 performed	16 performed	60 performed
Ploughing *de prece* .	36 ,,	All	36	All sold	44 performed	20
Harrowing .	54 ,,	?	All	All	44 performed	{ 9½ performed 17¾ sold
Harvesting per acre .	66 ,,					All
Harvesting *de prece* .	174 works	96	All	All	All	All
Manual works .	1470 ,, 399 ,, 882 ,, 488 ,, 784 ,,					
Total . .	4755 ,,	3841	3860	3924	1774	2264†
Sold . .	—	—	—	—	2119	1711
Defects . .	—	—	—	—		

* These services were owed by groups of customers and workmen ; the total cannot be definitely stated, but the maximum number of persons implied seems to be 168, the minimum 104. Similar tables could be compiled for all the Taunton manors.

† In 1354 the number sold had risen to 2,985 ; by 1376–7 it was over 3,000.

NAILESBOURNE. MANUAL WORKS.

	1345–6	1347–8	1348–9	1349–50	1350–1	1353–4	1376–7
Owed . . .	4755	4755	4755	4755	4755	4755	4755
Defects . .	—	—	None	2119	1711	505	?
Acquittances .	192	—	265	274	?	?	?
Sold . . .	3023	3860	3924	1774	2264	2985	3016
Performed . .	630	—	581	588	c. 520	?	?

THE MANORS OF WITNEY, BRIGHTWELL, AND DOWNTON

By A. Ballard

I. WITNEY

1. Early History

The manor of Witney lies on both sides of that tributary of the river Thames which is known as the Windrush, and consists of the three townships of Curbridge on the south and Hailey and Crawley on the north of the river ; the topographical features which require notice are the meadows lying on both banks of the Windrush, and the high land over the 400 feet contour line on the north where Hailey and Crawley touch the woods still known as Wychwood Forest : till the end of the eighteenth century both these townships had much woodland towards their northern boundaries, and till the end of that century the extreme southern part of the township of Curbridge was a heath known as Curbridge Heath.

The present area of these three townships is—

Curbridge	.	.	.	.	2,983 acres
Crawley	.	.	.	.	1,128 ,,
Hailey .	.	.	.	.	2,879 ,,

giving a total of 6,990 acres ; but the present Urban District of Witney is 192 acres in extent, and as it contains not only the old borough of Witney, but also an area recently annexed from the township of Curbridge, the extent of the manor must have been some 7,000 acres. Till the beginning of the nineteenth century, the whole manor together with the borough of Witney formed one ecclesiastical parish.

The earliest mention of Witney is found in a charter of 969,[1] by which King Edgar gave thirty cassates there to his minister Ælfhelm and his heirs ; but the estate seems to have reverted to the Crown, for in 1046 Edward the Confessor gave the same thirty manses to Ælfwin, Bishop of Winchester, to whose see the manor belonged till 1751, when it was leased to the Duke of Marlborough. Each charter gives the boundaries of the land affected by it, and a careful examination shows that the same points are mentioned in both charters ; but only a few of these points can be identified on the six-inch Ordnance map ; the Windrush and a field called the Moors are mentioned in both charters ; the meadow belonging to Shilton, the Ducklington mill weir, the Colwell brook, and the Nut Cliff are mentioned in one or the other ; and the boundaries in both charters agree with the boundaries on the map in passing along roads on the greater part of the north.

The Domesday entry is as follows :

' Episcopus Winton' tenet WITENIE.   Stigand archiepiscopus tenuit.   Ibi sunt xxx hidae.   Terra est xxiiii carucarum. Nunc in dominio v carucae et ix serui et xxxvi uillani cum xi bordariis habent xx carucas.   Ibi ii molini de xxxii solidis et vi denariis et c acrae prati.   Silua iii leugae longitudine et ii leugae latitudine.   Cum oneratur ualet L solidos.   T.R.E. ualebat xxii libras.   Modo xxv libras.' [2]

' The Bishop of Winchester holds Witney.   Archbishop Stigand held it.   There are 30 hides.   There is land for 24 plough teams.   There are now on the demesne 5 teams and 9 slaves, and 36 villains with 11 bordars have 20 teams. There are two mills of 32s. 6d., and 100 acres of meadow. The wood is 3 leagues in length and 2 leagues in breadth, when it is stocked it is worth 50s.   In the time of king Edward it was worth £22.   Now £25.'

It will be noticed at once that the thirty cassates of Edgar's charter and the thirty manses of that of the Confessor are reproduced in the thirty hides at which the manor was assessed.   We have already spoken of the meadows in the valley of the Windrush and of the woods in the northern

---

[1] Kemble 556.   [2] D. B. i. 155 a 1.

parts of Hailey and Crawley; but it is remarkable that although the Domesday Commissioners for Oxfordshire usually recorded the rough pasture, no rough pasture is recorded as belonging to Witney; possibly it was included in the statistics of the wood.

2. The Hundred Rolls

About two centuries after the compilation of Domesday Book, in the year 1279, another survey of the counties of Cambridge, Huntingdon, Bedford, Buckingham, and Oxford was taken by order of Edward I; this survey is known as the Hundred Rolls, and is far more detailed than Domesday Book, inasmuch as it records the names of the tenants and specifies the rents they paid and the services they rendered. The survey of Witney begins thus:

' Episcopus Wyncestr' tenet vii carucatas terre in dominico ut in dominico pertinente ad manerium de Wytteneye et habet liberum parcum set nescitur quo warranto, et habet visum franci plegii de hominibus suis, habet eciam liberum mercatum et feyriam in Wyteneye, et habet liberam piscariam et valet dimidiam marcam, et tenet de domino Rege in capite pro parte cujusdam baronie et habet liberam chaciam in bosco quod dicitur Bissopeswode, et tenet per cartas et con-firmaciones domini Regis set nescitur confirmacione cujus Regis.' [1]

' The Bishop of Winchester holds seven carucates of land in demesne as demesne belonging to the manor of Witney, and has a free park, but it is unknown by what warrant, and has the view of frankpledge over his men, and has a free market and fair at Witney, and has a free fishery which is worth half a mark; and he holds of our Lord the King in chief as a part of a certain barony; and he has a free chace in a wood which is called Bishop's wood, and he holds by the charters and confirmations of our lord the king, but of which king is unknown.'

Thus the five carucates in demesne at the time of Domesday Book had increased to seven two centuries later, and the bishop had received the grant of a market and fair since the

---

[1] Hundred Rolls, ii. 703.

date of Domesday Book ; [1] but apart from this reference to the market and fair, the Hundred Rolls contain no reference to the borough of Witney, which was formed by the amputation of a part of the township of Curbridge between the years 1209 and 1277; the Pipe Rolls for 1209 contain no accounts for the borough, but the borough accounts for 1277 are very full.

Although the Hundred Rolls omit all mention of the borough, yet they deal very fully with the three townships composing the manor, and give the names of the tenants in each township, the extent of their tenements, and their rents. First come the 33 freeholders in Hailey, of whom only two hold virgates, a fact which seems to indicate that only two held shares in the open fields ; Lucia de Wodes held four virgates at a rent of 8s. a year, and the Pipe Rolls tell us that these four virgates were originally held by villeins; Richard Young held half a virgate at a rent of 1s. and 6 acres of assarts at 3s. a year ; each of the other 31 freeholders held a messuage and a certain number of acres at 6d. an acre, and although nothing is said on this point, except in one or two cases, it seems probable that most of these acres were assarted from the woodland or the waste. Then follow the *servi*, of whom 17 were virgaters and 10 were semi-virgaters, all holding by money rent and works, and there were also 6 cottagers. Each virgater is said to have rendered 3s. 9d. for rent and 10s. 10d. for works when they were valued (*quando taxantur*), that is, when he paid the value of his works in order to be excused from his tenurial labour, this latter term being used to denote that labour which he performed as part of the consideration he rendered for his holding. The rents of the cottagers differed. The same order is followed in the other townships, or hamlets as they are called in the Hundred Rolls, and the whole may be tabulated as follows :

[1] The fair was granted in 1231 (Cal. Ch. Rolls, i. 140).

		Mes-suages.	Cottages.	Virgates.	Acres.*	Money Rents. £ s. d.
HAILEY.	Free .	32		4½	175½	5 2 3¾
	Servi .	17		17		
						4 2 6
		10		5		
					14	7 0
	Cotters		6			6 7½
CRAWLEY.	Free .	3		4½	33½	3 16 6
	Servi .	6		6		
						3 4 6
		2		6		
					36	
	Cotters		4			4 0
CURBRIDGE.	Free .	3		6	3	1 0 6
	Servi .	27		27		
						5 8 9
		4		2	.	
		104	10	78	262	23 12 3¼

Now, if we compare the extent contained in the Hundred Rolls with that of Domesday Book, we notice many differences: (1) the bishop's demesne farm had increased from 5 to 7 carucates, that is to say, its area had increased to such an extent that it was necessary to employ two teams more than two centuries before; (2) the 20 carucates in the possession of the tenants ‘had decreased to 78 virgates or 19½ carucates; (3) the nine slaves have disappeared; (4) if it is possible to equate the bordars of Domesday Book with the cottagers of the Hundred Rolls, they have decreased from 11 to 10; but, on the other hand, (5) the other inhabitants of the manor have increased from 36 to 104, as is shown by the number of messuages in the table. We must also remember that of the 78 virgates occupied by the tenants, 15 were occupied by freeholders and 63 by *servi*.

The existence of 175 acres of assarts* in the hamlet of Hailey is very suggestive : Curbridge and Crawley † are both

---

* These acres were assarts held by one or another of the servile tenants.

† In addition to these three hamlets, the Bishop had granted a messuage and six virgates in Caswell to Hugh de Scothorn at a rent of 19s. 1d. ; but the Pipe Rolls, as far as I have examined them, do not mention either Hugh of Scothorn or Caswell ; so I gather that Caswell did not form part of the manor of Witney : other six virgates in Caswell were held of the Abbot of Eynsham.

nucleated villages, to use Maitland's well-known phraseology :
Hailey contains one well-marked nucleus, and on its eastern
boundary there is a hamlet called New Yatt, evidently a
newer settlement than Hailey : about three-quarters of New
Yatt lies in the township of Hailey and the other quarter
in that of Northleigh.   But Davis's map of Oxfordshire
(1797) which distinguishes between the enclosures and the
open fields, reveals that New Yatt was surrounded by enclosures, while the rest of Hailey lay in open fields.   Whatever may have been the case elsewhere, it appears that at
Witney lands asserted from the waste were held in severalty
and not in open fields, as their area is reckoned in acres and
not in virgates ; and it would therefore appear that the 31
holders of asserts in the township of Hailey formed the
beginnings of this settlement at New Yatt.

Let us now proceed to check the Hundred Rolls by the
Pipe Rolls.   I have not been able to find the Pipe Roll for
the year ending Michaelmas 1279, the year of the Hundred
Rolls; but those for 1277 and 1278 have been examined
with surprising results : they show that in those years the
bishop received rents amounting to £41 ·17s. 10½d., or
£17 5s. 2d. above the amount shown in the Hundred Rolls.
And further examination shows another serious discrepancy :
the Hundred Rolls, as we have seen, record that each servile
virgater paid a money rent of 3s. 9d., but it is absolutely
clear from the Pipe Rolls that he paid a money rent of 5s. ;
for in every account the bailiff was allowed 5s. per virgate
as the acquittance of the rents of those permanent servants
of the manor who were employed all the year round, and in
the plague year the rents due at the Midsummer and Michaelmas quarters, amounting to 2s. 6d., were uncollected from
many virgates on account of the death of the tenants.   Now,
of our two authorities, the Pipe Rolls are to be preferred, as
they represent the accounts rendered to the bishop by his
bailiff, who, naturally, would not misrepresent the rents to
his own detriment ; the Hundred Rolls must be wrong, and
the bishop or his servants cannot be held guiltless of misleading
the king when they stated that the rent of a virgate was only

3s. 9d. But if we follow the Pipe Rolls and amend the extent contained in the Hundred Rolls by reckoning the rent of a servile virgate as 5s. a year, and therefore add to the rents shown by the Hundred Rolls a sum of £3 18s. 9d., representing the difference of 1s. 3d. a virgate on 63 virgates, the corrected total is £28 11s. 5½d., and there is still a deficit of over £13 from the rents accounted for in the Pipe Rolls.[1]

The Pipe Rolls also give information from which we may deduce the nature of the works performed by the servile tenants, which were valued by the Hundred Rolls at 10s. 10d. a year.[2] For in 1277 and 1278 the bailiff was allowed :

£3 10s. for the acquittance of the rents of 14 ploughmen working every other week throughout the year, i. e. 5s. each or the whole year's rent.

£1 for the acquittance of the rents of 8 harrowers working every other week from Michaelmas to Easter, i. e. 2s. 6d. each or a half-year's rent.

£2 15s. for the acquittance of the rents of 44 virgaters working every other day from Midsummer to Michaelmas, i. e. 1s. 3d. each or a quarter's rent.

And this list of acquittances is followed by the note :

'And, be it known, that by these same men, the corn is hoed and the meadows are mown and carried, and the corn is reaped and carried, and the dung is collected and spread, and other works are done as is necessary, and yet it is necessary to have so many (extra) works.'

It is fair to argue from the evidence of the list of acquittances and the note that the reason for the acquittance of their rents for the whole year, the half-year, or the quarter, as the case might be, was that as part of their tenurial labour these men worked on the demesne every other day throughout the year.

[1] I have found similar discrepancies between the total represented by the Hundred Rolls as being receivable from the sub-manors of the manor of Woodstock, and those actually received by the bailiff of the manor. Woodstock Manor in the Thirteenth Century, Vierteljahrschrift für Social- und Wirtschaftsgeschichte, 1908.

[2] The Rolls for 1376–7 contain accounts of the works of the customary tenants on most of the manors ; but there is no account for Witney in that year or in 1375 or 1377.

Seebohm has taught us that the render of the villein tenants was threefold, gafol or rent in money and kind, week work, and boon work ; the Pipe Rolls have therefore shown us that the gafol of the virgater at Witney was 5s. a year, and that his week work was three days a week, with probably the usual exceptions of feast days : they also give us some particulars from which it is possible to deduce the nature of the boon works at specially busy times. In 1277 there were 30 boon ploughings in winter and 31 during Lent ; in the following year there were 29 in winter and 31 in Lent : remembering that there were 63 servile virgaters in the manor, we may conclude that one of the boon works required from the virgater was one day's ploughing on the demesne.

The records relating to the autumn boon works are not quite so clear : in 1348 the bailiff charged for bread, beer, and cheese purchased for 485 men as it were for one day coming to four *precariae* ; at these four boon works labour equivalent to that of 485 men for one day was provided ; that is to say, on each day 121 men came to work. Apparently, each virgate provided two men at each of these four boon works, when the bishop supplied food ; there were also three other boon works with 2 men each, when no food was supplied.

It is well known that many of the extents contained in the Oxfordshire Hundred Rolls give the values of the particular services exacted from the servile tenants : Shipton-under-Wychwood (about ten miles north-west of Witney) is one of the manors where the services are thus valued,[1] and if the Witney labours, as deduced above, are valued according to the Shipton scale, the total works out to 10s. 7d., somewhat less than the valuation given in the Hundred Rolls.

		s.	d.
Between Michaelmas and the Gule of Autumn, 3 works a week at ½d. a work (43 weeks)		5	4½
Between the Gule of Autumn and Michaelmas, 3 works a week at 1½d. a work (9 weeks)		3	4½
One ploughing			2
Three boon works in autumn with 2 men each, without food .		1	0
Four boon works in autumn with 2 men each, with food . .			8
		10	7

[1] Hundred Rolls, ii. 734.

The Pipe Rolls further tell us the other liabilities of the
servi ; the bishop took the best beasts of the virgaters and
semi-virgaters as heriots at their deaths ; the heirs of those
who died paid heavy reliefs or fines on entering upon their
inheritances ; heavy fines were paid by purchasers on their
admission to the property they had purchased, and by those
who married women in possession of property, whether the
latter were widows or single.   But it is impossible to deduce
any scale on which these reliefs and fines were levied, and the
bishop's servants appear to have obtained the best bargain
they could.

Finally, we can make from the Pipe Rolls a calculation of the
number of the servile virgates in the manor, to act as a check
on the figures given in the Hundred Rolls ; in 1277 and
1278 4 permanent servants—the reeve, the swineherd, and
two shepherds—and 14 ploughmen were excused all their
rent in consequence of their permanent employment on the
demesne : to these must be added the 44 virgates, whose
occupiers worked on the demesne every day during the harvest
quarter, and we have a total of 62 servile virgates as compared
with the 63 shown by the Hundred Rolls.   The harrowers are
recorded as working from Michaelmas to Easter, and were
therefore included among those who worked every day during
harvest.

3. Before the Black Death

Hitherto we have been considering the manor as a machine
at rest ; but the accounts contained in the Pipe Rolls enable
us to form some idea of this machine in work ; and to ascertain
how the machine worked before the Black Death, let us
examine the Rolls for the years ending Michaelmas 1340, 1341,
1343, 1344, 1346, 1347, and 1348.   It will be noticed that
there is a break in this series : Adam, Bishop of Winchester,
died on July 18, 1345 ; his successor, William of Edington,
was consecrated on May 14, 1346 ; but when the temporalities
were restored, the king ordered the *custos* to account to him
only for the period from the death of Adam to December 9,
1345, so that the Pipe Roll for the period ending 1346 relates

only to nine months and a half, although all four quarter days are included.

The most important change in the interval between 1279 and 1340 is that the bishop's plough teams on the demesne had decreased in number from 7 to 5, and that the number of servile ploughmen had correspondingly decreased from 14 to 10. Historians have been in the habit of talking glibly about the carucate, the area of land ploughed by one team of eight oxen in the course of the year, and have roughly estimated this area as 120 acres. The Pipe Rolls record the number of acres sown with each kind of corn in each year and thus enable us to check this rough estimate. These respective areas may be tabulated as follows :

	1277	1278	1340	1341	1343	1344	1346	1347	1348	1349
Wheat	180	191	126	138	132	129	127	128	130	128
Barley	46	46	$40\frac{1}{4}$	$36\frac{1}{2}$	37	40	50	37	$42\frac{1}{2}$	$41\frac{1}{2}$
Oats	$153\frac{1}{2}$	146	74	$71\frac{3}{4}$	81	$80\frac{3}{4}$	51	63	64	56
Peas	1		10	$14\frac{1}{4}$	15	16	16	15	$12\frac{1}{2}$	16
Vetches	1									
Drage	16[1]		$21\frac{3}{4}$	$35\frac{1}{2}$	31	32		36	40	42
	$397\frac{1}{2}$	383	272	296	296	$297\frac{3}{4}$	244	279	289	$283\frac{1}{2}$

Some of this land, however, was ploughed by the boon works of the servile virgaters ; in 1277 there were 30 boon ploughings in winter and 31 in Lent, and in 1346 22 men did boon work with 11 ploughs ; but even without allowing for the boon works, it is clear that the utmost area ploughed by one team in one year at Witney was between 55 and 60 acres. The records give the names of the fields in which the various crops were sown, and show that as a general rule the manor was a three-field manor, and that each field was cropped for two years and lay fallow in the third year ; but one field, Smerehull, was under corn every year from 1346 to 1354. If, then, we add to the 55 or 60 acres actually under crop one-third to allow for the fallow in the other field, we shall see that the carucate at Witney was from 80 to 90 acres. It will be remembered that Walter of Henley said that a team could plough eight or nine score acres in the year.[2]

---

[1] Mixtilion.   [2] Ed. Lamond, p. 19.

Corresponding with the decrease in the bishop's demesne, was an increase in the gross rents from £59 0s. 7d. to £75 6s. 8¾d.; but the rent rolls were an old compilation, and from the gross rents recorded in these rolls were to be deducted certain sums for properties that had changed hands and had been let at lower rents : these were technically known as 'defects', and the defects reduced the net amounts to £41 17s. 10½d. in 1278 and £56 15s. 9¾d. in 1340. It seems probable that the area thus taken from the demesne was let to servile tenants : for in 1340 the tenants who were acquitted of the rents were the reeve, 3 shepherds, the swineherd, the smith, 10 ploughmen, and 53½ autumn workers, making a total of 69½ virgates occupied by servile tenants—an increase of 6½ on the number of servile tenants shown in the Hundred Rolls. But the lands thus let to *servi* would produce only an additional rent of 32s. 6d. a year, so that the greater part of the increase must be sought elsewhere. And it is found that there had been considerable assarting of the rough forest land ; in 1283 James of Crawley and Roger Hareng had paid a fine of £14 for entry upon 140 acres of new pasture, of which the yearly rent at 6d. an acre, the usual rent shown by both the Hundred and Pipe Rolls, would be £3 10s. a year. Although the Hundred Rolls record only 261½ acres of assarts and forlond, yet the accounts for 1353 mention 696 acres of assarts which were in the hands of the lord by death of the tenants during the pestilence : so that there must have been much assarting of which we have no record.

In the first half of the fourteenth century the demesne lands were cultivated by the five demesne ploughs, each of which had two men to work it, one to drive the oxen and the other to guide the plough : these ten ploughmen were rewarded by the remission of their rents ; eight servile virgaters acted as harrowers from Michaelmas to Easter, and were rewarded by the remission of their rents for these two quarters ; hoeing and weeding were done by the tenurial labour of the *servi*, who worked three days a week on the demesne without payment, and worked on the demesne from Midsummer to Michaelmas, during the hay and corn harvests, and for so doing were rewarded by the remission of their rents during this quarter. The actual reaping of the corn, or most of it, was done by the boon works, and in 1277 350½ acres were thus reaped, in 1346 the number was 285, and in 1348 the number was 292 ; the only operation for which labour was hired was the threshing and winnowing of the corn, for which £2 6s. was paid in 1277 and £2 14s. 7d. in 1278. But the yield of the crops was very poor, although better than in the neighbouring manor of Woodstock during the previous century.[1] The tables at the end of this essay will show the detailed figures ; suffice it to say here that between 1340 and 1349 the yield of wheat varied between 4¾ and 7½ bushels per acre, barley from 8 to 21, and oats from 6⅝ to 10¾. These figures should be compared with those quoted by the author of the anonymous ' Dite de Hosbandrie ', who says that wheat should yield to the fifth grain, barley to the eighth, and oats to the fourth.[2] As the seed sown at Witney was 2½ bushels of wheat to the acre, and 4 bushels each of barley and oats, the anonymous writer would have expected a yield of 12½ bushels of wheat, 32 bushels of barley, and 16 bushels of oats—crops which were never reached at Witney during the period under review. But in spite of the scanty yield, the proceeds from the sales of corn during these seven years averaged £20 a year.

A fair head of live stock was kept on the demesne : when Bishop Adam died in 1345, his executors removed most of the live stock as his private property, and it was therefore necessary for his successor to restock the manor as follows :

	£	s.	d.
2 Cart horses costing	1	2	0
13 Plough oxen	8	1	6
1 Bull		15	6
15 Cows and calves	8	2	9½
600 Sheep	56	10	11
2 Sows		8	4
Drake and 4 ducks		1	8
Cock and 5 hens			9
	75	3	5½

[1] See Woodstock Manor in the Thirteenth Century, p. 459.
[2] Walter de Henley, ed. Lamond, p. 71.

But it is remarkable that Bishop William of Edington kept no ewes at Witney, and that all the sheep kept on the demesne during his time were bred by and purchased from other farmers. For the five plough teams 40 oxen were kept, and there were usually a few in reserve; the flock of sheep averaged about 700. The surplus stock was sold from time to time, and during the seven years under review the sales of stock averaged £11 16s. a year. Occasionally, however, we find that some of the live stock was sent to the bishop for the supply of his household; thus in 1340 the bailiff was allowed 2s. 0½d. as the cost of driving 10 pigs to Farnham, and in 1349 two men were paid 1s. 6d. each for driving 11 pigs to London.

A large quantity of butter and cheese was produced in the dairy; but the only figures I have noted were £5 8s. 1½d. from this source in 1277 and £5 7s. 2d. in the next year. The wool from the flock of sheep was more valuable and produced £14 12s. 5d. in 1277 and £14 18s. in 1278; in fact, the clip was worth more than half as much as the flock of sheep; for the clip of 1278 was the produce of 370 sheep, which, at 1s. 4d. each, the price at which the bailiff sold sheep during that year, were worth somewhat less than £25. The sales of dairy produce and wool were included among certain receipts which were called ' Exits of the Manor ', and with them were grouped payments for grazing rights, for underwood, for fishing rights, and for other miscellaneous privileges. The receipts under this head were £63 13s. 5d. in 1348, but this amount is quite abnormal, as it includes a sum of £45 13s. 10d. from the sale of wool at £6 a sack: this was evidently the accumulated produce of several years; once or twice the accounts show that the wool was sent to Wolvesey, and in those years no sum was credited to the bailiff in respect thereof. Including this abnormal year, the ' Exits of the Manor ' averaged £24 6s. for the seven years under review. If all these averages are added together, corn sold £20, stock sold £11 16s., and exits £24 6s., we find that the receipts from the demesne farm averaged £56 2s. in the period before the Black Death.

The expenses were not very high; apart from the purchase

of stock and seed, the chief items were for the repairs to the ploughs, wagons, and houses, the necessary expenses on the dairy and fold, and those of the bailiff and steward; an abnormal year was 1346, when, as we have seen, a sum of £75 was expended on the purchase of new stock; but the average for the other six years was £25 10s.; deduct this from the receipts, £56 2s., and there remains an average profit of £30 12s. on the working of the demesne farm; as the area under crop averaged 282 acres, the accounts show a profit of a little over 2s. 2d. per acre. But this profit was obtained only because of the tenurial labour of the servile tenants: the only payment for labour on the farm was that for threshing and winnowing, a sum of about £3 a year.

The bishop, however, was not only the largest agriculturist in the manor; he was also the feudal lord of all the inhabitants, and from his feudal rights he received an income much larger than that from his farming operations. We have already spoken of the rents which he received as landlord: in addition to the rents of assize, he received large rents from the mills, of which there were four: in 1346, the corn mill and fulling mill known as Waley's Mill and the two corn mills at Woodford were let for £14 13s. 4d.; another fulling mill was let at £1 6s. 8d., and the corn mill at Crawley produced 13s. 4d. per annum, a total of £18; in 1277 there had been another fulling mill at Woodford, and the rent then paid for them was £22 11s. 8d.; the Hundred Rolls record that the fishery was worth half a mark, but in 1346 it had doubled in value and was let at 13s. 4d. As already noticed, whenever a servile holding changed hands a sum of money was paid to the bishop, and the fines thus levied were not fixed sums, but varied according to the financial position of the heir or the purchaser. The steward of the manor also held the manorial courts, at which were fined those who had broken the by-laws of the manor or had committed petty offences against the law of the land: for the Hundred Rolls record that the bishop had the view of frankpledge over his own men: the accounts for every year record the receipt of 26s. 8d. at the hundred of St. Martin and of a similar sum at the hundred of Hokeday; in 1285 these sums are said to arise from the eleven tithings for tithing. On his entering into possession of the manor in 1346 the new bishop received a gift of £19 5s. as 'recognition money from the free and native tenants of the manor'; of this sum, the free tenants paid 11s. 8d. The bishop was evidently entitled to certain regalities; for in 1346 the bailiff accounted for £40 2s. 4d. of the chattels of Richard of Standlake, forfeited by him because he had been condemned for the death of John the Fisher, and had fled. During the seven years under review, the fines of land and marriages averaged £11 3s. 6d., and the perquisites of the courts £3 4s. 3d. a year.

To sum up, the bishop's income for these seven years averaged :

	£	s.	d.
Farming profits	31	12	0
Rents	56	15	9
Rents of mills	18	0	0
Fines of lands	11	3	6
Perquisites of court	3	4	3
	120	15	6

But it cannot be repeated too often that the profit on the farming of the demesne was obtained only because the bulk of the labour was unpaid.

4. THE BLACK DEATH AND AFTER

On taking up the Rolls for the year ending Michaelmas 1349, we notice within the first few lines the rubric ' *Defectus per pestilentiam* '; then comes a long list of corresponding entries, of which the first reads :

' 2s. 6d. for the rent of one messuage and one virgate of Walter le Kene in Curbridge at Midsummer and Michaelmas, because the said Walter is dead, and there is no one who wishes to take the said land, and nothing from which the said rent can be levied.'

Altogether, there are 46 of these entries, relating to 18 messuages and 17 virgates in Curbridge, 6 messuages and

3 virgates in Crawley, and 18 messuages, 15½ virgates, and 6 cotlands in Hailey, a total of 42 messuages, 35½ virgates, and 6 cotlands, in respect of which rents were excused to the amount of £4 14s. 9d.; a further sum of £14 11s. 1d. was excused in defect of the rents of 586 acres of pasture and some assarts likewise in the hands of the lord through the death of the tenants. But these figures do not disclose the mortality: in the previous year five heriots had been received: in 1349 the number had risen to 57, showing that of the small tenants occupying one virgate or half a virgate each, 57 died of the Black Death. It would seem that from one property two heriots were paid during the year: John Hickes paid 13s. 4d. as a relief on succeeding to a messuage and virgate at Curbridge, late the property of his father, Thomas Hickes; but the list of heriots shows that the bailiff received a cow as a heriot on the death of Thomas Hickes and an ox on the death of John Hickes. The table on p. 185 shows that in 1279 the 63 servile virgates were held by 76 men, of whom 50 held a virgate each and 26 were semi-virgaters; the Pipe Rolls have shown that in 1340 the number of servile virgates had increased to 69½, and if the new virgates were distributed in the same proportion as the old, the tenants of virgates would be 55 and the semi-virgaters would be 29, or a total of 84 servile tenants; if so, the mortality would be 2 out of 3.

But during this year it was not all loss to the bishop; for there were some heirs who were prepared to take up the property of their deceased relatives, and the fines increased from £13 8s. 3¾d. to £30 3s. 1¼d.; in spite of the plague, they 'married and were given in marriage', for Simon Wykyn paid 10s. for licence to marry Alice, the widow of John Symonds, with one messuage and one virgate of land in Crawley, which had belonged to her late husband. The bailiff also took possession of the crops on the lands of those who had died and left no heir, and accounted for £4 12s. 10½d. for corn of deceased natives of Curbridge and Crawley that had been sold in the fields; besides, he retained unsold in the grange a quantity which he estimated at 12 quarters of wheat and 4 quarters of barley. Thus the increase in the fines and the receipts from corn seized more than balanced the loss on the rents. When we come to deal with the demesne farm we see another side of this great mortality: in 1348 the rents of the tenants of 53½ virgates were remitted in consideration of their work on the demesne during the harvest quarter; in 1349 only 21 virgates supplied workers during that quarter, and in 1350 the number had decreased to 2. In 1348 121 workers came to the Autumn boon works, at which food was provided; in 1349 the number was reduced to 60, and in the next year it was still further reduced to 28. Again, in 1348, 292 acres of corn were reaped by the boon works of the servile tenants; in 1349 only 130 acres were thus reaped, and in 1350 the number had decreased to 56. In 1348 no reapers were hired; in 1349 156 acres of corn were reaped by hired labour, and in 1350 the number of acres thus reaped had risen to 220½. No wonder, then, that the profit on the demesne, which was £88 in 1348, an abnormal sum owing to the great sale of wool, fell to £3 in 1349.

But although much information about the mortality and its effects is given in the account for 1349, it is the account for the following year that shows the full effects: the rent account for 1350 shows that 30 virgates, 15 half-virgates, and 7 cottages were in the hands of the lord through the death of the tenants during the pestilence, and still remained in his hands through failure of heirs; but although they were thus in the lord's hands, yet the bailiff accounted for 3s. a virgate under the rubric 'Exits of the Manor'; perhaps these 37½ virgates were let on yearly tenancies to persons unwilling to incur the responsibilities which would attach to them if they obtained them at the manorial court. It is noteworthy that in 1350 there was only one heriot, and no person paid a relief for entry into a virgate; the only reliefs were for entry into assarts and acres, all of which appear to have been freeholds, held at a money rent.

It would be tedious to trace the changes in every one of the next few years; a tabular statement is the best means of showing them:

	1348	1349	1350	1351	1352	1353	1354
Virgates supplying workers in the harvest quarter . . .	53½	21	2	11	11	6	8
Workers at Autumn boon works . . .	121	60	28	37	42	45	48
Acres of corn reaped at boon works . .	292	130	56	84	84	90	80
Acres of corn reaped by paid labour . .	—	156	220½	179	211	205	217
Paid for same . .	—	70/-	110/-	89/6	105/6	102/6	108/6
Total expenses (to nearest £) . . .	25	21	43	46	66	48	58

The labour bill on the demesne rose from £3 in 1348 to an average of £17 during the three years 1352-3-4; from 1350 onwards appears a charge for hoeing, which amounted to £1 in 1352, and £1 1s. 10d. and 84s. in the two following years. The farming profits fell from 2s. 1d. an acre for the seven years before the Black Death to 3d. an acre for the five years 1350-4, and in two of these years, 1351 and 1353, there was a small loss.

A further loss of £8 12s. a year was suffered in 1350 when the tenancy of Waley's Mill expired and a new tenant could not be found; and additional evidence of the difficulty in obtaining new tenants is afforded by the figures showing the decrease in the fines received by the bishop on the admission of new tenants; in 1349 these were over £30, in 1350 they were £15 19s., in 1351 they increased to £18, but in the next three years they were £11, £5 8s., and £6 16s. respectively.

In 1352 new tenants were found for 6 virgates and 2 half-virgates; but it would seem that they were excused from their tenurial labour, as the accounts for the next year state that no works were rendered from 11 virgates, a statement which had not appeared before. In spite of the admission of these new tenants, there were 32 virgates remaining in the hands of the lord in 1353, and in 1376-7 there were 35 virgates still in his hands. In 1353 there were also 696 acres of assarts in the hands of the lord on account of the death of the tenants during the pestilence—an entry which incidentally proves that the new pasture, to which reference was previously made, was assarted from the rough forest land. But the Rolls for the next year reduce the area of the untenanted assarts to 636 acres, as in the meantime it had been discovered that the bailiff had for five years been receiving the rent for 60 acres, but had not accounted for the same: he represented that the tenant had died and that a successor could not be found.

It is obvious that directly after the pestilence the bishop found himself face to face with a grave problem: before the plague the profits on his demesne farm had been 2s. 1d. an acre, owing to the supply of unpaid tenurial labour from his servile tenants; as the rent of a single acre of land at Witney was then 6d., we may reckon that the bishop received a profit equivalent to four times the rental value of his land; after the plague, owing to the failure of his tenurial labour, his profits fell to 3d. an acre, or only half the rental value of his land. He also found it impossible to let on the same terms the land which hitherto had been in the occupation of tenants; two-thirds of the population had died, and those who remained were not prepared to enter upon the tenancy of lands to which was attached the liability of working three days a week without pay.

The Pipe Roll of 1376–7 shows how the problem was met: in that year no tenurial labour was performed, the reason being that 'their works and the services of all the native tenants were commuted at fixed payments (*ad certos denarios*) by favour of the lord as long as the lord pleases, on account of the poverty of the homage'. And among the exits of the manor is a sum of £9 10s. from 14 tenants at Curbridge, 9 at Hailey, and 4 at Crawley, being a payment of 6s. 8d. a virgate in respect of 28½ virgates, for the release of their works for each virgate as long as the lord pleased, but they were all to join in haymaking and in washing and shearing the lord's sheep, to pay pannage for their pigs, to take their turn of service as reeve and tithingman, and to carry the lord's victuals and baggage on his departure from Witney as the natives were formerly wont to do. There was also a payment of 16s. 4d. from 11 tenants of 14 cot-lands: each cotland paid 14d. for the relaxation of all works, except that the lord reserved works similar to those reserved from the virgaters ; the only difference was that, instead of carrying the bishop's baggage, the tenants of cotlands served his writs. The problem of finding tenants was thus solved by allowing them to commute their tenurial labour ; services which the Hundred Rolls valued at 10s. 10d., and which were probably worth much more in 1376, were commuted for 6s. 8d. ; but, nevertheless, there were still 35 virgates in the hands of the lord, for want of tenants.

In that year the area of the demesne under crop had decreased to 164 acres, of which 16 acres were given to the servants of the farm, 2 carters, 6 ploughmen, 4 shepherds, a cowman, and a swineherd, and the other 148 acres were reaped, tied, and carried at the cost of 1s. an acre, while 124½ acres of meadow hay were cut and carried for £5 17s. 7½d. ; the only boon work recorded was that performed by 36 men coming with 18 wagons ' *de parte amoris* ' to assist in carrying the hay. The farming receipts this year were :

	£	s.	d.
Sale of stock	29	11	2
Sale of corn	19	4	6
Exits (omitting the payments for release of works) .	21	5	7½
	70	1	3½
The expenses were	49	0	3½
Showing a profit of	21	1	0

or a little less than 2s. 7d. per acre on the 164 acres under crop.   If this statement is compared with the farm accounts for the period after the pestilence, we notice a great increase in the receipts from the sale of stock and from the exits of the manor ; bearing in mind that the exits included the receipts from the sale of the wool and the products of the dairy, the changes may indicate that the bishop was increasing the stock on his farm.

This conclusion is confirmed by the roll for 1399 ; for then not a single acre was in the occupation of the lord of the manor : parts of the demesne had been let off previously, 17½ acres in Northmore Furlong for 8s. 7½d., and 40 acres, called Inland, for 15s. 4d. on a lease for ten years. But the

rest of the demesne had been let to William Gills for a term
of years, of which this was the first, at £11 per annum.

It will be remembered that in 1346 the bishop restocked
the demesne at a cost of £75, and in the days when the
ordinary tenant occupied only a virgate, it was not easy to
find a farmer who could command the capital necessary to
stock a holding of perhaps seven virgates : consequently the
bishop leased to his tenant not only the land, but the stock
necessary for its equipment. A schedule of the stock was
given in the Roll as follows :

	£	s.	d.
2 Horses at 6s. 8d. each		13	4
4 Horses at (?6s. 8d. each)	1	6	8
15 Oxen at 15s. each	11	5	0
2 Oxen at 13s. 4d. each	1	6	8
22 Cows at 10s. each	11	0	0
1 Cow at 6s. 8d.		6	8
7 Yearlings at 4s. 4d. each	1	10	4
2 Sows at 2s. 6d. each		5	0
27 Pigs at 2s. 2¼d. each	2	19	1
40 qrs. 2 bus. Wheat at 6s. per qr.	12	1	6
98 qrs. 5 bus. Barley at 3s. per qr.	14	15	10½
47 qrs. Drage at 3s. per qr.	7	1	0
32 qrs. Oats at 2s. 8d. per qr.	4	5	4
	£68	16	5½

The total value of the stock was therefore nearly £70,
and at the expiration of the term the lessee was bound to
return the same quantity of stock or its value.

The area of the demesne thus leased is not stated ; but
in 1376–7, out of the 164 acres under crop, 67 were planted
with wheat, and in 1399, when 56 acres of wheat were planted,
the area of the demesne under crop would appear, in proportion, to be about 140 acres ; add one-third for the fallow,
and it would seem that the area leased to the tenant was
about 210 acres.

It will be noticed that no sheep were included in the lease,
for the bishop had become a large sheep-farmer with a flock
which at the beginning of the year consisted of 1,335 wethers,
255 ewes, and 8 rams : during the year a serious murrain
carried off 215 wethers before shearing, and 25 wethers after
shearing, and 47 lambs were added to the flock, so that at the

end of the year he had 1,485 sheep on the pastures: for their winter keep he retained the meadows, but the tenant of that part of the demesne which was called Inland, was bound to find a shepherd for the sheep which lay on his land and to provide a fold as often as was necessary. Sheep-farming did not, however, bring a profit to the bishop in that year: his receipts were:

						£	s.	d.
Rent of demesne	.	.	.	.	.	11	0	0
Sale of stock	.	.	.	.	.	14	0	0
Exits .	.	.	.	.	.	36	17	5¾
						£61	17	5¾

while the expenses were £75 4s. 7¾d.; of this, £36 was spent in the purchase of stock.

The last Pipe Roll is that for the year 1453. It shows that the bishop had ceased to farm at Witney: all the demesne and all his sheep were leased to tenants; part of the demesne and 300 sheep were leased to one tenant for £18 3s. 4d., another part and 160 sheep were leased to another tenant for £2 3s. 4d., while a third man had a lease of 45 sheep at a rent of 15s. a year. In this year the tenants commuted their tenurial labour for 6s. a virgate.

5. CONCLUSIONS

Let us now summarize the facts: before the Black Death, the bishop of Winchester, the lord of the manor, had kept a large proportion of the manor in his own hands and cultivated it by his bailiffs; his labour was provided by the servile tenants, who were obliged to work on the demesne three days a week all the year round as part of the consideration for which they held their lands; payments for labour were few, and so the farming was carried on at a profit.

The Black Death comes: two-thirds of the population of the manor dies; sufficient forced labour cannot be found to cultivate the demesne; paid labour has to be employed, and the profits are reduced or turned into losses. More than that, much of the land which had previously been let to tenants is thrown on the lord's hands, and cannot be let again on the same terms as before. How can these losses be met?

The servile tenants willingly pay an increased rent that their forced labour may be remitted, and others are found who are willing to take leases of the demesne and the stock at money rents; the bishop ceases to cultivate the demesne and becomes merely a receiver of rents.

Hence we see that at Witney the Black Death marks the change between a barter economy and a coin economy: formerly the occupation of land had been given in exchange for services, and services had been requited by tenancies of land: henceforward, land would be let for money rents, and services would be requited with money.

I. Yield of Corn Crops (in Bushels).

Year.	*Wheat.*	*Barley.*	*Drage.*	*Oats.*	*Peas.*
1277 . .	8½	15½		10½	7
1283 . .	8½	12		16½	
1284 . .	10½	20		11¾	
1285 . .	7¼	16		10¾	
1340 . .	5½	15¾	13	7¼	2
1341 . .	7½	20¼	10½	8¾	10
1342 . .	6	18	11	6	7½
1346 . .	5½	19¼		17	4¼
1347 . .	6½	20¾	11	8	4¼
1348 . .	6¾	21¼	13	10¾	4½
1349 . .	4¾	8	8	6½	
1350 . .	5¼	10	4	6	
1351 . .	6½	11¾	9	11¼	
1352 . .	8½	7½	5¼	4¾	4
1353 . .	5	8½	7¼	8	1

II. Abstracts of Accounts.

A. Farm	1340	1341	1342	1343–4	1346	1347	1348
	£	£	£	£	£	£	£
Sale of stock . .	15	10	12	10	2	19	16
Sale of corn . . .	13	16	25	22	14	21	30
Exits of manor . .	12	24	30	14	9	15	64
Additional sales . .	1	1	1	1	2	4	4
Total receipts from farm	41	51	68	47	27	59	114
Expenses	23	21	34	18	101	33	25
Net profits from farm .	18	30	34	29		26	89
B. Seignorial							
Net rents	57	57	57	57	58	58	57
Fines and marriages .	10	11	14	11	8	12	13
Perquisites of court .	3	2	2	3	2	3	5
Mills	19	19	19	19	19	19	19
Net income from manor	107	119	126	119	13	118	183

A. FARM	1349	1350	1351	1352	1353	1354	1376-7
	£	£	£	£	£	£	£
Sale of stock . .	4	14	10	13	16	31	30
Sale of corn .	8	11	12	46	22	19	19
Exits of manor . .	10	10	10	11	6	8	21
Additional sales . .	1	12	11	1	2	9	
Total receipts . .	23	47	43	71	46	67	70
Expenses . . .	20	43	46	66	48	57	49
Net profits from farm .	3	4	—	5	—	10	21
Loss from farm . .	—	—	3	—	2		
B. SEIGNORIAL							
Net rents . . .	40	58	59	43	43	45	55
Fines and marriages .	30	16	18	13	5	7	8
Perquisites of court .	2	2	1	—	—	—	2
Sale of works . .	—	—	—	—	—	—	10
Mills	18	10	11	12	12	12	19
Net income from manor	93	90	86	73	58	74	115

II. BRIGHTWELL

The manor of Brightwell lies in Berkshire on the southern bank of the Thames, at about the same distance from the City of Oxford as the manor of Witney, to which it has, indeed, certain resemblances. In the first place the manor of Brightwell contains three townships, Brightwell, Sotwell, and Mackney, corresponding to the three townships of Curbridge, Crawley, and Hailey in the manor of Witney; again, as at Witney, the three townships were united to form one ecclesiastical parish; thirdly, it is mentioned in pre-conquestual charters in which the boundaries are given; but my local knowledge is not sufficient to enable me to identify any point on the boundaries with the present ordnance survey, except the river Thames. The first of these three charters is a gift by King Eadred in 945 to his minister Aethelgeard of 10 manses in Brightwell, 15 in Sotwell and 5 at Maccanig (Mackney) together with 36 acres of arable land and 10 acres of meadow on the north of the 'port' of Wallingford, and other land within the town which was described as '*binnan porte fram eastgeate on norðhealf strete on ðaene broc; and vii heorðas buton ðam*, and *þreo cyrican*', 'within the town from Eastgate to the brook on the north side of the street, and seven houses

therein and three churches '.[1] Of the other two charters, one
is dated 947 and the other 948; they are gifts by the same
king to the same man, the one of 10 manses at Brightwell,[2] and
the other of 5 manses at Sotwell and 5 at Mackney, together
with the land at Wallingford as in the first deed.[3] Apparently
the king had overestimated the lands at Sotwell in the first
deed, and granted the two others to correct his mistake. The
area of the present parish is 2,063½ acres. La Rocque's map of
Berkshire (1761) shows that then Mackney had a separate
set of open fields, and that a hedge was the only division
between the fields of Sotwell and those of Brightwell. The
Domesday entry reads as follows :

' Ipse episcopus (Wintoniensis) tenet BRISTOWELLE de
episcopatu suo. Stigandus episcopus tenuit T.R.E. Tunc pro
xx hidis modo pro x hidis. Terra est xvi carucarum. In
dominio sunt iiii carucae et xvii uillani et xvi cotarii cum ix
carucis. Ibi xv serui, et molinus de xx solidis. Ibi aecclesia et
de placitis terrae que in Walingeford huic Manerio pertinet xxv
solidi. T.R.E. et post ualebat xx libras. Modo xxv libras.'[4]

' The same bishop held Brightwell as pertaining to his see.
Bishop Stigand held it T.R.E. Then it was assessed for
20 hides, now for 10. There is land for 16 plough teams.
In demesne are 4 teams, and 17 villeins and 16 cottars have
9 teams. There are 15 slaves, and a mill of 20s. There is
a church, and 25s. from the pleas of the land in Wallingford
which pertains to this manor. In the time of King Edward
and afterwards it was worth £20, now £25.

Here, as at Witney, the 20 manses of Eadred's charters
appear as the assessment of 20 hides before the Conquest; the
favour of the Conqueror had reduced the assessment to
10 hides. But while the Brightwell record speaks of 25s. as
arising from the pleas of the land in Wallingford, the Wallingford record states :

' Walchelinus episcopus habet xxvii hagas de xxv solidis
et sunt appreciatae in Bricsteuuelle Manerio ejus.'[5]
' Bishop Walkelin has 27 haws of 25s. and they are valued
in his manor of Brightwell.'

[1] Kemble 1154. [2] Ibid. 1156. [3] Ibid. 1161.
[4] D. B. i. 58 a 2. [5] Ibid. i. 56 a 2.

One of these houses was destroyed for the castle ditch, for as late as 1453 the bailiff was allowed a defect of rent of 3¾d. for the rent of Andrew of Wallingford in the castle ditch.

As Brightwell is situate in Berkshire, no extent of the manor is contained in the Hundred Rolls; but luckily, the Pipe Roll for 1376-7 incorporates an account of the works due from the various tenants in the manor, from which, with the assistance of the other Rolls, the deficiency can, in a measure, be supplied.

A messuage and 2 carucates at Mackney were held by military service, and a relief of £5 was paid in respect of this tenement in 1349. Then there were 25 virgates held by *nativi*, 4 at Brightwell, 7 at Mackney, and 14 at Sotwell; there were also 20 semi-virgaters, and of them 10 are recorded as living at Brightwell, while there is no record of the situation of the other ten; altogether there were 35 servile virgates within the manor, a figure which is almost equal to the 9 carucates occupied by the tenants in 1086: there were also 19 cotlands within the manor.

Possibly it will be best to follow Seebohm's example, and set out the services of the tenants in tabular form.

THE VIRGATER AT BRIGHTWELL AND SOTWELL.

1. Rent, 5s. a year.
2. Week work. To work every day on the demesne with his cart between the Feast of SS. Peter and Paul (June 29) and Michaelmas 65 works.
    97 manual works between Michaelmas and June 29.
3. Boon work. To plough and harrow one acre.
    To plough ¼ acre as Churchshot.
    To make two journeys to Winchester with his horse, carrying 3 bushels of wheat each journey.
    To carry one load of underwood.
    To mow for one day in Northmede.
    To load hay for one day.
    To join with another virgater in carrying one load of corn.
    To make one quarter of malt.
    To find two men for all the autumn boon works required by the lord.
    To carry all necessaries for the lord's victuals to the nearest manor.
    To do all the carrying service required for the grange and fold.

The virgater at Mackney did all the boon works required of the other virgaters, and also the work with the cart in the thirteen weeks before Michaelmas, but he performed no manual week work.

The services of the semi-virgater were as follows (we have no information as to the amount of his rent):

1. Week work. 65 manual works between SS. Peter and Paul and Michaelmas (i. e. every day except Saturday).

    117 manual works between Michaelmas and SS. Peter and Paul (i. e. 3 days a week).

    To plough 2 acres for Graserth.

2. Boon work.

    To mow for one day in Northmede.

    To load hay for one day.

    To toss hay for one day.

    To find two men for every autumn boon work required by the lord.

    To carry 10 hens to Winchester.

    To carry the lord's writs (or possibly letters, *brevia*) to the nearest manor.

The cottager's rent is not recorded, but he was bound to wash and shear his lord's sheep for 2 days and to work for one day at haymaking. The number of works in the autumn was 1,155 with carts and 1,300 manual works, and during the rest of the year 3,407 manual works; and in 1376–7, 390 autumn boon works were due from the tenants.

The demesne lay in two fields, Eastdon and Westdonne, but the area under crop differed from year to year: that in the West field varied from 152½ to 186 acres, and that in the East field from 137 to 168 acres: this land was ploughed by the boon works of the *nativi*, and by five demesne ploughs. The greater part of this land was sown with wheat and barley: the oat crop was always disappointing, not to say a failure, as it only once exceeded 10 bushels to the acre, and in 1352 and 1353 the yield was less than the seed. But the yields of wheat and barley were good, averaging 9½ and 23½ bushels to the acre respectively in the period 1346–53.

The mortality from the Black Death was not so severe at Brightwell as at Witney: in 1348 there were two admissions to virgates of heirs on the death of their relatives. In 1349 there were similar admissions to 4 virgates at Sotwell, to 3 at Mackney, and to 1 virgate and 4 half-virgates and 4 cottages at Brightwell, one of the cottages being in the hands of the lord for default of heirs, as were one virgate at Brightwell and two at Sotwell. But the cottage was taken up in 1349, the Brightwell virgate in 1350, and the two Sotwell virgates in 1351. Altogether there appear to have been 19 deaths in the manor in 1349 out of 66 tenants, a mortality of less than 30 per cent., against the death-rate of 66 per cent. at Witney. Moreover, while at Witney half the servile tenements remained in the hands of the lord for many years after the Black Death for want of persons willing to take them up, at Brightwell all the tenements vacated by the pestilence were taken up within two years. These figures can be checked; 15 heriots were received in 1349, which is the number that would be expected if the cottagers did not pay heriots.

It was probably on account of this difference in the death-rate that the economic history of Brightwell after the Black Death was so different from that of Witney. A glance at the abstract of accounts printed at the end of this chapter will show that there always was a considerable profit on the demesne, although in the plague year that profit was only about one-third of that in the preceding and following years : this small profit is to be attributed to the small quantity of corn sold in that year, a decrease which was probably due to a short harvest in the previous year. Moreover, the Pipe Rolls show that up to and including the year 1399 the *nativi* of the manor rendered at least part of their tenurial labour as they had done in the days before the Black Death. But as early as 1350 one or two of the tenants began to commute their services ; for in that year John Adams paid a fine of 5s. to be allowed to commute the services arising from one virgate at Mackney for 9s., and Robert Hunlok paid 3s. 4d. to be allowed to commute the service from one half-virgate in Brightwell for 5s. 6d. But in the course of time the charges for commutation increased, 13s. 4d. being paid for the commutation of the services of a virgate in Mackney in 1376-7, and 10s. for those of a half-virgate in Brightwell in the same year.

Reference to the abstract of accounts will show that the financial results of the working of the estate for the year 1376 were practically the same as for the year 1354 ; but, as has been pointed out before, the Pipe Roll for the later year is especially valuable, as it contains an account of the works due from and performed by the customary tenants of the manor.   That account may be abstracted as follows :

	Due.	Performed.
Ploughing and harrowing when the lord provides food	25 acres	0
Ploughing for Graserth	40 ,,	2
Do. Churchshot . . .	6¼ ,,	0
Carriage of wheat	50 works	48
Do. underwood	25 ,,	0
Malt to be made	25 qrs.	0
Washing and shearing sheep . . .	38 works	34
Making hay in Northmede . . .	48 ,,	43
Carriage of hay	67 ,,	61
Loading hay	39 ,,	31
Autumn boon works	390 ,,	108 (36 acres)
Carriage of hay	12½ ,,	12
Works in summer and autumn . . .	2496 ,,	962½
Manual works	3047 ,,	636

No less than 202 autumn boon works were allowed to the persons from whom they were due, on the ground that they were not required by the lord, and 970 manual works were released to 10 virgaters who paid rent during that year. And an addition sum shows that out of a total of 6,212½ works due, only 1,937½ were performed during that year, or less than one-third of the number that was due.

In 1453, however, we find a greater change, for then the bishop was not cultivating a single acre in the manor, and all the tenants had commuted their services, the virgaters at Brightwell and Mackney paying 8s. each, those at Sotwell 4s. each, the semi-virgaters paying 10s. each and the cotlands paying 1s. each. But there were excepted from the commutation of the virgaters, their mowings in Northmede, 5 days each carrying corn in autumn, one day each collecting stubble, and half a day each carrying manure to the fields. Altogether the tenants paid £16 10s. for the release of their labour services.

As far back as 1399 certain lands, which had formerly belonged to native tenants, had been let by the lord for terms of years : and the tendency to substitute terms of years for grants at the manorial court is more pronounced in 1453, for the Roll for that year shows that two half-virgates, the one at Brightwell and the other at Sotwell, were demised for terms of years at a rent of 13*s*. 4*d*. But the changes on the demesne were the most important: during and after the Black Death, it employed five ploughs; in 1376–7 the acreage under crop was reduced to 107 acres and the number of ploughs was reduced to three. In 1399, 112½ acres were sown with corn, but in 1453 the whole demesne with certain stock was let for a term of twenty years at £18 13*s*. 4*d*. a year. The Terra Warecta (fallow land) was stated to consist of—

42	selions in	Street Furlong.
7	,,	Pykes.
22	,,	Gavesbreche.
17	,,	Church Furlong.
26	,,	White Furlong.
42	,,	Bright Furlong.
9	,,	Nine Lands.

There were left in the barn 13½ quarters of wheat, 22 quarters of barley, 9 loads of peas, and 18 loads of hay; and the live stock consisted of 3 horses (valued at 12*s*. each), 6 carthorses, *affri* (5*s*), 16 oxen (12*s*.), 5 rams (1*s*. 3*d*.), 115 ewes (1*s*. 3*d*.), and 3 pigs (3*s*.); at the end of the term the lessee was bound to leave the same stock or to pay at the valuation for whatever was not forthcoming. And it is to be noticed that the tenant of the demesne was appointed the reeve of the manor.

Hence the manor of Brightwell was practically unaffected by the Black Death: the bishop continued his dominical farming, the servile tenants rendered their tenurial labour as before, and new tenants were found to take the vacant lands: a comparison of the history of Brightwell with that of Witney warns us against hasty generalizations.

I. Yield of Corn Crops (in Bushels).

Year.	*Wheat.*	*Barley.*	*Drage.*	*Oats.*	*Peas.*	*Rye.*
1346 . .	10¾	25½	22	5¼		
1347 . .	6¼	28	12	5½		
1348 . .	—	25	22½	10½	—	10
1350 . .	9¼	18½	5½	4	10½	4
1351 . .	8½	20¼	7¼	—	3¼	4
1352 . .	8½	17	4¾	2½	3½	8
1353 . .	13½	29¾	6	2½	5½	11¾

II. ABSTRACT OF ACCOUNTS.

A. FARM	1346	1347	1348	1349	1350	1351	1352	1353	1354	1376–7
	£	£	£	£	£	£	£	£	£	£
Sale of stock .	1	16	2	5	5	2	3	9	13	8
Sale of corn .	48	68	64	22	46	57	78	40	49	45
Exits of manor	3	7	6	4	6	7	6	6	6	10
Additional sales . .	2	—	—	2	2	3	4	4	3	4
Total receipts from farm .	54	91	72	33	59	69	91	59	71	67
Expenses . .	29	22	29	21	18	15	24	26	16	13
Net profit from farm . . .	25	69	43	12	41	54	67	33	55	54
B. SEIGNORIAL										
Net rents . .	12	12	12	12	12	13	13	12	12	12
Fines and marriages . .	15	16	32	41	20	7	5	5	2	2
Perquisites of court . .	2	3	3	2	1	2	2	2	2	3
Mill . . .	—	8	9	3	1	—	4	4	3	—
Net income from manor . .	54	108	99	70	75	76	91	56	74	71

III. DOWNTON

Downton lies in the valley of the Wiltshire Avon, about six miles south of Salisbury; part of the manor lies in the valley, but part stretches up the sides of the hills on both sides of the valley, and the highest land on the eastern side was, in the time of Domesday Book, within the borders of the New Forest. It is one of the oldest possessions of the see of Winchester, for the Winchester cartularies contain a grant of 100 manses at Downton to the church at Winchester by Coenwalha of Wessex in about the third quarter of the seventh century,[1] and there are before the Conquest seven other deeds dealing with this estate, of which four give its boundaries.[2] Domesday Book tells us that in the time of Cnut, two hides were taken away from the church and the bishop, and that of the remainder, he had granted 28½ to various knights (*militibus*), and three hides were held by the church of the manor.

[1] Kemble 985.   [2] Ibid. 342, 421, 599, 610, 698, 1036, 1108.

The agricultural statistics are as follows :

'Terra est xlvi carucarum et dimidiae. De hac terra sunt in dominio xxx hidae et ibi xiii carucae et xl servi. Ibi lxiiii uillani et xxvii bordarii habentes xvii carucas. Ibi vii molini reddentes lx solidos et lx acrae prati. Pastura ii leugae longitudine et una leuga latitudine. Silua una leuga et dimidia longitudine et dimidia leuga latitudine ... Modo quod habet in dominio ualet lxxx libras.' [1]

'There is land for 46½ plough-teams. Of this land there is in demesne 30 hides, and there are 13 ploughs and 40 slaves. There 64 villeins and 27 bordars have 17 teams. There are seven mills yielding 60s., and 60 acres of meadow. The pasture is two leagues in length and one league in breadth. The wood is one league and a half in length and half a league in breadth .... Now what he has in demesne is worth £80.'

As at Brightwell, so at Downton, we have to deduce an extent from the account of the works of the customary tenants in the Pipe Roll of 1376–7, and this roll introduces us to two classes of tenants who were not found at either Witney or Brightwell, the *ferlingarii*, who held the fourth part of a virgate, and the *custumarii*,[2] who seem to have held a position intermediate between the ferlingers and the cottagers. There were six or seven townships in the manor of Downton, and the numbers of the various tenants in each of these townships may be tabulated as follows:

	Virgaters.	Semi-virgaters.	Fer-lingers.	Custo-mers.	Cot-tagers.	Total.
East Downton .	—	4	4	11	7	26
Barford . . .	1	6	1	—	—	8
Nunton . . .	—	13	5	10	3	31
Wyke and Walton	8	9	16	—	6	39
Charlton . . .	27	1	—	—	—	28
Witherington .	8	7	3	2	—	20
	44	40	29	23	16	152

The works rendered by the tenants varied from township to township; the 29 ferlingers each worked two days a week all the year round, except in the three festal weeks of Christmas,

[1] D. B. i. 65 b. 1.

[2] On other manors the term *customarii* appears to have a more general meaning.—A. E. L.]

Easter, and Whitsuntide, and the two customers at Withering-
ton each worked one day a week. Apparently the only works
executed by the cottagers were the spreading of 50 loads of
manure every year, and the provision of two men each for
washing and shearing the bishop's sheep; the latter work
was also required from each ferlinger. But while at Witney
and Brightwell week work was required from the virgaters,
none was required of them at Downton, and it was only at
ploughtime and harvest that the virgaters and semi-virgaters
performed any work. At Charlton each virgater ploughed
three acres, and mowed half an acre of hay every working
day during hay harvest, and half an acre of corn every day
during corn harvest, an average of 18 days during each
harvest; he performed also a few minor works. The services
of the virgaters and semi-virgaters varied from township to
township, but the work in hay and corn harvests was exacted
from all alike. The rent seems to have been 5s. a virgate. With
regard to the ploughing services, it was provided that those
who did not possess a full team (*carucam integram*) should
join with the lord in ploughing and harrowing according to
the number of their animals (*secundum quantitatem animalium*),
and in 1376–7 no less than 88 acres of ploughing were excused
because the persons who were liable for their performance
had no cattle. Part of the ploughing was done by the free
tenants.

The demesne lay in the townships of East Downton and
Wyke only, and the area under crop varied from 327 acres
in 1347 to 248½ in 1353.

In the year 1349, the bishop received 106 beasts as heriots
from his ' native ' tenants, who, according to the extent that
we deduced from the roll of 1376–7, numbered 152 (including
the cottagers), so that the death-rate was about 66 per cent.
of the population, the same as at Witney: but, contrary to
his experience at Witney, the lord had little difficulty in
finding tenants for the premises thus vacated. In the plague
year itself new tenants were found for 15 virgates, 8 half-
virgates, and 18 cottages (41). In the following year
there were admissions to 9 virgates and 5 half-virgates (14),

and the bailiff reported that 9 virgates, 21 half-virgates, 14 ferlings, and 12 cottages were still in the hands of the lord for defect of tenants: but in 1376–7 this number was reduced to 6 virgates, 9 half-virgates, and 17 ferlings. It should be remembered, however, that even in the plague year the bailiff obtained from the exits of the lands of the deceased natives, not only their accustomed rent, but also a sum of £6 6s. 9¼d., which was to be refunded to their representatives; in later years there was a regular entry, in the accounts, of 'Exits on account of the pestilence', which shows that the bailiff secured some income from these lands, probably by letting them from year to year, as we have suggested in dealing with this item at Witney. And at Downton, as at Witney and Brightwell, there were large increases in the fines paid by new tenants in the years 1349 and 1350: at Downton, the fines in 1349 were almost four times the amount in the previous year, while at Witney and Brightwell they were double. The lord might have congratulated himself in 1349 and 1350 on the large increase in his income from the fines paid by the incoming tenants, which far out-balanced the losses that he suffered through his dominical farming: in order to show these losses at Witney, we have had to rearrange the accounts ; but the accounts in the Pipe Rolls are not distinguished : the items of the farming and seignorial accounts are added together, and show a large profit on the whole estate ; the profit being shown, it is probable that the bishop would not trouble to inquire how it was made up.

In spite of the large death-roll, the bishop proceeded with his dominical farming at Downton in exactly the same manner as he had done before the Plague : and the account of the works in the roll of 1376–7 shows that the tenurial services of the tenants supplied more labour than was required on the demesne farm ; for he sold 116 acres of ploughing at 7d. an acre, and 288 autumn works at 2d. each, and released to the tenants 677½ other autumn works because they were not required: all the manorial servants were excused their works, and many more works could not be exacted because of the number of tenements in the hands of the lord.

For instance, if all the manual works had been exacted, they would have numbered 2,940, but 784 were excused to the manorial servants, and 1,666 were ' *in defectu* ', as 17 ferlings were in the hands of the lord, through default of tenants, and there were other allowances. Altogether only 224 manual works were performed. The following table will show the works due and those actually performed :

	Due.	Performed.
Ploughing	425 acres	98 acres
Harrowing	205 works	105½
Making malt	94 quarters	0
Carrying manure . . .	1624 works	1292
Spreading manure . . .	725 ,,	500
Hurdles to be made . . .	139 ,,	105
Washing and shearing sheep . .	332 ,,	324
Repairing mill weir . . .	136 ,,	97
Making fences	167 perches	107
Haymaking	1197 works	669
Weeding corn	156 ,,	123
Cutting corn	1818 ,,	342 (171 acres)
Acres to be mown . . .	7 ,,	6
Autumn boon works . . .	205 ,,	28½ (9½ acres)
Carrying corn	57 ,,	55
Manual works	2940 ,,	234

Thus out of a total of 10,227 works, 3,535½ were actually performed in 1376–7. Only 172 acres were under crop in that year, so that more than half the ploughing was done by the unpaid labour of the tenants, by whom all the corn, in extent 186½ acres, was reaped. But 88 acres of the demesne had been let at farm to eight persons at a rent of 52s., or about 7d. an acre.

The accounts for 1399 show very little change from those of 1376–7, except in three particulars : (1) the area under crop had increased by 25 acres to 197 ; (2) a sum of £29 was expended in the erection of new buildings ; and (3) the amount received from sale of works had decreased from £5 15s. 8d., in 1376–7, to £2 9s. 2d.

But, as at Brightwell, a great change had come over the manor in 1453, for then the whole manor known as the New Court, with its live and dead stock, was let to a farmer at £50 a year, apparently an exorbitant rent if compared with the rent of £18 13s. 4d. for the demesne at Brightwell : true, the area under crop at Brightwell in 1399 was only 112½ acres, while at Downton there were 197 acres : but at Downton, with the demesne, the tenant had acquired the bishop's rights to the tenurial labour of the native tenants, and for that reason was prepared to pay a high rent : the bishop, however, retained in his own hands the perquisites of the court, and the right to require labour from the tenants for the repair of the mill weir.

Comparing then our three manors, we find that labour services were entirely commuted at Witney in or before 1376, at Brightwell in or before 1453, and at Downton probably not till after 1453—another warning against hasty generalizations.

YIELD OF CORN CROPS (IN BUSHELS).

	Wheat.	Barley.	Drage.	Oats.	Pease.	Vetches.
1346	5¼	14		8½	8¼	7
1347	3½	10		8¼	8	5¼
1348	3¾	10¼		16	8	6¼
1349	3¼	7¼		8¼	3¾	2¾
1350	9¾	16		7¾	2	3
1351	4½	13	9	9½	3	2½
1352	14	8¼	14½	9	6½	8
1353	7	12	—	5		

ADDENDA

P. 32, l. 18. On the other hand, labour might be hired for special reasons, where the villein services were commonly sufficient. E. g. at Twyford, in 1212–13, 4s. was paid to extra harvesters, hired *pro timore pluvie*.

P. 33, l. 15. *Benhurche* is not ' boon-harrowing ', as one might imagine, but a corruption of Benerthe, a ploughing service. *Forhors* would seem to mean supplying a man to lead the team, a *fugator*, but in one case it is said to be due only ' when the lord comes '.

P. 37, l. 32. A marginal note on the Waltham account for 1301–2 directs that services shall be commuted (sold) to the poor and the old, while they shall be performed by the rich and the strong. Although the charitable principle hardly seems to have been acted upon, it shows that the rate of commutation was considered beneficial to the tenant.

P. 50, l. 27. At Morton, in 1212, fines of £14 and £17 6s. 8d. were paid by Robert and John de la Berie, but the size of their holdings is not given. At Sutton in the same year a fine of £4 was paid.

l. 31. A cursory examination of lists of fines in the sixteenth and even in the eighteenth century suggests that on the Winchester estates the rates at which fines were levied had increased very slightly ; small sums of less than £5 are the most common.

P. 54, l. 22. At Nailesbourne, 1301–2, £6 13s. 4d. was paid for a messuage, one virgate and eight acres of free land, but it is not clear whether the whole tenement or only the eight acres, was free. At Woodhay a fine was paid for one-fifth of a knight's fee.

P. 80. The Rental referred to on p. 10 shows that early in the fourteenth century Waltham proper contained 238 holdings, many of them houses and gardens, while seven of the outlying tithings contained 367 holdings, and the totals for two tithings are partly illegible. Of course some of these tenements were held in groups, but there are very few virgates.

INDEXES

I. PLACE-INDEX

Names marked with an asterisk are not episcopal manors; the unmarked names form a complete list of the episcopal manors as entered in the Pipe Roll; names marked † are apparently subdivisions of episcopal manors.

II. SUBJECT-INDEX

X

RURAL NORTHAMPTONSHIRE UNDER THE COMMONWEALTH

A STUDY BASED PRINCIPALLY UPON THE PARLIAMENTARY SURVEYS OF THE ROYAL ESTATES

BY

REGINALD LENNARD, M.A.

LECTURER IN MODERN HISTORY AT WADHAM COLLEGE, OXFORD, AND LECTURER TO THE WORKERS' EDUCATIONAL ASSOCIATION

PREFACE

I wish to express my gratitude to those who have helped me with advice in the preparation of this essay. To the Editor of this series I owe not only my first acquaintance with the Parliamentary Surveys but much guidance in their study. Professor C. H. Firth very kindly read the manuscript of the first chapter and gave me valuable advice. On some philological points I have had the advantage of advice from Dr. Henry Bradley, and I am also indebted for help in various ways to Mr. A. E. Bland and Mr. C. Hilary Jenkinson of the Public Record Office, and to the Librarian at Lambeth Palace. Some of the earlier surveys of Grafton and Hartwell were transcribed for me; but in the case of all the Parliamentary Surveys and most of the other MSS. I have been my own scribe.

The pressure of other work has somewhat delayed the correction of proofs.

REGINALD LENNARD.

October 18, 1915.

CONTENTS

CHAPTER I

THE ORIGIN OF THE PARLIAMENTARY SURVEYS

1. The financial exigencies of the Puritan Government

THE Parliament which wrested sovereign power from Charles I soon found itself embarrassed by financial difficulties at least as serious as those which had brought ruin upon the King. Even he had been troubled not only by the obstinate repugnance to his policy exhibited by Parliament, but also by the extraordinary expenditure which that policy involved. Parliament tried to cut off supplies; but the ordinary supplies, if they had been forthcoming, would have been quite insufficient for the royal needs; and it may be argued with some plausibility that it was the heavy expenses of the wars which caused the breach of 1629, and induced the fatal experiment of despotism, and that the crisis of the reign was precipitated by the financial strain of the two 'Bishops' Wars'.[1] The ordinary revenue was quite incapable of supporting any unusual expenses; and it is quite clear that in the subsequent period the chief embarrassments of the Long Parliament were produced not so much by any failure in the ordinary sources of revenue, or by any insufficiency in the control exercised by the executive over them, as by the rising tide of expenditure. The financial history of the Great Rebellion and the Commonwealth is still unwritten, so generalizations on the subject must be tentative; but there can be no doubt that the maintenance of enormous armaments, which the state of affairs necessitated, was the great source of difficulty for the Government and the real cause of the novel and manifold devices for raising money to which it had recourse, though, on the other hand, some allowance must be made for the disorganization of the

[1] v. G. W. Prothero, Cambridge Modern History, vol. iv, ch. viii, pp. 269, 274.

Exchequer,[1] and for the reaction of civil strife and foreign war upon the prosperity of the country and the yield of the older taxes.[2] Gardiner, writing of the situation in 1647, says ' there had been an enormous increase of the public burdens, though it is impossible to calculate, even conjecturally, what that increase was '.[3] He adds that ' the greater part of the increase was upon the army and navy', and says ' it appears from a report from the Committee of Accounts . . . that before the formation of the New Model Army, the expense of the

[1] v. W. A. Shaw, Cambridge Modern History, vol. iv, ch. xv, p. 454. He says that ' many of the Exchequer officials had followed the King to Oxford, carrying with them the mysterious knowledge which was necessary for the working of that ancient institution'.

[2] An interesting statement about the decay of trade produced by the Civil Wars was made in 1650 to a Parliamentary Committee by Thos. Violet, v. Calendar of State Papers (Domestic), 1650, p. 178, no. 61, quoted by W. Cunningham, Growth of English Industry and Commerce in Modern Times (1907), p. 190. This may be compared with the evidence afforded by the tract called The Mournful Cryes of many thousand Poore Tradesmen who are ready to famish through decay of Trade, which belongs to the beginning of the year 1647 and is quoted by Cunningham, ibid. pp. 182–3, footnote ; cp. F. C. Montague, Political History of England, vol. vii (1907), p. 322. The output of literature about agriculture, so plentiful in the period 1635–42 and after 1651, seems practically to have ceased in the years between 1642 and 1650 ; and Mr. R. E. Prothero points out that ' between 1640 and 1670 not more than six patents were taken out for agricultural improvements ', though he mentions nine such patents which belong to the period 1623–40 : v. English Farming Past and Present (1912), pp. 104–5. But other factors besides war affected the economic situation : corn was cheap during the first Civil War and it is the six bad harvests from 1646 onwards which make the decennial average price of wheat, barley, and oats higher in the period 1643–52 than in any other decade from the death of Elizabeth to the death of Anne (1603–1702), v. J. E. Thorold Rogers, History of Agriculture and Prices, vol. v (1887), pp. 203–9, 276. One piece of evidence witnesses to the surprising fact that luxury was increasing. Lady Verney, in May 1647, wrote in a letter to her husband : ' As long as I have lived in London I never in my life saw half that bravery amongst all sorts of people as is now. Truly I think they have a greater vanity for clothes and coaches than I think was ever in the world. .There are those that make every week or fortnight a new gown.' v. S. R. Gardiner, History of the Great Civil War, vol. iv (1905), p. 78. It is none the less certain that the receipts from customs declined in the time of trouble. Gardiner gives some figures which he obtained from the Audit Office Declared Accounts : it appears that ' in 1635 the customs brought in £328,000 ', but the annual average revenue from this source during the five years 1643–47 was only £224,000 ; v. op. cit., vol. iii, p. 193. After the King's death there was, however, an improvement and the net customs revenue from all sources amounted in 1654–5 to £501,000 ; v. Hubert Hall, The Customs Revenue of England (1885), vol. ii, Appendix, p. 246 ; cp. ibid., vol. i, p. 184.

[3] v. S. R. Gardiner, Great Civil War, vol. iii (1905), p. 192.

navy was about £235,000 a year, and that of the army about £440,000 ', though ' this result is . . . far from being complete, as ordnance stores and money spent on local forces are left out of the account, more than 10,000 soldiers, for instance, being employed in garrisons '.[1] Dr. G. W. Prothero and Colonel E. M. Lloyd consider that even at the beginning of the Civil War the cost of the army amounted to a million a year and that of the navy to £300,000.[2] With regard to the expenditure of the Commonwealth, Professor Firth writes that, ' taking the whole period from the King's death to the Restoration, it is clear that the cost of the army ran from £1,200,000 to about £2,000,000 per annum '.[3] The expenses of the navy, apparently for a year, were estimated in 1651 at £589,317, in 1652 at £985,000 (in addition to £300,000 spent in building new frigates), and in 1655 at £903,532.[4] That the ordinary sources of supply were incapable of producing such enormous sums as these is abundantly evident. ' In 1651', writes Professor F. C. Montague, ' the public expenses amounted to £2,750,000, or thrice the total revenue of Charles I in his most prosperous years.' [5]

2. The inadequacy of the revenue raised by taxation

In facing its extraordinary obligations, the Parliamentary Government, even before the King's death, showed both energy and ingenuity. ' In the taxes imposed by the parliamentary ordinances ', says Dowell, ' we find the germs of our subsequent fiscal system.' [6] But no amount of energy and no degree of ingenuity could overcome the obstinate fact that, as years passed, the hold of the Puritan Government upon the sympathies of the nation was becoming more and more feeble. As the need for increased expenditure became

[1] v. S. R. Gardiner, op. cit., vol. iii, p. 192, footnote.
[2] v. Cambridge Modern History, vol. iv, ch. x, p. 310.
[3] v. C. H. Firth, Cromwell's Army (1902), p. 185.
[4] v. S. R. Gardiner, History of the Commonwealth and Protectorate (1903), vol. ii, p. 21, footnote, and p. 200, and vol. iii, p. 238, footnote.
[5] v. F. C. Montague, Political History, p. 382 ; cp. S. R. Gardiner, Commonwealth and Protectorate, vol. ii, p. 21.
[6] v. Stephen Dowell, History of Taxes and Taxation in England (1884), vol. ii, p. 4.

greater, so also the reluctance of the taxpayers to bear additional burdens became more pronounced. The Smithfield riot against the excise in February 1647, and the opposition offered to the renewal of the monthly assessments in the debates of the Nominated Parliament in November 1653, illustrate the public hostility to taxation.[1] It was impossible for the Government to pay its way merely by raising fresh taxes. Dr. W. A. Shaw has calculated that ' on an average there was a deficit of from £400,000 to £500,000 yearly on the total expenditure of the three kingdoms ',[2] and even the most casual survey of the political history of the period reveals the tremendous consequences which ensued from the fact that the pay of the army was constantly in arrears. It was in order to make some headway against the annual deficit, and especially to allay the discontent of the army by the payment of arrears, that recourse was had to the sale of the various estates which passed into the hands of the legislature.

3. The policy of selling land

The policy of living on capital readily commends itself to those in financial distress, and the particular forms which this policy assumed under the rule of the Puritans had little that was really novel about them. Just as the sale of the King's pictures can be paralleled by the use the Royalists made of melted plate, so in the sale of the Crown Lands the Parliament followed a precedent which had been set by Charles himself.[3] Indeed, it is not impossible to trace some phases of the policy to much more venerable antecedents. The Parliament was following the example of William the Conqueror, who treated his opponents in England as rebels : opposition to the new Government was treason and the King was beheaded on the

[1] v. S. R. Gardiner, Great Civil War, vol. iii, p. 216 ; Commonwealth and Protectorate, vol. ii, pp. 311–13.

[2] v. Cambridge Modern History, vol. iv, ch. xv, p. 457.

[3] ' Charles I,' writes Mr. S. R. S. Bird, ' in his endeavour to support the expenses of his Government without the aid of Parliament, sold many of the estates of the Crown.' v. Hubert Hall and S. R. S. Bird, Notes on the History of the Crown Lands, in the Antiquary, vol. xiii (1886), p. 195. As regards the principle of confiscating the lands of rebels, a precedent had been set by Charles I when he gave his consent to the Act of 1640 [16 Ch. I, ch. 33], which was directed against the Irish rebels.

theory that he was guilty of high treason. Such a theory naturally led to the confiscation of the Crown Lands and the estates of delinquents; and the financial strain forced the Government to realize what it could by sales instead of merely drawing rents. As regards the episcopal and capitular estates, the use which Henry VIII made of the lands of the dissolved monasteries may perhaps be quoted as almost parallel.

4. The policy of Parliament with regard to the estates of Delinquents

Even before the imposition of the excise, the principle that the estates of the delinquents should be sequestrated to help pay for the war found acceptance with the Parliament. It was foreshadowed in a Declaration of the Houses on September 2, 1642, partially enforced in October, and made applicable to all delinquents by an Ordinance of March 27, 1643.[1] As yet, however, only the revenue of the sequestered lands was to be touched. But soon delinquents judged worthy of mercy were allowed to compound for their estates—a change which indicates, on the one hand, a desire to win over deserters from the King, and, on the other hand, a tendency to prefer the realization of a capital sum to the receipt of a regular income derived from rents. Compounding was authorized in the case of some of those who had taken part in the ' late Rebellious Insurrection in the County of Kent ' by an Ordinance of August 16, 1643 ;[2] and a basis for the extension of the policy during the two succeeding years may be found in the ' Declaration of Both Kingdoms ' of Jan. 30, 1644, which asserts that those authorized to compound with delinquents ' will be as careful to prevent their ruin as to punish their Delinquencies ', and that ' the time of their returning and offering themselves, the reality of their affections and intentions, and readiness, to joyne in the common Cause, and Covenant, will be taken into speciall consideration '.[3] Another merciful provision

[1] v. S. R. Gardiner, Civil War, vol. i, pp. 17, 37, 100 ; C. H. Firth and R. S. Rait, Acts and Ordinances of the Interregnum (1911), vol. i, pp. 106–17.
[2] v. Firth and Rait, op. cit., vol. i, pp. 247–8.
[3] v. Calendar of the Committee for Compounding, Part V (1892), Introduction, pp. v to ix.

occurs in the Ordinance of Aug. 18, 1643, which empowered
the Committees for Sequestrations to make allowance for the
maintenance of delinquents' families, provided such allowance
did not exceed one-fifth of the goods and estates seized.[1]
A good deal is said in this Ordinance about the sale of goods
and estates ; but the language used is vague and hard to
interpret, and it is impossible to regard this Ordinance as
initiating a definite policy of sale, for the sales of land contemplated may have been simply in the way of distraint when
the revenue of the sequestered lands was not forthcoming.
The Ordinance states that those classed as delinquents shall
' forfeit as Papists within this and the said former Ordinances ;
and Seizure and Sequestration of two-thirds parts of all their
Goods and Estates Real and Personal, and Sale of such
proportion of their Goods so seized and Sequestred, shall be
made and their Rents and Estates disposed of, in such manner
and proportion, and by such Persons as by the said Ordinance
of Sequestrations is appointed for Papists '. But the ' Goods '
here appointed to be sold may be goods other than landed
property, especially as the former Ordinance of March 27
had instructed the Sequestrators to ' let, set, and demise '
two parts of all the lands of Papists. And though in another
place the ordinance of Aug. 18 speaks of the ' sale of all such
goods and estates as are and shall be seized, and are appointed
to be sold by this or the said former Ordinance ', this passage
immediately follows a paragraph which is concerned with
sales of a delinquent's ' goods and estate ' by way of distress
for rents, debts and so forth.[2] At all events, a later Ordinance
—one of May 25, 1644—provides that all sequestered Houses
and Lands ' now standing void and unlet, shall forthwith be
Let, Tenanted, or improved ' ;[3] and there is a long series of
Ordinances, down to the very eve of the Restoration, which
contemplate the receipt of rents from the estates of delinquents.
On the other hand, it is clear that the sale of delinquents'
estates was occasionally resorted to. On July 10, 1644, the
House of Commons issued an order that a Committee at

[1] v. Firth and Rait, op. cit., vol. i, p. 258.
[2] v. ibid., pp. 256, 107, 258.   [3] v. ibid., pp. 438-9.

Goldsmiths' Hall should consider the feasibility of raising
a month's pay for the Scottish army out of delinquents'
estates either by sale or otherwise, and should draw up a list
of delinquents' estates fit to be sold and report at how many
years' purchase the sales were to be effected.[1] In the same
month of the following year, it was decreed that the money
to be levied for the troops needed to relieve ' the Counties of
Oxon, Bucks, Berks, and Southampton ' should be repaid
' to all and every person and persons disbursing the same
respectively, out of the Moneys to be raised by the sale of
Delinquents' Estates, next and immediately after the Two
hundred thousand pounds already charged thereon shall be
paid '.[2] Again, in October 1645 it is expressly stated that
the settlement of a revenue out of delinquents' estates upon
the Elector Palatine shall not be a bar to the sale of the
pledged estates, provided that the sum of £6,000 per annum
charged on the land is made good in some other way.[3]

On the whole, the policy of the Government seems to have
been to draw a revenue from the lands of ordinary delinquents,
to raise a capital sum from those who could be induced to
compound,[4] and at length to inflict the full penalty of forfeiture for treason, followed by sale of their estates, in the
case of peculiarly contumacious opponents of the Commonwealth. The process of compounding often led to more
drastic measures, for, according to Miss M. A. E. Green, the
sale of part of an estate ' was frequently necessary before the
second half of the fine could be paid '.[5] A more severe policy
can be traced in an Ordinance of June 9, 1646, which passed
the House of Commons but failed, so it seems, to receive the

[1] v. Calendar of the Committee for Compounding, vol. i, p. 6 (12).
[2] v. Ordinance of July 18, 1645, Firth and Rait, op. cit., vol. i, p. 736.
[3] v. Ordinance of October 8, 1645, Firth and Rait, op. cit., vol. i, p. 786.
[4] ' The fines ', says Miss M. A. E. Green, ' varied in amount from two-
thirds to a tenth of the value of the compounder's estate, according to
the more or less aggravated circumstances of his delinquency ; ' but, she
adds, the ' difference in the rates of fine was not quite so great as *prima
facie* it appeared to be, because there was a different mode of calculation
for the different classes of compounders ', and those ' fined at a tenth paid
at the rate of 20 years' purchase, or 2 years' value of their estates ', while
' those fined at two-thirds paid only at 12 years' purchase ' : v. Calendar
of Committee for Compounding, Part V, p. x.
[5] v. ibid., Part I, Preface, p. x.

assent of the House of Lords. This Ordinance was to the effect that those who had not come in to compound before the preceding first of May should forfeit, in some cases all, and in others two-thirds, of their estates. It appears that a modified form of this decree was actually passed : forfeiture was to be the penalty if delinquents did not compound before Oct. 3, 1646.[1] As a matter of fact, however, compounding went on long after that date ; so the decree must be regarded as being of the nature of an inoperative threat. At the same time, it indicates a wish for a more rapid receipt of money than the process of compounding, unstimulated by threats, was likely to afford. This wish showed itself in a more definite shape in October 1649. ' The present mode ', it was said, ' cannot conduce to the end, which is to raise considerable sums in a reasonable time, whereas now it comes in by driblets, passes through many hands, and comes in a dilatory way.'[2] Administrative changes followed, which form part of a general and much needed movement to reduce the unmanageable complications of the numerous financial committees of the Puritan Government.[3] At length, too, the policy of confiscation and sale was definitely adopted. On July 16, 1651, an Act was passed declaring the estates of 73 delinquents to be forfeited for treason, and providing that these estates should be surveyed and sold—the immediate tenants being allowed pre-emption and a minimum price of ten years' purchase being fixed.[4] This was followed on Aug. 4, 1652, by a second Act of a similar nature containing 29 names,[5] while a third Act, of Nov. 18, 1652,[6] contains 678 names, being those ' of all sequestered delinquents who had not compounded, or had not paid the remainder of their fines.'[7] Yet compounding was still permitted in the case of those who had not committed ' any Act of Treason or Rebellion ' since the King's death.[8]

[1] v. Calendar of Committee for Compounding, Part I, Preface, p. xi.
[2] v. ibid., p. 160.
[3] v. W. A. Shaw, Cambridge Modern History, vol. iv, ch. xv, pp. 455–6.
[4] v. Firth and Rait, op. cit., vol. ii, pp. 520–45.
[5] v. ibid. vol. ii, pp. 591–8.   [6] v. ibid., vol. ii, pp. 623–52.
[7] v. M. A. E. Green, Calendar of Committee for Compounding, Part I, Preface, p. xix.
[8] v. Firth and Rait, op. cit., vol. ii, pp. 644–6 and p. 650. Miss Green

5. The treatment of the episcopal estates

Meanwhile, the policy of raising money by the sale of land had been developing in other directions. The abolition of episcopacy, which had been approved by both Houses of Parliament so early as September 1642,[1] was accomplished by an Ordinance of Oct. 9, 1646, and this same Ordinance provided that the bishops' lands should be vested in trustees —the immediate object being to get some security for the remuneration of the Scots.[2] Surveyors were to be appointed ; and a subsequent Ordinance of Oct. 13 initiated the practice of ' doubling '—' my dear friend Dr. Burgess's singular invention ', as Baillie calls it.[3] Any old creditor of the Government might, by advancing a further sum equal to his original loan and any arrears of interest due upon it, have both the old and the new debt secured out of ' the Receipt of the Grand Excise ' and ' the sale of the Bishops' Lands '. There was to be a ' speedy sale ' of the bishops' lands, advowsons and impropriations excepted ; [4] and a lengthy and detailed Ordinance of Nov. 17, 1646, provides for the sale of these lands at not less than ten years' purchase ' of the full values they were at in the year 1641 '.[5] Dr. W. A. Shaw gives a list of 23 later Ordinances relating to the episcopal estates, the last being that of Oct. 12, 1652 ; [6] but the policy of selling and doubling dates back to the time when the lands were first seized by the State on the abolition of episcopacy, and the subsequent explanations and modifications need not be discussed here.

suggests that lack of purchasers caused the continuance of compounding, though on severe terms. Presumably she is speaking of the case of persons who had been guilty of ' treason ' since January 30, 1649. v. op. cit., Part I, Preface, pp. xix–xx. [1] v. Gardiner, Civil War, vol. i, p. 19.

[2] v. Firth and Rait, op. cit., vol. i, pp. 879–83 ; cp. Gardiner, Civil War, vol. iii, p. 145. Long before this the estates of some bishops had been sequestered as those of individual delinquents. v. W. A. Shaw, History of the English Church, 1640–60 (1900), vol. ii, p. 206.

[3] v. Baillie's Letters, II, 411, quoted by W. A. Shaw, op. cit., vol. ii, p. 212, footnote. For the whole subject of the treatment of episcopal and capitular estates, Dr. Shaw's book is invaluable.

[4] v. Firth and Rait, op. cit., vol. i, p. 884.

[5] v. ibid., vol. i, pp. 887–904. Besides advowsons and impropriations, certain other exceptions were made: e. g. the *jura regalia* of the bishoprics of Durham and Ely.

[6] v. W. A. Shaw, op. cit., vol. ii, pp. 211–12, footnote.

6. The treatment of the lands of Deans and Chapters

What was sauce for the bishop was sauce also for the dean.
' The Ordinance for dean and chapter lands ', says Dr. W. A.
Shaw, ' had been ordered to be brought in at the same time
as the Bill for bishops' lands ', but he adds that ' as the sale of
the bishops' lands had served its turn it was not for two years
and more that the Commons turned to the capitular lands
again with the idea of raising money from them, although
they were specially referred to in the propositions for the
King in October 1647.'[1] Gardiner calls attention to a letter
which Fairfax wrote to Lenthall on Nov. 9, asking that the
payment of the soldiers might be provided for by the sale of
the estates of the deans and chapters.[2] But perhaps the
possibility of an arrangement with the King postponed the
adoption of extreme measures ; for though an Ordinance for
the abolition of deans and chapters was introduced into the
House of Commons some months before the King's death,[3]
it was not until April 30, 1649, that an Act was passed
providing at one blow for the abolition of the deans and
chapters of cathedrals and collegiate churches, for the
surveying of their estates, and for the sale of the estates
at not less than twelve years' purchase. Reservations were
made similar to those in the Ordinance of Nov. 17, 1646, for
the sale of the episcopal estates, and ' doubling ' was provided
for.[4] Further Ordinances were issued from time to time with
regard to the treatment of the capitular estates, and of these

[1] v. W. A. Shaw, op. cit., vol. ii, p. 213, footnote, and S. R. Gardiner,
Constitutional Documents of the Puritan Revolution, 2nd edition (1899),
p. 343.   [2] v. Gardiner, Civil War, vol. iv, p. 12.
[3] On September 6, 1648 ; v. W. A. Shaw, op. cit., vol. ii, p. 213, footnote.
[4] v. Firth and Rait, op. cit., vol. ii, pp. 81–104, and Shaw, op. cit., vol. ii,
p. 213. Ludlow definitely connects the policy of selling the capitular
estates with military exigencies. ' The Parliament ', he writes, ' having
an army ready to send to Ireland, a formidable fleet to put to sea, another
army to keep at home for their own defence, and a considerable force to
guard the north against the Scots, who had declared themselves enemies,
and waited only an opportunity of showing it with advantage, thought
themselves obliged to expose to sale such lands as had been formerly
possessed by Deans and Chapters, that they might be enabled thereby to
defray some part of that great charge that lay upon the nation.' v.
Ludlow's Memoirs [ed. C. H. Firth, 1894], vol. i, p. 231.

Ordinances Dr. W. A. Shaw gives a list. The last of them
was issued on Sept. 2, 1654.[1]

7. The treatment of the Royal Estates

The prophecy of James I, ' No Bishop, no King', received
its fulfilment in the execution of his son and the Act of
March 17, 1649, abolishing the kingly office. And as the
monarchy had followed the episcopate, so the royal lands
were soon subjected to treatment similar to that applied to
the estates of the bishops, and the Parliament was thus able
to make a logical and consistent virtue of what was really
a stern financial necessity. So early as Sept. 21, 1643, an
Ordinance had been issued for the appropriation of all the
royal revenues,[2] and less than six months after the King's
death the sale, first of the personal estate,[3] and then of the
lands of ' the late King, Queen, and Prince ' was decreed.
The Act dealing with the landed estates is dated July 16, 1649.[4]
It begins by rehearsing the great need of the Parliament, and
mentions the ' very great Debts ' contracted for the Army
and the arrears due to the officers and soldiers ; and states
that ' whereas the late King, the Queen and their eldest Son,
have been the chief Authors of the late Wars and troubles '
it follows ' in all Justice and Equity ' that they ' ought to
bear the burthen of the said Debts, and their Estates in the
first place to be applyed to take off and discharge the same,
it being the duty, and especial care and endeavor of the
Parliament, that the people should not in any sort be taxed
and charged, but in cases of inevitable necessity, and when
other ways and means are wanting '. In its administrative
arrangements, the Act bears considerable resemblance to the
Ordinance of Nov. 17, 1646, for the sale of the episcopal lands.
The estates were to be vested in trustees, who were authorized
to appoint surveyors and stewards of manors. Contractors
were also appointed to arrange the sales : none of them was
to be himself a purchaser, and each was to take an oath that

[1] v. W. A. Shaw, op. cit., vol. ii, pp. 213-4, footnote.
[2] v. Firth and Rait, op. cit., vol. i, pp. 299-303.
[3] v. ibid., vol. ii, pp. 160-8.   [4] v. ibid., vol. ii, pp. 168-91.

he would discharge his trust without favour. The surveyors
were also to take an oath, in the case of the royal lands, that
they would make true surveys according to their ' best skill
and cunning ', and take no gift or reward other than the
allowance made for their pains and expenses by the trustees ;
and the Ordinance for the sale of the bishops' lands, the
rules of which in regard to surveyors were to be observed
by the surveyors of the Crown lands, had provided that ' no
Surveyor, or any his Child or Children, or any in trust for
him or them, shall be admitted to be a Purchaser of the
Lands surveyed, or to be surveyed by himself, upon pain of
losing his or their purchase Money and the purchase to be
void '.[1] The surveyors were authorized to hold courts of
survey and to examine witnesses upon oath. Both in the
provisions for the bishops' lands and in those for the Crown
lands, treasurers, a ' comptroller ', and a ' register and keeper '
were appointed. Another official to be appointed by the
trustees under the Act of July 16, 1649, was the ' register of
debentures ', whose duties seem to have been similar to those
of the ' register accomptant ' in the case of the bishops' lands.
Yet all was not repetition : experience had taught Parliament
new administrative needs. An Ordinance of Nov. 21, 1648,
had appointed a committee for the removal of obstructions
to the sale of the episcopal lands ;[2] but in regard to the royal
lands, as in the case of the capitular estates, the appointment
of a similar committee was contemplated in the initial Act
for the sale of the lands.[3] Another point in which the Act
of July 16 follows the precedent set in the Act for the abolition
of deans and chapters in preference to that of the Ordinance of
Nov. 17, 1646, is in the appointment of Colonel William Webb
as surveyor-general. In both cases this appointment was
made because of the ' many neglects and imperfections in

[1] v. Firth and Rait, op. cit., vol. i, p. 902 ; vol. ii, p. 172.
[2] v. ibid., vol. i, pp. 1227-33.
[3] v. ibid., vol. ii, pp. 97, 187. An Act of June 20, 1649, appointed the
committee for the capitular estates, and this committee apparently took
over the work of the committee which had been appointed on November 21
to deal with the bishops' lands, while the same persons were authorized to
deal with the royal lands by an Act of February 18, 1650 ; v. Firth and
Rait, op. cit., vol. ii, pp. 152-4, 338-42.

the surveys of the late Bishops Lands', by which ' the sale of the same hath been much retarded '.[1]

For the sale of the Crown lands other than castles, houses, and palaces, a list of minimum prices was fixed.[2] The lands were not to be sold out and out for less than 13 years' purchase. For the sale of reversions of the lands on leases the minimum price was six and a half years' purchase when the lease was for one life, three and a half years' purchase when it was for two, and two and a half years' purchase when it was for three lives. In the case of leases for years, six and a half years' purchase was to be the minimum price for the sale of a reversion upon a lease for seven years, while 4¼ years' purchase was fixed when the lease was for 14 years, and 3 years' purchase when it was for 21 years. It was enacted that ' all other Reversions upon Leases for more or fewer yeers, shall be sold proportionably to this Rule '.[3]

[1] v. Firth and Rait, op. cit., vol. ii, pp. 93, 173.
[2] An Ordinance of December 2, 1647 had allowed ' any Castles, Places, or other Houses ' belonging to the bishops to be sold by the contractors ' as they shall conceive most conducing to the advantage and benefit of the Commonwealth, though at lower rates then their materials are valued by the Surveys returned thereof'. This exception was extended to royal castles, houses, and palaces other than those reserved from sale altogether. v. Firth and Rait, op. cit., vol. i, p. 1030 ; vol. ii, p. 176.
[3] v. Firth and Rait, op. cit., vol. ii, pp. 176-7. The changes in the minimum prices fixed for the sale of lands are many and hard to account for. In 1646, ten years' purchase was the minimum for the bishops' lands; v. supra, p.15 ; Firth and Rait, op. cit., vol. i, p. 902. On April 30, 1649, 12 years' purchase was fixed for the capitular estates, and creditors of the State who wished to receive lands in discharge of the debt owed them could only take the land at 15 years' purchase unless they first advanced a further sum of money by way of doubling ; v. ibid., vol. ii, pp. 87, 103. It seems, however, that this scale of prices proved too high, and on June 25 the Parliament, ' taking into consideration how expedient it is for this Commonwealth, that speedy Sale be made of the premises, for the present raising of moneys ', reduced the minimum rate for the capitular estates to ten years' purchase for ready money and to 13 years for purchase by transference of debt without doubling ; v. ibid., vol. ii, pp. 155-6. In July, 13 years' purchase was the minimum established for the royal lands, and creditors might deduct the amount owed them from the price, if they paid in money the percentage of the gross price due as fees to the officials, v. ibid., vol. ii, pp. 176, 184-5. This last requirement was made inoperative in the case of soldiers on February 18, 1650, v. ibid., vol. ii, p. 339. For the estates forfeited in 1651 and 1652, ten years' purchase was the minimum, v. ibid., vol. ii, pp. 528, 594, 644. For sales under the Deafforestation Act of November 22, 1653, it was 14 years, v. ibid., vol. ii, p. 796. In the case of the fee farm rents, 8 years' purchase was the minimum established at

The Act provided that the immediate tenants should have a right of pre-emption for 30 days from the return of the surveys. After that, liberty of pre-emption was reserved for a further period of ten days to 'such of the Original Creditors, their Heirs, Executors and Administrators or any of them, who shall desire to become Purchasers of any the Lands mentioned in this Act, with Debentures given immediately to them the Original Creditors, and not by way of assignment from others'.[1] Any lands which were not already leased were in the interval before sale to be let on lease 'for one year or less, and so from year to year or less', at the best rent that could be got. Copyholds were to be demised 'by Copy of Court-Roll'.[2]

The Act did not extend to certain castles, palaces and manors which were mentioned by name, nor to the royal forests, nor 'to any Timber Trees fit for the use and service of the Publique Navy of this Commonwealth, which are now growing or being within fifteen miles of any River fit for conveyance of such Timber'. Again, it was provided that the Act should not extend to 'any Fee-farm Rents, or other Rents now due and payable to the Commonwealth out of any such Manors, Lands or other Hereditaments, where there hath not been reserved in the Crown any Right or Propriety in or to such Manors, Lands or Hereditaments, other then the Rents reserved.'[3]

But these various exceptions were not long maintained. An Act of March 11, 1650,[4] followed by others on Aug. 13, 1650;[5] Feb. 6, 1651;[6] June 3, 1652;[7] Sept. 9, 1652;[8] and Sept. 8, 1653,[9] provided for the sale of the fee farm rents. Certain castles, parks and the like, specially exempted in 1649, were delivered over for sale by an Act of Dec. 31, 1652.[10]

---

first (March 11, 1650) ; but later enactments, the terms of which suggest that the law was not being kept, fix it at 10 years ; v. ibid., vol. ii, pp. 360, 499, 584, 616.

[1] v. Firth and Rait, op. cit., vol. ii, pp. 176, 191.
[2] v. ibid., vol. ii, p. 180.   [3] v. ibid., vol. ii, pp. 188–91, 171.
[4] v. ibid., vol. ii, pp. 358–62.   [5] v. ibid., vol. ii, pp. 412–19.
[6] v. ibid., vol. ii, pp. 498–500.   [7] v. ibid., vol. ii, pp. 583–8.
[8] v. ibid., vol. ii, pp. 614–18.
[9] v. ibid., vol. ii, pp. 720–2.   [10] v. ibid., vol. ii, pp. 691–6.

An Act ' for the Deafforestation, Sale and Improvement of the Forests and of The Honors, Manors, Lands, Tenements and Hereditaments within the usual Limits and Perambulations of the same ' was passed on Nov. 22, 1653.[1]

8. The policy of Sale in its political aspects

By such stages and in such ways the policy of selling land developed. The political wisdom or unwisdom of that policy might be discussed at length. On the one hand, it made the new order of things one which many could never be expected to accept. It filled the ranks of the irreconcilable opponents of the Commonwealth. On the other hand, it should be remarked that in the case of ordinary delinquents, compounding and not sale was the primary aim of Parliament and that the opportunity of compounding did detach considerable numbers from the Royalist cause, while the sale of lands created strong vested interests pledged to the support of the revolutionary system. ' Every acre of land sold ', says Gardiner, ' was a bond attaching the purchaser to the Commonwealth.' [2]

It was no doubt this aspect of the matter which appealed to Baillie, who, after praising the efficacy of 'doubling' as a means of attracting purchasers, says : ' By this means we gett the bishops' lands on our backs without any grudge and in a way that no skill will get them back againe.' [3] In this relation, too, the Puritan policy can be compared with many historical parallels—with the disposal of the monastic estates by Henry VIII, which formed an effective obstacle to restoration in the reign of Mary, and with the policy of Revolutionary France in regard to the estates of the Crown, the Church, and the émigrés.[4]

---

[1] v. Firth and Rait, op. cit., vol. ii, pp. 783–812.
[2] v. Gardiner, Commonwealth and Protectorate, vol. i, p. 251.
[3] v. Baillie's Letters, II, 411, quoted by W. A. Shaw, History of the English Church, 1640–60, vol. ii, pp. 212–13, footnote.
[4] The French *assignats* may be compared with the ' debentures ' of the Commonwealth. In regard to the former Mirabeau said : ' Partout où se placera un *assignat-monnaie*, là sûrement reposera avec lui un vœu secret pour le crédit des assignats, un désir de leur solidité ; partout où quelque partie de ce gage public sera répandue, là se trouveront des hommes qui

9. The financial aspects of the policy

But whatever may be thought of the political aspects
of the policy of sale, there can be no doubt that it was
really moulded by financial needs, and it is primarily
on financial grounds that it must be judged. And, in
the first place, there is no denying the fact that the
sales did relieve the pressing necessities of the Government.
Of the money brought in by the sale of the episcopal lands
nothing seems to be known; but a sum of £1,993,951 was
realized on the Crown lands by sales and doubling, and the
estates of the deans and chapters produced by similar methods
£980,724 between 1649 and Aug. 31, 1650, and possibly
£503,178 after that date.[1] As has already been mentioned,
Dr. W. A. Shaw estimates that on the total expenditure of
the three kingdoms the annual deficit, due to the excess of
expenses over the regular revenue, amounted under the
Commonwealth to between £400,000 and £500,000. But
he adds : ' It may be very roughly reckoned that the extraordinary sources of income (viz. the sale of Bishops' lands,
Royalist compositions, and the sales of Crown lands and of
Dean and Chapter lands) made up this yearly deficit and
kept the Commonwealth fairly solvent till about 1654, from
which time onwards the deficit became an accruing and ever-
increasing debt.'[2] At the same time, it is obvious that the
policy was financially unsound, and that it can only be
justified, if justified at all, on the ground of emergency.
The conditions of the sales must have caused the lands to be
sold at a price below their proper value. So great an amount
of land must have glutted the market ; while no doubt the
risks attaching to purchases which a restoration of Church
and King might make invalid further tended to depress the

voudront que la conservation de ce gage soit effectuée, que les assignats
soient échangés contre les biens nationaux, et comme enfin le sort de la
Constitution tient à la sûreté de cette ressource, partout où se trouvera un
porteur d'assignats, vous compterez un défenseur nécessaire de vos mesures,
un créancier intéressé à vos succès.' The passage is quoted by Leroy-
Beaulieu, Traité de la science des finances (7th edition), t. II, p. 699.
[1] v. W. A. Shaw, Cambridge Modern History, vol. iv, p. 457.
[2] v. ibid., pp. 457-8.

price. Moreover, the proceeds were used for current expenses :
the Government in selling land was living on capital. In order
to avoid taxation, Parliament got rid of estates which would
have produced an income in perpetuity and have lessened
the burden of taxation in the future. An irreplaceable fund
was drained to meet expenses which showed few signs of
diminishing and were likely to recur with every war.[1] And
not only so. Not only was the fund bound to come to an end.
It was hardly satisfactory even as a means for raising money
rapidly to meet immediate needs. Purchasers hung back, as
was only to be expected ; and the Acts and Ordinances are
noisy with complaints of delay and incitements to greater
speed. A minor obstacle to rapid sale was the necessity of
surveying and valuing the estates before offering them to
buyers.

10. The art of surveying in the sixteenth and seventeenth centuries—The Parliamentary Surveys

The application to rural economy of the undeterred
intelligence and intrepid commercialism of the Tudor age had,
among other consequences, the effect of developing the art
of land surveying. It was by no accident that the author of
the book which, more than any other, marks the advance
made in English agriculture in the first half of the sixteenth
century, was also the writer of a treatise on ' Surveying '. And
while the ' Boke of the Measurynge of Lande ', by Sir Richard
de Benese, which was first published in 1537, shows that

---

[1] The speech which Cromwell made to the first Parliament of the Protectorate on September 4, 1654, is instructive on these points. ' Ay ' ; he
is reported to have said, ' and then all your treasure was exhausted and
spent, when this Government was undertaken : all *accidental* ways of
bringing in treasure " were " to a very inconsiderable sum, consumed ;—
That is to say, the " forfeited " lands are sold, the sums on hand spent ;
rents, fee-farms, King's, Queen's, Prince's, Bishops', Dean-and-Chapters',
delinquents' lands sold. These were *spent* when this Government was
undertaken. I think it 's my duty to let you know so much. And that 's
the reason why the taxes do yet lie so heavy upon the people ; of which we
have abated £30,000 a-month for the next three months.' v. Carlyle's
Letters and Speeches of Oliver Cromwell, ed. S. C. Lomas (1904), vol. ii,
pp. 357–8. Similar criticisms to those in the text have been made by
Mr. Henry Higgs in regard to French finance at the period of the Revolution,
v. Cambridge Modern History, vol. viii, p. 701.

Fitzherbert's 'Surveying' did not stand alone, the plentiful crop of similar literature which appeared in the reigns of Elizabeth and James I witnesses to the continued interest that was taken in the development of estates and helps to throw doubt upon the contrast between the two periods which has been drawn by some modern historians.[1] However this may be, it is clear that the progress made in the theory of surveying had important practical results. The surveys of Crown lands made by order of Parliament at the time of the Great Rebellion are at once the test and the triumph of the contemporary surveyor's art. They are well and carefully made, and that this should be so is an indication that a tough tradition of professional efficiency in surveying had already been established. For the chief care of the Government was for speed. In the instructions for surveyors laid down in the Ordinance of Nov. 17, 1646, for the sale of the bishops' lands, it is expressly provided that ' nothing in the Instructions, Oath, or in this present Ordinance, shall be construed to compel the Surveyors to make any admeasurement of the Lands, or any particular Survey of the number of Acres, unless they in their discretion shall think fit ; the intention of the Houses being, that the said Surveyors should make a speedy return of their several surveys, to the end that a speedy sale may be made thereupon.'[2] These instructions were afterwards applied to the surveyors of the capitular[3] and royal[4] estates ; and though in these latter cases, as has

---

[1] Editions of Fitzherbert's Surveying were issued in 1523, 1526, 1539, 1545 (?), 1546, 1567, and 1587 (?). The dates of the various editions of Richard de Benese's book are uncertain ; but they are supposed to be 1537, 1540, 1562, 1564. Among the treatises on surveying which appeared in the later period may be mentioned : (1) Leonard Digges, Tectonicon, 1556, re-issued 1592, 1625, 1634, 1637, 1647, 1656 ; (2) Valentine Leigh, Most Profitable and Commendable Science of Surveying of Landes, Tenements &c., 1577, re-issued 1578, 1588, 1592, 1596 ; (3) John Norden, The Surveyor's Dialogue, 1607, reissued 1610, 1618 ; (4) W. Folkingham, Feudigraphia, the synopsis or epitome of surveying methodized, 1610 ; (5) Aaron Rathbone, The Surveyor, in foure bookes, 1616. For my knowledge of most of these books I am indebted to M. F. Moore, Two Select Bibliographies of Medieval Historical Study (1912), and to the bibliography in R. E. Prothero, op. cit., pp. 419–30. The dates of editions have been obtained from the catalogues of the Bodleian and British Museum Libraries.

[2] v. Firth and Rait, op. cit., vol. i, pp. 902–3.

[3] v. ibid., vol. ii, pp. 85–6.   [4] v. ibid., vol. ii, p. 172.

already been noticed, a Surveyor-General was appointed to supervise the work and see to the correction of imperfect surveys, the ' neglects and imperfections ' in the surveys of the bishops' lands seem to have been regretted chiefly because they caused a delay in the sale.[1]

The various Parliamentary Surveys which have survived form a most valuable store of information for the economic historian. Of the surveys of episcopal and capitular estates the most important collection is that at Lambeth Palace. The Library there contains 24 large volumes of Parliamentary Surveys, but one of these (volume C) consists of duplicates, while along with the surveys of capitular estates made for the purpose of sale are bound a large number of ' parochial surveys ' made under commissions of April 3, 1650, to discover the value of livings. These latter, however, have an interest of their own, for they ' afford the means of judging of the actual value of the different benefices, and of their relative values as they stood in the middle of the seventeenth century ; and when they speak of the advantage of dividing parishes, of raising chapels to the rank of parish churches, or of connecting neighbouring parishes, they admit us to a view of the distribution of population at that period, and sometimes to the state of the country generally.' [2] A list of all the Lambeth surveys is given in Mr. Hunter's Report in an Appendix (R. 3. b.) to the Report of the Commissioners on the Public Records (1837). The volumes numbered A, B, and C contain ' sale surveys ' of the archbishop's estates ; and the remaining 21 volumes [Lambeth MSS., 902–22] contain, along with ' parochial surveys ', ' sale surveys ' of estates belonging to the deans and chapters of a large number of cathedrals and apparently to several bishops.[3] Besides the Lambeth collection, ' sale surveys ', apparently of capitular estates, were reported to the Committee on Public Records of 1800 to be in the possession of the deans and chapters of Chichester, Ely, Lichfield, St. Paul's, Westminster, Salisbury,

---

[1] v. *supra*, p. 19.

[2] v. Report of Commissioners on the Public Records (1837), p. 395.

[3] v. ibid., pp. 397–411 ; W. A. Shaw, History of the English Church (1640–60), vol. ii, pp. 603–6.

Wells, Winchester, and Worcester, and a MS. 'appearing to be a copy' of a Parliamentary Survey of the lands of the Arch-bishopric of York was reported to be in the custody of the deputy registrar of the archbishop's consistory and prerogative courts.[1] Some surveys of lands belonging to the dean and chapter of Chester are preserved in the British Museum [Addit. MS. 14415].[2] But the documents best known under the name of Parliamentary Surveys are those of the royal lands, together with those made under the Act for the Sale of Fee Farm Rents. The largest group of these surveys is to be found among the records of the late Augmentation Office preserved in the Record Office; but the Record Office also contains a few distinct surveys, along with a considerable number of duplicates of the Augmentation Office surveys, among the records of the Duchy of Lancaster and among the Land Revenue Records [Miscellaneous Books, vols. 276–304], as well as a duplicate of a survey of Hanbridge Manor, Cheshire, among the Miscellaneous Records of the King's Remembrancer in the Exchequer. Another series, mostly duplicates of Augmentation Office surveys relating to Corn-wall, are deposited in the Office of the Duchy of Cornwall.

There is a Calendar of the Augmentation Office surveys and lists of those belonging to the Duchies of Lancaster and Cornwall in the Appendices to the Seventh and Eighth Reports of the Deputy Keeper of the Public Records.[3] Some of the documents in these series are not surveys but short certificates of value, and some are 'copies of various Evidences apparently submitted to the Surveyors', but most of them are surveys signed by the surveyors. According to the Introduction to the above-mentioned Calendar, the 'series throughout is uniformly written on paper of foolscap folio size, each page being 15 inches long and 12 inches wide', and 'with trifling exceptions, the whole series is in perfect

---

[1] v. W. A. Shaw, History of the English Church (1640–60), vol. ii, pp. 605–6, and Report of Commissioners on the Public Records (1837), p. 396.

[2] v. Shaw, op. cit., vol. ii, p. 606.

[3] v. 7th Report (1846), Appendix II, pp. 224–38; 8th Report (1847), Appendix II, pp. 52–81.

condition '. Some idea of the bulk of these records and of the wealth of information which they contain may perhaps be gathered from the fact that the documents of the Augmentation Office series which refer to Northamptonshire are 49 in number and contain 831 leaves. These Northamptonshire documents are the chief source of information used in the succeeding chapters.

CHAPTER II

THE ECONOMY OF THE MANORS OF GRAFTON AND HARTWELL IN NORTHAMPTONSHIRE AS DESCRIBED IN THE PARLIAMENTARY SURVEYS

1. The Surveys and their interpretation

THERE are in all seven Parliamentary Surveys relating to the Manors of Grafton and Hartwell in Northamptonshire. Of these much the longest and most important is the first.[1] It was made in April, 1650, under authority of the Act of July 16, 1649, ' for the sale of the Honors, Manors, Lands heretofore belonging to the late King, Queen and Prince ', and it is entitled ' A survey of the Mannor or Lordship of Grafton being the principalle seate of the Honnō with the Mannor of Hartwell annexed '. It consisted of 102 numbered leaves, one of which appears to be missing.[2] The survey is written, as the Parliamentary Surveys of the Augmentation Office series usually are, on one side of the paper only ; but the backs of some leaves are used for corrections and for reports of actions taken by the Committee ' for the removal of obstructions '.[3] The first entry is a brief statement of the Quit-rents due to the Lord of the Manors of Grafton and Hartwell from the freeholders in the townships and parishes of Hartwell, Hanslope, and Bugbrook. Next come an account of the Rents of Assize, a list of cottages erected on the waste, and a survey of the ruins and premises of Grafton House, ' the principal seate of the Hōnoř ' which ' was by the Parliament fforces demolished '. After this we get the

---

[1] v. P. S. Northants, 20. It is not the earliest in date, but the first of the Grafton Surveys according to the present numbering.

[2] The missing folio is No. 101.

[3] The Act of July 16, 1649, provided for the appointment of a Committee for the Removal of Obstructions as provided in the case of the bishops' lands by the Ordinance of November 21, 1648. Further provision was made in an ' Act for Removing of Obstructions ' of February 18, 1650.

' particulars of all such landes tenements and hereditaments belonging to the Manor of Grafton and Hartwell as are under demise or Graunts either for lives or yeeres '. These form the great bulk of the survey, which concludes with a statement as to the remuneration of the Bailiff and Hayward, a note on the Court Baron and Court Leet, an abstract of the rents and valuations, a ' Rent roll of all tenants belonging to the Manors of Grafton and Hartwell ', and particulars of the ' ffree rents in Hanslopp ' and the ' ffree rents in Hartwell '. The descriptions of holdings let on lease for the most part follow a common form. They begin with an account of the house and its premises, and where there are subordinate tenements attached to the holding a notice of them follows. Then, in order, come the pasture, the arable land and the meadows, each class of land, and sometimes the individual parcels, being separately valued. Lastly there is an account of the lease, its terms and conditions, a statement of the difference between the rent and the total annual value of the holding ' as by the pticulars before appeareth ', and a note as to the number and value of the trees on the premises. The handwriting of the survey is generally easy to read and, except for some errors in arithmetic, great care seems to have been taken to make the work accurate. The survey appears to have received personal revision at the hands of Colonel William Webb, the Surveyor-General. His signature occurs at the end, and corrections and notes signed or initialed by him appear in the margin.[1]

In many respects the other Grafton surveys resemble the first, but they are much shorter, and the information they contain is much less important for the historian of rural economy. The second [2] was made in April, 1656, and contains 22 leaves. It gives an account of 148 acres odd which had apparently been omitted from the first survey and were claimed as part of their purchase by those who had bought certain farms named in that survey. The surveyors reported that the Trustees did not intend to convey to any purchaser any land not surveyed and particularly mentioned in their

---

[1] v. e. g. folio 32.   [2] v. P. S. Northants, 21.

contracts, and that the reversion of the 148 acres was still saleable. The third survey[1] is merely a Feodary of the Honour of Grafton, and throws no light upon agrarian conditions. The fourth[2] is much more important. It is a survey of Grafton and Pottersperry Parks, and was made in December, 1649. The fifth of the series[3] consists of two leaves only, and contains an account of a tenement and 4½ acres of land which were ' claymed by the Inhabitants of the Towne of Grafton '. The surveyors reported that ' nothing appeared unto us to make good there clayme although wee somoned them thereunto ', and the case was therefore left to ' the further consideracon of the hon^{ble} the Trustees '; but a marginal note states that the claim was to be made good. The sixth survey[4] is classed in the printed ' Lists and Indexes ' as a survey of Paulerspury, but the title on its cover is ' An adicõnall Survey belonging to the Manor of Grafton '. It was made in January, 1650, consists of one folio only and refers only to two cottages of unspecified area in Paulerspury parish which were attached to a farm that is dealt with in the principal survey. Lastly there is the ' Parcell of A S'vey of ẙ Manõ of Hartwell ', which contains an account of a holding of 10¼ acres including two cottages.[5]

On the whole, the interpretation of these surveys presents few difficulties; but there is one particular of some interest wherein the surveys completely fail to present a clear picture. The treatment of the land described as ' Leyes ' is curiously ambiguous. In general it seems probable that on the ' leyes ' some kind of convertible husbandry or *Feldgraswirthschaft* was practised. But whatever may be the right interpretation of the word ' ley ', the error caused in the interpretation of the Grafton surveys by a wrongful understanding of it is not likely to be great. Apart from certain parcels of land which the evidence indicates to be arable, though perhaps lying fallow for a longer period than usual, the total amount of land classed as or named leys in the principal survey of Grafton does not seem to have exceeded about 31 acres.

---

[1] v. P. S. Northants, 22.   [2] v. P. S. Northants, 23.
[3] v. P. S. Northants, 24.   [4] v. P. S. Northants, 25.
[5] v. P. S. Northants, 30.

If the extent to which convertible husbandry was used can be measured by the area of the leys, there would seem to be very little justification at Grafton for the prominence given to this type of agriculture by Nasse and some of his successors.[1]

Besides the entries regarding ' leys ', a little difficulty arises from the occasional appearance of grass-land among the strips of arable. For instance, among the ' Acres of Arable land in coṁon fields ' we get two ' ridges of Green Swarth yt be comonable as ye fformer ',[2] and in another place [3] among the acres of arable land ' in Westwell Field ' there is a ' little Sydeling of Greene-swarth ' of 20 poles. The amount of land of this kind, however, seems to be negligibly small, and though I cannot hope to have been always consistent in my treatment of such doubtful cases as these, the amount of error and variation must be infinitesimal.

2. The Leases : their terms and conditions

Nearly all the land described in the Grafton surveys was let on lease. The account of each holding concludes with particulars of the lease by which it was demised and of former leases which fix the date for the commencement of the most recent. Though the leases were for various terms, the latest leases, the conditions of which are described, seem to have been almost uniform in their general nature. The lands were held at an annual rent, half of which was paid at Michaelmas and half at Lady Day. Great trees, woods, underwoods, mines, and quarries were generally reserved to the lessor. The lessee had to keep and leave the premises in repair, but frequently he was allowed ' all necessary Bootes to be spent

---

[1] The evidence relating to the meaning of the word *ley* is considered in Appendix I. Besides the 31 acres mentioned above, a certain amount of land is described as ' arable land lying in that ffeild called the Towne ffeild by severall pcells well knowne the wholl ffeild being Lease land ' [v. for instance P. S. Northants, 20, folio 15]. Though it is impossible to regard the difference in spelling as significant because of the definite equation of ' Lease ' and ' Leys ' in another entry [v. ib., folio 13], I am inclined to think that the surveyor only intended to indicate that the ' Towne ffeild ' was lying fallow, perhaps for a longer period than usual, at the time when the survey was made. At all events I have classed this land as arable in all the statistical tables, and have treated similarly a ' pcell of arable land called Nan leyes ' which amounted to 15 acres [v. ibid., folio 57].

[2] v. ibid., folio 31.　　　　　　　　　　　　[3] v. ibid., folio 36.

uppon the premises and not elsewhere '. In this expression ' necessary bootes ' we have doubtless a descendant of the old English word *bōt* [= amends], and the meaning would seem to be that the lessor had to find the materials with which repairs had to be executed. In one case the usual phrase is varied, and the lessee is ' allowed sufficient House-Boote ' to be spent on the premises.[1]

If the conditions of the leases tended towards uniformity, the periods for which they ran were very various. It must be remembered, however, that the survey only describes the *conditions* of the latest leases, whereas the *terms* of former leases are often mentioned as well. Taking all the leases mentioned, it is clear that during the first half of the seventeenth century there was a tendency to substitute leases for terms of years for leases for lives, and, in the later part of this period, a rather less marked tendency to shorten the terms of years and to make leases for 31 years general. In estimating the force of these movements, I have thought it best to reckon all leases that were made on the same day for the same period as one lease. Otherwise, the grants of several holdings to the same individuals on the same day—of which there are some remarkable instances from the reign of Charles I— would unduly weight the statistics. But, even when this precaution is taken, the figures are striking. Taking all the seven Grafton surveys together, there are 20 leases which date from the reign of Elizabeth.[2] Of these, 15 are leases for 3 lives, 2 for 21 years, one for 30 years, one for 31 years, and one for 50 years. The earliest lease for years is the longest, and dates from the 27th year of the reign : the latest lease for years belongs to the 42nd year and is the latest of all the leases of this reign. The earliest lease for lives is of the 21st, and the latest of the 38th year.

There are 25 distinct leases belonging to the reign of James I.[3]

---

[1] v. P. S. Northants, 20, folio 28.

[2] This is not counting two undated leases for lives which probably belong to her reign, nor two undated grants for three lives which are definitely specified to belong to it, nor one other grant of Elizabeth for a period unspecified.

[3] A lease for an unspecified period is not counted.

None of these is for lives alone; but one—a lease of the 21st year—is for 3 lives or 90 years, whichever shall determine first. Six of the leases are for 60 years, 3 for 50, one for 41, 7 for 40, 5 for 31, one for 30, and one for 21 years. With the exception of two leases for 60 years, one of which dates from the 12th and the other from the 18th year, none of the leases for 40 years or more is of later date than the 8th year of the reign. Of the 7 leases for 31 years or less, 4 belong to the 21st year, 2 to the 8th, and one—the lease for 21 years— to the 4th year. The earliest of all the leases is one for 40 years, which dates from the 2nd year; the latest are those of the 21st year, and all of these—except, of course, the one for mixed lives and years—are for 31 years.

From the reign of Charles I we have 12 leases that may be counted as distinct. This includes two grants made by Sir Francis Crane, one of which certainly and the other probably dates from the 9th year. It does not include a grant for seven years made to Sir Francis Crane in continuation of a former lease and in confirmation of a sublease which he had made.[1] Of the 12 leases, 10 are for 31 years. One, made in the 2nd year, is for 3 lives or 80 years, whichever should determine first; and the remaining lease made by Sir Francis Crane, probably in the 9th year, is for 21 years. All but three of the leases for 31 years belong to the 13th, 14th, and 15th years. There is only one instance of a grant made under the Commonwealth. This is a grant of a cottage to Christopher Merrey and is for one year only, in accordance with the Act of July 16, 1649, which required that lands out of lease should be leased for a year or less and so on from year to year until the land should be sold.[2]

In the case of most of the leases the land is said to be

[1] v. P. S. Northants, 20, folios 18–19.
[2] If leases of the same date and for the same terms are *not* counted as the same lease, but all leases mentioned are reckoned as distinct, we get the following results: Elizabeth, 26 leases, 19 for 3 lives, 2 for 50 years, 1 for 31 years, 1 for 30 years, 2 for 21 years, and 1 for an unspecified period; James I, 45 leases, 1 for mixed lives and years, 15 for 60 years, 3 for 50, 1 for 41, 13 for 40, 7 for 31, 2 for 30, 2 for 21 years, and 1 of unspecified period; Charles I (including Crane's leases), 31 leases, 1 for mixed lives and years, 1 for 21 years, and 29 for 31 years.

demised by Letters Patent. One holding is described as demised by Letters Patent ' as well under the Great Seale of England as und^r the Dutchy Seale of Lancaster ',[1] while there is a single instance of a lease ' made by King James under the Seale of the Courte of Exchequer '.[2] But frequently mention is made of a ' lease ' or a ' grant ' without indication of the formalities with which it was issued.

The lessees appear to have enjoyed full power to sublet. Of the 51 holdings, which are described in the principal survey under the heading of lands ' under demise or Graunts for lives or yeeres ', only seven were certainly in the actual tenure of the lessee or of a person whose name suggests that he was the heir of the lessee. In one of these cases, too, the lease was not forthcoming and was reported not to have been held from the Crown.[3] In one additional case, however, the tenant seems to have been related to the lessee who was the last survivor to hold under a lease for lives and probably was a woman.[4] Identity of surnames, again, indicates that the tenants of three holdings were relatives of former lessees of the land continuing to rent it from the new lessees.[5] The lessee of one of these three holdings, moreover, is not named in the survey, so it is possible that he was the same person as the tenant. Indeed this uncertainty attaches to eleven other cases, where the holders of the leases actually in being are unnamed. But it is clear that most of the holdings were sublet.

Of the process by which subletting was arranged we can learn very little from the surveys. We are told that land ' in the Tenure and present occupačon of Richard Wardley Gent.' had been demised to John Eldred and William Whitmore, but that on the very next day these persons had by an ' Indenture of Lease ' of 12 May, 8 James I, ' bargained and sould there estate of the premises and Terme of three-score yeeres to Nicholas Windmill of Grafton '.[6] But this statement apparently concerns a transfer of the lease and cannot be regarded

---

[1] v. P. S. Northants, 20, folio 16.
[2] v. ibid., folio 68.
[3] v. ibid., folio 50.
[4] v. ibid., folios 91–2.
[5] v. ibid., folios 15–6, 40–2, 95–6.
[6] v. ibid., folio 8.

as casting any light upon the subletting of the land, unless it can be proved that Richard Wardley was the heir of Nicholas Windmill. There is, however, a passage in the survey of 1656 which lends probability to this last hypothesis. It concerns some land also held by Richard Wardley and also under a lease of 11th May, 8 James I, which was made to Eldred and Whitmore, and the passage is to the effect that this lease ' by assignment is now come to Richard Wardley gentleman.'[1] This seems to suggest that 'subletting' may be an inexact description of the process by which control over the land passed from the original lessee to the actual tenant. But we cannot be sure whether this case was typical or exceptional. Similarly unsatisfying is the entry which states that the ' King's Arms ' and some pasture attached to it—both ' now in the Tenure or occupačon of Mrs. Marthana Wilson or her assignes '—were in the fifth year of James I ' demised to William ffaldow and John ffaldow for fforty yeeres which said demise was assigned to Sir ffrancis Crane Kt in the third yeere of King Charles which said Sir ffrancis Crane uppon the surrender of the lordship of Grafton had another Graunte for seven years by way of confirmačon of a Lease yt. Sir ffrancis Crane had made to [blank] for XXI yeeres '.[2]

On the whole I am inclined to suspect that much of the land was leased, probably for a ' consideration ', to persons who only took it with a view to arranging profitable sub-tenancies. Several facts make me incline to this belief. In the first place we find large groups of holdings demised to two pairs of lessees. The surveys show that 17 distinct holdings, comprising nearly 450 acres of land, were at different times in the reign of James I demised to John Eldred and William Whitmore, and that 19 holdings, which contained altogether nearly 500 acres, were during the 14th and 15th years of Charles I leased to John Chew and Richard Fitzhugh.[3]

Again there is ground for believing that some of the lessees

[1] v. ibid., 21, folios 1–5.   [2] v. ibid., 20, folio 18.
[3] If a divided messuage is counted as one, the total is 18. The two parts of this farm are described as if they were separate holdings, but are asserted to be parts of a divided messuage [v. P. S. Northants, 20, folios 61–2, 69–70].

were not local men. William Whitmore is described as 'of the Citie of London', and we are told of two holdings which were, in the third year of Charles I, leased to 'James Elliot and Wm. Loving of London gent.'[1]

Another fact which seems to suggest that the lessees were often speculators rather than intending farmers is the frequent granting of leases long before the expiration of their predecessors. Sometimes leases lay two deep. For instance, in 1650 a certain farm was held by the last survivor of a lease for lives granted under Elizabeth. This lessor was only 67 years old, and a lease for 40 years made in the 8th year of James I had still to run after the expiration of the lease for lives, but this had not prevented the reversion from being leased to John Chew and Richard Fitzhugh so early as the 15th year of Charles I.[2] In another case, these same individuals had in that same year received a lease of a farm, though a lease for lives, which eventually expired in 1642, was still in being, and though the reversion had already been granted on lease for 40 years by James I.[3] Of this dealing in reversions we find a trace in the reign of Elizabeth, for the reversion of a holding which was leased for 21 years in the 30th year of her reign was granted out for a further period of 21 years in the very next year.[4]

The evidence of the Grafton surveys is quite compatible with the hypothesis that this system was largely developed under the impecunious Stuarts, and indeed that conclusion would seem to be definitely suggested by the facts recorded; but it is important to remember that the information given by the surveys is, as one would expect, much more complete for recent than for far-gone years.

That money was advanced to the Crown in return for the grants of leases seems more than probable in view of the lowness of the rents when compared with the Parliamentary valuation. In the abstract at the end of the principal survey

----

[1] It is added that this was done 'in nominacõn of Robert, Earle of Monmouth' [v. P. S. Northants, 20, folio 16, cp. P. S. Northants, 21, folios 13–17].   [2] v. P. S. Northants, 20, folio 90.
[3] v. ibid., folio 79.   [4] v. ibid., folio 52.

of Grafton the ' present rents ' are reckoned as amounting to
£89 3s. 1d. and the value of the lands over and above this
amount is estimated at no less than £881 19s. 6d. per annum.[1]
But it is impossible that the actual value of the land can have
risen to this enormous extent in so short a time, and it is
hardly likely that monarchs so badly in need of money as
the first two Stuarts would have granted beneficiary leases
without requiring any return or have managed the Crown
estates so uneconomically as these figures would suggest if
the rent represents all that was received.   It is much more
likely, on the face of it, that a draft was drawn on the future.
Besides, we have only to turn to the Parliamentary Survey of
Ashton to find definite evidence of the process.   One William
Hocknell had in 1634 ' compounded ' with Sir Miles Fleetwood,
Deputy Steward of the Honour of Grafton, for a lease of eleven
acres of pasture.   The lease was for 31 years and was to
commence on the determination of a lease for 30 years made
in the 26th year of Elizabeth, previous leases being one of
30 July, 14 Elizabeth, for 31 years [?], and one of 10 April,
31 Henry VIII, for 40 years.   The rent to be paid under
Hocknell's lease seems to have been 12s. a year, but it is
expressly stated that he paid a fine of £87 for the lease.
The annual value of the premises was estimated in 1650 at
£7 6s. 8d.   Mrs. Judith Dorrell was then the occupant.[2]

Though there seems good reason for believing that the
lessees of a great part of the lands in the Honour of Grafton
were merely speculators or dealers, some lessees were clearly
local men and some actual farmers.   Apart from the cases
already quoted where the lands were actually in the ' tenure

[1] v. ibid., folio 99.   Apparently nearly £26 should be deducted from this
total for the value of lands not let on lease and of lands in which an estate
was claimed by the occupier ; but some small deduction ought also to be
made from the total of ' present rents '.

[2] v. P. S. Northants, 16, folio 26, and a memorandum of the proceedings
of the Committee for the Removal of Obstructions which is written on the
back of folio 25.   The process of leasing and subletting may further be
illustrated from a survey of Grafton of the year 1619.   There we read of
a certain holding *Et revercio conceditur per contractoř*, and of another
*Ricardus Church modo Thomas tenet per dimissionem ex concessione Eldred
et Whitmore per literas patentes datas.*   v. Land Revenue : Miscellaneous
Books, vol. ccxxi, folios 112–19.   For further evidence on these points
v. Appendix II.

and occupation' of the lessees, there are instances of the occupying tenants of certain holdings leasing and subletting other holdings. Thomas Smyth, Peter Browne, and Richard Church each it appears farmed one or more holdings, but each had leased and sublet another holding.[1] Again the occurrence of the names England and Foster in the list of those owing [free?] rents, which is found at the end of the principal survey of Grafton, makes it probable that two lessees who bore those names were local men.[2] Thomas England, who dealt largely in leases of Crown Lands both at Grafton and elsewhere, is described in the Parliamentary Survey of Pottersperry as 'of Stittlanger', Northants.[3] John Chew, who so frequently appears as a co-lessee with Richard Fitzhugh, seems to have lived at Ashton, which is quite near Grafton, for the Parliamentary Survey of Ashton mentions a tenement which was 'bounded on the north side with yᵉ house of John Chew.'[4] Richard Fitzhugh also seems to have lived in the county: he is described as 'of Heathencoate'.[5] Yet another lessee, one Alexander Travell, was clearly a local man, for there are entries relating to him in the parish register of Roade.

The subtenants as well as the lessees appear to have had power to sublet. Holdings are commonly described as 'in the tenure or occupačon of A. B. or his assignes'. One farm was 'in the Tenure of Anthony Whalley, Gent and in the p'sent occupačon of Widdow Goodman';[6] and Anthony Whalley, though curiously enough he seems to have been a relative of former leaseholders, was only a subtenant himself, since a lease to Elliot and Loving had been in being since 1630. Probably from the mention of the occupier's name in this case we may conclude that the tenant and occupier were the same person in the case of all the other holdings mentioned in the principal survey, though no doubt the farm-tied cottages were sublet by the farmer.[7]

---

[1] v. P. S. Northants, 20, folios 32, 39, 20, 67, 91, 93.
[2] v. ibid., folios 23, 24, 300, 102.   [3] v. P. S. Northants, 40, folio 17.
[4] v. P. S. Northants, 16, folio 6.   [5] v. P. S. Northants, 40, folio 17.
[6] v. P. S. Northants, 20, folio 15.
[7] I can neither rid myself of the belief that this is the most probable interpretation, nor hide from myself the fact that the mention of the

3. Mediaeval survivals : the size of holdings and the treatment of the lands

The holdings described in the Parliamentary Surveys of Grafton have more vestiges of mediaeval uniformity about them than appears from a mere comparison of their areas. Thus holdings of $44\frac{1}{2}$ acres, $42\frac{1}{2}$ acres, 42 acres, $52\frac{1}{2}$ acres, and $43\frac{1}{2}$ acres respectively are alike in that each contains just 36 acres of arable land.[1] Again, though the comparison of the holdings in respect of arable land is made difficult by the frequent failure of the surveys to distinguish between arable and leys, it is probably just to see traces of a normal area of 36 acres of arable in a holding of 70 acres 2 roods 4 poles which contains 37 acres of arable and in a holding of 46 acres 2 roods 20 poles with 36 acres 3 roods of arable and leys.[2] It is possible too that vestiges of holdings of half the normal area should be seen in arable allotments of 16 acres, 17 acres [two cases], and 19 acres which appear on holdings of various sizes.[3] Nor is it only in regard to arable land that the survival of the mediaeval tendency towards uniformity shows itself. On four out of the five holdings which contain 36 acres of arable we find $2\frac{1}{2}$ acres distinguished as leys and $2\frac{1}{2}$ acres of meadow. On the fifth holding there are 2 acres of leys and 2 acres of meadow.

As regards the size of the holdings in general, if we exclude Grafton and Pottersperry Parks from the calculation,[4] it appears that, out of the total of 65 holdings reported on in the various Parliamentary Surveys of Grafton and Hartwell, only one was more than 100 acres in extent and only three

occupiers of *subordinate* tenements on one farm makes it illogical [v. P. S. Northants, 20, folio 51]. It assumes that the mention of a distinct occupier in the case of one whole farm means that the silence of other entries implies a negative, while precisely the opposite is concluded with regard to subordinate tenements. Yet this is only to accuse the survey of a not improbable inconsistency in the case of a single entry.

[1] v. P. S. Northants, 20, folios 7–8, 10–11, 12–13, 15–17, 25–6. In the case of the last holding, however, some leys seem to have been included in the total of 36 acres. It is true $2\frac{1}{2}$ acres are distinguished in the survey as leys, but apparently some other leys were classed with the arable.

[2] v. ibid., folios 51–2, 53–6.

[3] v. ibid., folios 91, 86–7, 93–4, 95.

[4] These parks are surveyed in P. S. Northants, 23.

contained more than 60 and less than 100 acres.[1] On the other hand 13 holdings contained between 30 and 60 acres each,[2] and 13—or 14 if a holding that consisted entirely of wood is included—contained between 15 and 30 acres each. Fifteen cottages had less than an acre of land attached to them : six others had less than 5 acres each or, on an average, just under 3 acres. Six holdings contained between 5 and 10 acres : six contained between 10 and 15 acres.

It is, however, possible and perhaps more just to classify the holdings in another way. Some of the farms, though let under separate leases and separately reported on in the survey, appear to have been held by the same individuals who held other farms, and if this 'engrossing' and the opposite process of subdivision, which appears on 2 holdings, be taken into account, the total number of holdings is reduced to 52.[3] The following table shows how they are grouped in regard to size :

100 acres and over	.	.	.	.	.	.	.	. 3 [?2]
60 acres and over but less than 100 acres				.	.	.	8 [?10]
30 ,, ,, ,, 60 ,,				.	.	.	5
15 ,, ,, ,, 30 ,,	.			.	.	.	6 [?5]
10 ,, ,, ,, 15 ,,	.			.	.	.	2
5 ,, ,, ,, 10 ,,	.			.	.	.	7
1 ,, ,, ,, 5 ,,	.			.	.	.	7
Under one acre	.	.	.	.	.	.	.	. 14

[1] The areas of these three are respectively about 85 acres, 74 acres 3 roods 26 poles, and 70 acres 2 roods 4 poles. The uncertainty about the exact area of the first of these is due to the fact that the particulars and totals given in the MS. do not agree.

[2] This includes an area of $36\frac{1}{2}$ acres of 'leaze' or 'pasture ground' claimed as a common shared by 5 farms and 4 or 5 cottages, but treated as a distinct holding in P. S. Northants, 21, folio 22.

[3] In obtaining these figures I have assumed that 'Thomas Church' and 'Mr. Thomas Church' are the same person and distinct from 'Thomas Church of Wootton', and that 'John Maninge' and 'John Manning' are the same and different from 'John Maninge of Horton'. I have not counted as a case of subdivision one mention of distinct tenants of two cottages on a third man's holding [v. P. S. Northants, 20, folio 51]. The further identification of T. Church and T. Church of Wootton and of J. Maninge and J. Manning of Horton would only affect the figures to the extent of reducing by one each the numbers of holdings of 5 to 10 and 30 to 60 acres. Difficulty also arises with regard to farms described in P. S. Northants, 21, for this survey was made 6 years after P. S. Northants, 20. In the former we read that Samuel Goodman occupied lands of which A. Whalley was tenant : according to the latter 'Widdow Goodman' occupied other lands of which Whalley was tenant, and Ann Goodman was tenant and occupier of other

One warning, however, must be given with regard to this table. It cannot be regarded as a measure of the extent of engrossing, for some of the tenants of the Crown at Grafton may also have cultivated land elsewhere, or as freeholders they may have cultivated in Grafton itself other lands besides those surveyed. The evidence in regard to these possibilities will be considered later.

Perhaps it may fairly be looked upon as a sign of affinity with the mediaeval economy that there was very little *specialization* on the farms reported on in the Parliamentary Surveys of Grafton. If we take the principal survey by itself and exclude the 15 holdings of less than one acre and one holding of two acres where the land is undescribed, we are left with 41 holdings. Now if we disregard the uses to which the gardens and premises of the homesteads were devoted, we find that out of these 41 holdings no less than 33 contained both arable and either pasture *or* meadow. On 13 of them— or 14 if one counts as pasture an enclosed assart which is not definitely so described [1]— both pasture *and* meadow were reported. Of the remaining 8 holdings, 5 appear to have consisted of grassland, while one was a wood. Only 2 holdings can be regarded as really specialized to arable uses and one of these contained a close of pasture ground attached to the premises of the house,[2] and was moreover apparently in the occupation of a man who had a little meadow land as part of another farm held by him.[3] Yet arable predominated in most cases. It amounts to more than 75 %, almost certainly of 13 and, probably, of 9 other holdings.[4] Besides

lands. I have assumed (1) that Ann Goodman and ' Widdow Goodman' are identical, (2) that S. Goodman held in 1656 all the lands previously held by Ann Goodman. But one Anthony Goodman appears as a tenant in 1656 and *he may* have held part or all of Ann Goodman's farms. Hence the queried figures in the table.   [1] v. P. S. Northants, 20, folio 85.
    [2] v. ibid., folio 93.   [3] v. ibid., folios 91–2.
    [4] The uncertainty, which is, I think, negligibly slight, is due to the doubtful sense of the word ' ley ' in the survey and to the frequent confusion of arable and leys. In calculating the amount of arable I have deducted the leys as best I could, with the exception of the 'arable land . . . in . . . the Towne ffeild . . . being Lease land ' and the 'pcell of arable land called Nan leyes ' to which I have referred in a previous note. Here the assertion that the land was arable seems too emphatic to be ignored.

these it appears to reach over 50 %, though less than 75 %, in the case of 11 or possibly 12 holdings.[1] Excluding the cottages which had only an acre or less attached to them, it seems that more than half the holdings had over three-fourths of their area in arable, while on over 80 % of them the arable exceeded half the whole.

A similar condition of things shows itself if we turn to the Grafton Survey of 1656,[2] but in this the land is less precisely described. In it 7 distinct portions of land are mentioned: 5 of these portions consisted entirely of arable and ' leazes ' in the three fields of Grafton, and the remainder comprised (i) a ' pcell of Leaze land ' of 2 roods and (ii) a ' prcell of Leaze or Pasture Ground ' of 36 acres which was in the possession of the occupiers of the above-mentioned 5 farms and 4 or 5 cottagers and was claimed by them as a cow pasture ' belonging to their farms and cottages according to their several proportions '.[3] The total area reported on in this survey was 148 acres 20 poles and the five farms varied in size from 19¼ acres to 24 acres 1 rood 20 poles. Apart from the survey of Grafton and Pottersperry Parks, the only remaining Parliamentary Survey of Grafton which tells us anything about the uses made of the land is concerned with a single tenement and 4½ acres of land. Of this land 2 acres were arable.[4]

On the whole then it is clear, firstly, that there were very few instances of real specialization on the farms at Grafton in the middle of the seventeenth century, and, secondly, that on most of the farms arable predominated. But these facts, though they serve to illustrate the survival of mediaeval features in the Grafton economy, may easily be misunderstood and given undue prominence. It is important to notice that specialization, where it does occur, is generally specialization in grazing, and that it occurs on the largest holdings. It follows that on all the lands surveyed, if taken together, the ratio of pasture to arable is very much greater than it is

[1] In the case of one holding it is doubtful whether a piece of pasture contained 4 or 14 acres, v. P. S. Northants, 20, folio 95.
[2] v. P. S. Northants, 21.   [3] v. ibid., folio 22.
[4] v. P. S. Northants, 24.

on the majority of the holdings taken separately. The total area reported on by the parliamentary surveyors of Grafton was as nearly as possible 1,760 acres, in addition to 1,003¼ acres in Grafton and Pottersperry Parks.[1] This is excluding the premises of houses and 5½ acres attached to the ruins of Grafton House. Now out of this total of 1,760 acres, 961¼ acres are described as arable or leys. So far as I can tell after a careful examination of the surveys, about 72 acres would be a fair allowance for those leys which are not definitely described as arable and for such grassland as was mixed with the arable. Practically then we may say that the arable reported on in the Parliamentary Surveys of Grafton amounted to 890 acres, or 50·57 % of the cultivated area. But perhaps the area of Grafton Park, which amounted to 622¼ acres, ought to be counted in the total. Presumably none of this was arable, so its inclusion in the calculation will bring down the proportion of the arable to 37·36 %.[2]

It is interesting to compare these figures with the modern statistics of Northamptonshire. In 1913, the county of Northamptonshire, exclusive of the Soke of Peterborough, contained 516,745 acres under crops and grass, and of this total 159,513 acres were arable.[3] This works out at 30·87 %.

On the whole, then, the Grafton figures, so far as they go, seem to indicate that the process of conversion by which the mediaeval uses of the land were changed was by no means complete in Northamptonshire in the middle of the seventeenth century. It remains, however, an open question

[1] I make the exact total 1,759 acres 1 rood 20 poles, but there is uncertainty about some of the areas, so I have preferred a round number as making the arithmetic simpler and as avoiding a deceptive appearance of exactness.

[2] v. P. S. Northants, 23. All we are told is that in the two parts there were 341 acres of coppice, and the presence of 200 deer is mentioned. Obviously the area of Pottersperry Park must be excluded from the calculation, since the arable at Pottersperry is not dealt with in the Grafton surveys. In 1660 there were 1,061 acres 3 roods 40 poles of arable at Pottersperry and only 291 acres 33 poles of pasture and meadow. v. Land Revenue, Miscellaneous Books, vol. ccxxii (summary at the beginning of the volume). The presumption that no arable lay inside Grafton Park in 1650 may possibly be unjustified, for according to a survey of 1558 there were then 42 acres of arable in the park [v. *infra*, ch. iii, p. 75].

[3] v. Agricultural Statistics, 1913, vol. xlviii. Part I, Cd. 7325, p. 41.

whether Grafton can be regarded as a typical case ; and that question must be dealt with in the following chapters. But it may be noted here that the neighbourhood of forest creates a presumption that enclosure and conversion would be easier and would therefore come earlier at Grafton than elsewhere in the county, though, on the other hand, the general policy of the Tudors may have delayed the process of change on the royal estates.[1]

In the arrangement of the arable land at Grafton, as well as in its predominance on the majority of the farms, the survival of mediaeval features is apparent in the Parliamentary Surveys. In each of the two parishes of Grafton Regis and Roade, which contained most of the lands reported on in those surveys, we find the three fields of the typical mediaeval economy. The great bulk of the ploughed land clearly lay in scattered parcels in the common fields.[2] Acre, half-acre, and quarter-acre strips seem to have been the rule ; but sometimes the *morcellement* of the land went further, as when 33½ acres of arable were made up of 136 ' ridges ' and 3 'headlands', and 13 acres of 54 'ridges'.[3] On the other hand there are signs of consolidation, to which I shall refer later.

Another mediaeval feature shows itself in the lot meadows. In the parish and manor of Grafton there seem to have been two common meadows, called respectively the Mill Holmes, or the Holme Meadow, and the Fen Mead. The former of

[1] With regard to the effects of the neighbourhood of forests and woodland upon enclosure, v. E. C. K. Gonner, Common Land and Inclosure (1912), pp. 111–13, 142–3, 231, 282–9, and E. M. Leonard, Transactions of Royal Historical Society [New Series], xix (1905), pp. 137–9.

[2] In connexion with this fact it is interesting to notice that in Ogilby's Britannia (1675), Pl. 21, the road from Stony Stratford to Towcester is marked as enclosed to within 1½ miles of the latter place, and, though in Pl. 40 some unenclosed road is shown near Grafton, the road in Grafton itself is marked enclosed and the same is true of the greater part of the road in the neighbourhood. Unless therefore it is assumed that there was extensive enclosure in this district between 1650 and the time when Ogilby made his investigations, the state of things revealed by P. S. Northants, 20, makes me doubt whether Professor Gonner is justified in considering that Ogilby's maps can even ' very roughly represent the average ' of enclosure ' throughout the county ' [v. E. C. K. Gonner, op. cit., pp. 172–3, footnote].

[3] v. P. S. Northants, 20, folios 77–8, 82.

these was certainly and the latter probably a lot meadow.
This appears from such entries as the following : [1]

Meadow belonging to the p'emises as itt falleth yeerely by
  Lott In the Meadow called the Mill Holmes by esti-
  maċon. . . . . oi : 02
Itm. in the Meadow called the ffen Meadow by estimaċon oi : oo

Lot meadows were also to be found in the parish of Roade
and manor of Hartwell. Thus ' one lott in Ash meadow '
consisting of one rood is mentioned, while another holding
in Roade contained a rood of meadow in ' Ash Mead lotts
as the lott falls ' and also a second rood in ' Ash Mead lotts '.[2]
It seems, however, that particular parcels of lot meadow were
permanently attached to some holdings : it is difficult to
know how else to explain the fact that the meadow belonging
to Sir John Wake's holding in Roade consisted of a ' pcell in
Ashton mead next Mr. John Cooke west butting on the
river south being lott meadow '.[3]   Clearly the opposite should
be concluded with regard to a parcel of meadow in ' broade
mead ' which is described as ' changable ' and distinguished
from another parcel in the same meadow ' joyning Ash Mead
lots ' and therefore, it would appear, of fixed locality.[4]   One
is reminded of the permanent and changeable allotments in
the common meadow at Stratton in Dorset.[5]   Possibly in
permanent allotments of this kind we have an instance of
individualistic invasion of an older communal system ; but
it is difficult to imagine how land once subject to the lot
could be disentangled and held in severalty without a complete destruction of the custom.   Perhaps the process may
have been assisted by the division of the common meadow
into ' shots ' or ' furlongs ', for a particular ' shot ' could be
withdrawn from the lot without affecting the customary
treatment of other parts of the meadow.   The lot meadows

---

[1] v. P. S. Northants, 20, folio 16.   [2] v. ibid., folios 39, 46.
[3] Perhaps a parallel to this may be found in the meadow called Pixey
at Yarnton in Oxfordshire, for only 60 acres of it, out of some 200, come
under the lot [v. R. H. Gretton, Economic Journal, xx (1910), p. 43 ;
B. Stapleton, Three Oxfordshire Parishes, Oxford Hist. Soc. (1893),
pp. 307–11].   [4] v. P. S. Northants, 20, folio 46.
[5] Gilbert Slater, The English Peasantry and the Enclosure of Common
Fields (1907), pp. 24–8.

at Yarnton in Oxfordshire are thus divided into 'shots', and probably an indication of a similar arrangement should be seen in an entry in the principal survey of Grafton which speaks of a parcel of land in Broad mead ' being Lot meadow in ye ffurl. called 7 acres '.[1]

Apart from meadows asserted to be subject to lot, the arrangement of a meadow holding in scattered strips is revealed by the entry which states that John Manning had attached to his farm with some other meadow, four parcels ' in Chall (?) mead lying intermingled with the meadow of Luke Barrett '.[2]

With regard to the activity of the manorial communities of Grafton and Hartwell and of the functioning of the Courts, the surveys naturally tell us little. We are, however, informed that 40s. a year was paid out of the rents and profits of the manors as the Bailiff's fee and that a small cottage and an acre of meadow belonging to the Lord of the Manor and valued at 24s. a year were by custom allowed to ' the Towne Heiward '.[3] The ' Towne Herd-House ' is mentioned in the description of a farm in Grafton parish.[4] It is stated that the Court Baron for the Manor of Grafton was usually held at the King's Arms and the Court Leet at the usual times : the tenants of the Manor of Grafton owed suit and service to the Lord and the said Court according to custom.[5] The various fines of the Courts together with all other royalties and privileges were estimated as worth £3 a year.

4. Modern features in the economy of Grafton

Though the Parliamentary Surveys of Grafton reveal considerable mediaeval survivals, they none the less bear witness to the existence of changes and forces making for change. The scaffolding of the modern village stands beside the ruins of the manor. Already in 1650, the process which was to

[1] v. P. S. Northants, 20, folio 96. Another lot meadow, distinct from those mentioned in the text, is referred to, ibid., folio 56.
[2] v. ibid., folio 79.
[3] v. ibid., folio 98. I have followed the survey in treating this holding separately and have not included its area in any of the statistical tables.
[4] v. ibid., folio 7.   [5] v. ibid., folio 98.

lead to the conversion of arable land into pasture, to the growth of large farms and to the development of a landless class of labourers had gone some way.

The surveys expose two distinct *strata*, so to say, in the history of 'engrossing'. In the first place, holdings which are described as units and let under a single lease betray indications of their composite origin. Eleven such holdings contain, besides the farm house, some other tenement or tenements.[1] Thus the farm-tied cottage appears to have been a well-established institution in the manors in the middle of the seventeenth century. It would probably be a mistake, however, to consider all these cases as precisely similar. Possibly a distinction should be made between those cases where the subordinate tenement appears to be adjacent to the farmhouse[2] and those where they seem to have only a tenurial connexion. In these last instances, the origin of the system in engrossing can hardly be doubted. It is a significant fact that a small detached tenement on Sir John Wake's farm had a little barn as well as 'a little fould yard and close' attached to it, for these seem to point to its having been once the centre of an independently cultivated holding.[3]

A more recent stage in the process of engrossing is revealed by the occupation of distinct holdings by the same individual. Though it is sometimes difficult to determine whether the surveyors are speaking of one person or of two persons bearing the same name,[4] it appears that Thomas Church was tenant and occupier of 4 holdings while Thomas Church of Wootton, Richard Church, John Manning, Sir John Wake, Francis Arundle and Robert Brooks had 2 holdings each.[5] This is

---

[1] v. P. S. Northants, 20, folios 40–2, 43–6, 51–2, 57–9, 71–2, 75–6, 77–9, 86–7, 93–4, 94; also ibid., No. 30. All these belong to the parish of Roade. There was also a small tenement, clearly subordinate, on Sir Robert Osborne's large grazing farm, but to this no farmhouse or mansion was attached. The figure in the text does not include two cottages surveyed in P. S. Northants, 25, which were attached to Thomas Burton's farm [v. P. S. Northants, 20, folios 53–6].

[2] e. g. v. P. S. Northants 20, folios 75, 77, 93.

[3] It is puzzling to find that subordinate tenements were attached to two very diminutive holdings—one of less than 10 acres and one of less than an acre [v. ibid., folios 71, 97].   [4] v. *supra*, p. 40, note 3.

[5] The case of Robert Brooks is peculiar and similar to that mentioned in

exclusive of all doubtful cases. A slightly different form of engrossing was practised by the Widow Goodman. She was in 1650 tenant and presumably occupier of a farm of 42 acres, which had been leased from the Crown by Eldred and Whitmore, but she was also occupier of another farm of 52½ acres which is described as in the tenure of Anthony Whalley and of which the lessees were James Elliott and William Loving.[1]

That engrossing really went further than these facts show may possibly be argued from the occurrence in the list of those liable to pay free rents of the names of 5 or perhaps 6 persons who also farmed land let under lease. Mrs. Marthana Wilson, who held the King's Arms at Grafton—a holding of 7 acres in all—was almost certainly the same person as the Marthana Wilson who was tenant of a holding of 87½ acres in the neighbouring manor of Pottersperry.[2] Again, the farms of two tenants whom we should not otherwise suppose to be engrossers contained no house, and it is not perhaps too bold to guess that they lived on other farms which are not included in the Grafton Surveys.[3] One of these tenants is described as John Clarke of Ashton [a neighbouring parish], and this would lead one to hazard the conjecture that possibly John Manning of Horton had land in that parish as well as the holding reported on in the survey, but the existence of another man bearing the same name is more probably the reason why he is thus described.[4]

But if engrossing was not uncommon, subdivision was not

note 3, for Brooks's two holdings consisted of two cottages and the total area he is reported to have held only amounted to 2½ acres.
[1] v. P. S. Northants, 20, folios 15–17. I assume that Ann Goodman and Widow Goodman were identical. [2] v. P. S. Northants, 40.
[3] v. P. S. Northants, 20, folios 29, 33. Perhaps Sir Robert Osborne's farm should be classed with these two, though it contained one small tenement, for Grafton House seems at the time of its destruction, in 1643, to have been occupied by Sir Francis Crane's widow.
[4] This is almost certainly the case with Thomas Church of Wootton, for in one place he is described as 'late of Wootton'. v. ibid., folio 73. From the Parliamentary Survey of Ashton it appears that in 1650 John Clarke occupied a holding of nearly 50 acres there, and that 5 tenements (including one in Hartwell) were attached to this farm: v. P. S. Northants, 16. In the Grafton Survey he is assigned 20½ acres of land without a house.

unknown in the district covered by the surveys. One farm
of 14 acres, though described and let on lease as a unit, had
evidently been divided among 3 subtenants by the lessees.[1]
Again, two holdings of some 10 and 11 acres respectively,
though separately described in the survey, are stated to be
parts of a divided messuage.[2]   Yet the tenant of one of these
parts also held another farm of 41 acres; [3] and there can be
no doubt that the tendency to engross was much stronger
than the tendency towards subdivision.

The other side of the story of engrossing tells of the divorce
of houses from land and of the unsettlement of families who
had lived on the small farms that were amalgamated.   Indications of these changes can be discerned in the surveys.
In the account of lands demised for lives or years in the
principal survey we find nine cottage holdings of not more
than 3 roods of land, while in the case of six of them the
land attached to each cottage, including the area of the house,
did not exceed 10 poles.   One of the holdings contained
another 'small tenement' besides the cottage, though its
total area was only 2 roods 8 poles.   That these cottages had
not always been in this unendowed condition is, I think, shown
by the fact that barns were attached to three of them and
a large stable of seven bays to one.[4]   Two other facts naturally
connect themselves with these phenomena.   Not counting
a holding that consisted entirely of wood, and excluding (as
possibly attached to other farms and not really distinct) the
lands reported on in the survey of 1656, we find three holdings
which contained no house, while on Sir Robert Osborne's
pasture farm of 585 acres odd there was only one small
tenement.[5]   Again, six cottages or tenements had been
erected on the waste, and if this can be regarded as a result
of the unsettlement produced by engrossing or the conversion
of arable to pasture, some light can perhaps be obtained on
the date of the changes, for three of these houses are said to

[1] v. P. S. Northants, 20, folios 36–7.   [2] v. ibid., folios 61–2, 69–70.
[3] v. ibid., folios 77–79.   [4] v. ibid., folios 48, 67, 97 and 22.
[5] An instance of a decayed house is provided by one of Sir John Wake's
holdings, where was a subordinate tenement described as ' lately burnt '
and ' not repaired '.   v. ibid., folio 57.

be 'newly erected', and a fourth to have been built by the
licence of the Steward of the Honour at the expense of the
man who was still occupying it in 1650.

The existence of cottages with very little land attached to
them seems to point to the failure of the Act of 1589.[1] Apart
from subordinate or farm-tied tenements, the Grafton surveys
yield no less than 19 instances of cottages with less than the
statutory minimum of 4 acres of land. It is impossible to
suppose that these were all lawful exceptions and occupied
by such people as quarrymen, brickmakers, workers in lime-
kilns, keepers in the forest, the 'comon Herdman or Shep-
parde for keepinge the Cattle or Sheepe of the Towne ', or
' poore lame sicke aged or ympotent' persons. Even if these
cottages were maintained under the licences from the Justices
of the Peace for which the Act makes provision, that would
only show that it was the Justices who were failing to adminis-
ter the law properly. One of the cottages, however, was in
all probability privileged under the Act, for a close called
the 'Lyme yard' parcel was attached to it.[2] Another had
a smith's forge attached to it.[3] Again, three cottages mentioned in one or other of the surveys had just over 4 acres of
land appended, and it is tempting to consider these instances
as survivals of a time when an attempt had been made to
enforce the law.[4]

There is some reason for supposing that the extension of
pasture farming had been the greatest or at least a principal
force making for the disturbance of the mediaeval order at
Grafton. The one really large farm among those described
in the surveys consisted, it seems, entirely of grassland.
Besides this, there were three farms of more than 80 acres, if
one counts as a single farm two or more holdings occupied by
the same individual. On these three farms taken together
the arable seems to have amounted to under 74 % of the
whole. On all the smaller farms taken together the arable

[1] v. 31 Eliz. c. 7.
[2] v. P. S. Northants, 20, folio 35.   [3] v. ibid., folio 20.
[4] v. ibid., folios 34, 60, and P. S. Northants, 24, folios 1–2. It should be
noticed, however, that the tenant of one of these cottages was Sir John
Wake, who also held a farm of 38½ acres.

appears to reach more than 80 % of the whole.[1] Thus pasture
farming was apparently developed to a greater extent on the
larger than on the smaller and medium-sized holdings. This
is not, however, true of the very small holdings, which cannot
be regarded as farms at all, for no arable is mentioned in connexion with any holding of less than one acre, while on the
seven holdings of 1 to 5 acres taken together the arable was
less than 59 %.

That pasture farming had tended to destroy the survivals
of mediaeval uniformity in holdings is illustrated by the farm
of Anthony Whalley, which is described in the principal survey
as occupied by the Widow Goodman. In respect of every
other variety of land this farm was an exact replica of William
Smith's holding as it is described in the same survey, but it
contained 10 acres of pasture land which were lacking in the
case of the latter farm. Richard Wardley's holding, too,
resembled William Smith's in the amount of arable it contained and in the area of the house and its premises : it
differed in that 3 acres of pasture were attached to it, while
it had an acre less meadow and leys than the other.

Of the extension of the area under grass there is evidence
in some entries concerning assarts. We read of a parcel of
pasture ground ' called an Assarte ' which was bounded on
the south by Ashton Wood, of another piece of pasture ' called
Asarte ' which lay in the parish of Greens Norton and was
bounded on the south ' with the land called munks [?] wood ',
and of a third pasture described as ' an Assarte ' which was
in the parish of Piddington and had the forest of Salcey as its
western boundary.[2] The mention of these woodland boundaries is important : it shows that the land most recently
cleared in three distinct directions was used for grazing.

[1] In making these calculations I have excluded the 36½ acres of 'leaze'
and pasture ground described in P. S. Northants, 21, folio 22, because this
land was claimed as a common by the occupiers of farms of various sizes
and some cottagers. I have assumed that the lands occupied in 1656 by
Samuel and Anthony Goodman were in 1650 held by Widow Goodman :
it was necessary to choose between uncertainties, and I have chosen the
alternative *least* favourable to the argument in the text. As usual the
failure to discriminate leys precisely and the doubtful sense of the word
introduce an element of inexactness into the figures.

[2] v. P. S. Northants, 20, folios 28, 53, 95.

The connexion between grazing and enclosure is apparent.
I have noted in the principal survey fifty entries which refer
to closes. Thirty-three of these speak definitely of closes of
pasture, and in the case of fourteen out of the remainder there
is nothing at all to suggest that the absence of definite description of the land as pasture was intentional. I have only
noticed three instances of closes where there is any reason to
suspect an enclosure of arable land. One is an ambiguous
entry which, under the heading of ' Severall pcells of arable,
meadow lying in the comon ffeild ', speaks of a parcel of
land ' called Ley Close being 7 ridges '.[1] The second refers,
under the heading of arable in common field, to two parcels
of 1 rood and 2 roods respectively which lie ' in Larason [?]
close ', one of them being ' next the hedge '.[2] The third, in
a list of arable lands in the common fields, mentions a ' close
next the Highway '—an entry which leads one to guess that
perhaps it was the need of keeping beasts from straying into
the field from the road rather than any appreciation of the
general advantages of enclosed arable which led to the fencing
of this close.[3] Possibly one ought to reckon along with these
cases several entries where arable land is described as being
on ' Kettle Hedge ' furlong, or ' on Long Patch hedge ', on
' Nuttedge [=Nut-hedge ?] furlong ', ' at Longthorne Hedge ',
or ' in Acre Hedge furlong '.[4] But there is really nothing at
all to show that these furlongs were enclosed : each may have
derived its name from the hedge of some close of pasture
which bounded the furlong on one side but did not separate
it from the open field.

Of the conversion of arable into pasture, there is practically
no evidence in the surveys except the mention of a close of
pasture ' called fallow corner ', unless indeed it is possible to
see a sign of such conversion in the fact that the Rector of

---

[1] v. P. S. Northants, 20, folio 29.   [2] v. ibid., folio 75.
[3] v. ibid., folio 94. This tends to throw further doubt upon Ogilby's
Britannia as an authority for the extent of enclosure. And indeed Prof.
Gonner, though he attaches ' very great importance to Ogilby's testimony ',
admits that ' hedges and walls would often occur along a road and not on
the land ', v. op. cit., pp. 170, 173 notes.
[4] v. P. S. Northants, 20, folios 78, 86, 93.

Grafton claimed a tithe out of Grafton Park.[1] Only one entry tells of the confusion of rights which might 'accompany enclosure. It is a marginal note with reference to a close of pasture on Anthony Whalley's farm, and it informs us that ' this Close is claymed to belong to the Inhabitants of Alderton as being exchanged for some Lande of theirs now impaled within Grafton park and therewith sold '.[2]

The valuation of the different kinds of land in the principal survey is very instructive, and in particular illustrates the importance of pasture. Excluding doubtful cases, the amount of pasture which is valued in this survey apart from buildings, meadows, or other sorts of land is 337 acres 3 roods 10 poles. The value of this amounts to £321 9s. 2d. per annum, or about 19s. an acre on an average.[3] The least valuable of these pastures was a close of 9½ acres valued at £2 6s. 8d. per annum, or slightly less than 4s. 11d. an acre.[4] The most valuable apparently was the piece called the Old Park, which contained 36¼ acres, and was estimated to be worth £48 7s. 4d. per annum, or slightly more than £1 6s. 8d. an acre.[5]

The average value of meadow land seems to have been less than that of the pasture. The total amount of meadow separately valued in the principal survey is 165 acres 3 roods 12 poles, and the total value of this land was £128 10s. 7d. per annum, which works out at about 15s. 6d. an acre. A certain amount of meadow was valued at £1 an acre, which is the highest figure found, while, on the other hand, we find some that was only worth 10s. an acre per annum.[6]

[1] v. P. S. Northants, 20, folio 60, and P. S. Northants, 23. On February 6, 1641, Thomas Austen, the parson of Grafton, made complaint about proceedings which had been taken against him in the High Commission Court. It is stated that litigation first began in the matter sixteen years before about the tithe of Grafton Park. But on June 24, 1641, some parishioners of Grafton complained that Austen used to vex his neighbours with frivolous and idle suits, that he stirred up suits between them, and uncharitably affirmed that lawing kept him alive. The petitioners enumerated many instances of his profanity and want of reverence during the services of the Church, and begged that he might be removed from the living. v. Calendar of House of Lords MSS. in Appendix to 4th Report of Royal Commission on Historical MSS., Part I (1874), pp. 47, 78, 80, 82.
[2] v. P. S. Northants, 20, folio 16.
[3] For the particulars v. Table II at the end of this chapter.
[4] v. P. S. Northants, 20, folio 27.   [5] v. ibid., folio 4.
[6] For the particulars see Table III at the end of this chapter.

Excluding doubtful cases, the arable land separately valued in the survey amounts to 322 acres and is valued at £67 14s. per annum, or just over 4s. 2d. an acre on an average. The most valuable arable was assessed at 6s. an acre, and the poorest at 3s.[1]

The great difference in the values of arable and pasture sufficiently explains the tendency to increase the area of pasture; and in the light of the valuations it is only surprising that the surveys do not reveal more definite traces of the conversion of arable land.

Great as was the importance of pasture farming, we are not without evidence that even in tillage there had been some innovation and some disturbance of the mediaeval order on the lands reported on in the Grafton surveys. As I have already pointed out, there is some reason for supposing that a little ploughed land, though only a very little, was enclosed. There are more definite indications of the consolidation of strips, though here too the area affected seems to have been small. On Mrs. Fleetwood's farm most of the arable was consolidated, lying indeed in three contiguous fields of 13, 14, and 14¾ acres respectively. But the names of these fields—Hall Field, Middle Hall Field, and Nether Hall Field—make one suspect that the farm was once a demesne, and in that case the consolidation is less noteworthy.[2] In the case of another holding—that in the tenure of John Waite—the arable seems to have lain in scattered strips in one of the three fields, but to have been consolidated in the other two. At least, that appears the most natural interpretation of the survey, for it speaks of eight parcels lying in south field ' severally ', of eleven parcels lying in Roade field ' severally ', and of nine parcels in the mill field ' divided in the comon feild '[3]. Sometimes a portion of a man's land would be consolidated, while other portions even in the same field lay scattered. This was probably so on one of the holdings of

[1] For particulars see Table IV at the end of this chapter.
[2] v. P. S. Northants, 20, folio 27. It is interesting to notice that these lands were still subject to common of shack : that at least seems the proper deduction from the fact that they are described as ' lying in common fields '.
[3] v. ibid., folio 47.

Thomas Church, who, besides other pieces of land in the same
' common field ', had ' 13 ridges butting on the common leane
the land of Luke Barrett west '.[1]   It is, however, just possible
that these 13 ridges were not contiguous, and that only the
end of each adjoined the lane, which in that case would be
in the position of a headland towards them.   This possibility
seems excluded, however, in the case of another holding of
' Mr. Thomas Church '.   Besides several pieces of one to six
roods in Wallis's Field, this holding contained in the same
field ' one parcel in Addington corner called the 15 ridges ',
the area of the parcel being 3 acres 3 roods.[2]   In a good many
cases it is possible, but not certain, that consolidation is indicated.   When we read that Thomas Church of Wootton had
as part of the arable held by him in Windmill Field ' 7 ridges
next John Manning west and Sir John Wake east ', are we to
conclude that seven strips lay together, or merely that each
of these strips was flanked by strips belonging to Manning
and Wake ? [3]   Perhaps some light on this problem of interpretation may be obtained from the description of some
arable in the tenure of John Manning.[4]   We read of two
ridges in a certain furlong which were flanked on both sides
by some land belonging to John Haines.   Immediately afterwards comes a duplicate entry ; and one is tempted to suppose that each pair of strips lay together, for otherwise it
would seem that a single entry speaking of four ridges must
have commended itself to the draughtsman of the survey as
the simplest means of expressing his meaning.   And from this
one could argue by implication that all the entries which
speak of 2, 3, 4, 5, 6, or more ' ridges ' or ' lands ' with the same
neighbours are evidences of a certain measure of consolidation.
But, unfortunately, it is possible that the duplicate entries
which contain the name of John Haines may have originated
in a careless repetition, and that each may refer to the same
two strips.   In that case a large number of entries which otherwise would afford evidence of much piecemeal consolidation
may have to be put aside as barren of certain conclusions.

---

[1] v. P. S. Northants, 20, folio 63.   [2] v. ibid., folio 75.
[3] v. ibid., folio 80.   [4] v. ibid., folio 78.

More interesting are some cases where we find that the strips which a man held as part of one holding were contiguous with other strips held by him from some other source. For instance, attached to one of John Manning's holdings as part of the arable belonging to him in the town field in Roade parish, were ' eleven ridges in Gorecraft John Manning E '.[1] Apparently John Manning had contrived to get two holdings with some adjacent strips ; and on turning to the description of the other holding in his tenure, which is reported on in the survey, we find that along with other arable in the town field he held ' 2 lands on Cley furlong John Maninge west and Tho. Saxbey senior east '.[2] But if these two entries can be considered complementary, they enormously strengthen the case for the interpretation of other entries which was suggested by the doubtful references to John Haines's land quoted above. For obviously *eleven* ridges cannot be adjacent to *two* lands without being themselves more or less consolidated. But even here doubt assails one. There seem to have been two John Mannings. At least there was a third holding which is described as in the tenure of ' John Maninge of Horton '.[3]

Another farmer who appears from the principal survey of Grafton to have held adjacent but tenurially heterogeneous strips was Richard Church. An acre and a half of the arable which he held in the Town Field in Roade parish was adjacent to some more land of his which lay to the south of it.[4] On another farm he had in Ashton Field, along with other arable, two roods ' at Birch Bush Rd. Church west Jo. Manning E.', and three acres ' at Hartwell parke gate next Rd. Church east '.[5] As neither of these entries corresponds to the first, it may be concluded that Richard Church held other land besides the two holdings described in the survey. Of this,

[1] v. P. S. Northants, 20, folio 77.   [2] v. ibid., folio 61.
[3] v. ibid., folio 73.   [4] v. ibid., folio 93.
[4] v. ibid., folio 91. Similar instances might be quoted in regard to holdings of Thomas Church ; but the question of identity is in this case so doubtful as to make conclusions worthless. Besides ' Thomas Church ' and ' Mr. Thomas Church ', we read of ' Thomas Church of the Greene ', ' Tho. Church of Wootton ', ' Tho. Church of Brinton ', ' Tho. Church de Benington ', and ' Tho. Church son of Will Church '. Even the hypothesis made above in estimating the size of holdings seems risky.

other evidence may be found in the appearance of his name among those owing ' ffree rents in Hartwell '.[1]

It is impossible, in the face of the various uncertainties mentioned above, to estimate the extent of piecemeal consolidation which had taken place. But however far the gathering together of small groups of strips may have gone, it is quite clear that the great bulk of the arable land described in the survey lay in scattered parcels. Though little groups of strips may have been formed in this furlong or that, ' mingle-mangle ' was still the rule, and, in each great field at least, if not in every furlong, nearly every holding had its share made up of numerous divided portions. Nor does this seem surprising when we consider the valuation of the consolidated arable fields on Mrs. Fleetwood's farm. The three consolidated fields together contained 41¾ acres, and their total value was assessed at £7 3s. 7d. per annum. But this is appreciably less than the average value of the arable land reported on in the principal survey.[2]

APPENDIX I

THE MEANING OF THE WORD *LEY* IN THE PARLIAMENTARY SURVEYS OF GRAFTON

In the sixteenth and seventeenth centuries the words *leye, ley, lay, lea* and *leaze* seem to have borne a fluctuating and uncertain meaning. For one thing, it appears that two words of distinct origin were confused.[3] A reference to the literature of the age makes one despair of attaching any precise meaning to the word *ley* as used in the parliamentary surveys of Grafton. Fitzherbert in one place speaks of ploughing ' leys ' for fallow or to sow oats upon.[4] In another passage, he remarks that ' leye hey is good for shepe '.[5] In his ' Surveyinge ' he

---

[1] v. P. S. Northants, 20, folio 102.
[2] v. ibid., folio 27. It should be remembered that these fields, though consolidated, were still subject to common of shack, v. *supra*, p. 54 footnote.
[3] The plural of lea (O.E. *lēah*) has been confused with lease (O.E. *læs*) and also with an elliptical use of the adjective lea (=fallow). v. A New English Dictionary (Oxford, 1908), vol. vi, pp. 136–7. I am indebted to this work for several of the references which follow.
[4] v. Husbandry, § 8.   [5] v. ibid., § 25.

distinguishes between the fallow field, the ley field, and the pasture field, and says that the farmer may ' plough up his close that he had for his layse '.[1] The language of Shakespeare is similarly puzzling. On the one hand we read that—

> Her fallow leas
> The darnel hemlock and rank fumitory
> Doth root upon.[2]

On the other hand, there are the lines,

> Ceres most bounteous Lady thy rich Leas
> Of Wheate, Rye, Barley, Fetches, Oates and Pease ; [3]

and the line,

> Dry up thy marrows, vines and plow-torn leas.[4]

The ballad ' Now-a-days ' clearly opposes ' lays ' to arable land in the couplet,

> The towns go down, the land decays
> Of corne-fieldes, plaine lays ; [5]

and similarly, in the seventeenth century, Drummond of Hawthornden spoke of the husbandman turning his ' acres into leyes '.[6] Again, Sir William Forrest, a versifier of the reign of Henry VIII, speaks of ' Cow Leys ',[7] while Aubrey, in his ' History of Wiltshire ', defines ' Leghs ' as pastures.[8] On the other hand the sense of ' fallow ' seems given to the word ' lay ' in Evelyn's ' Terra ', which dates from 1676,[9] while Folkingham, writing in 1610, asserts that 'rapes require a broken-up lay '.[10]

Modern dialectal uses are not much more definite ; but occasionally the word seems to be used with a precise sense in reference to arable land temporarily under grass. Thus in Caithness ' lea ' signifies ' cultivated land under a second year's crop of grass '. In Northamptonshire it is said to be a ' very common name for pasture fields ', though it ' will never be found in connexion with meadow land proper, but it will usually denote land once arable but now " laid " down '.[11]

---

[1] v. Fitzherbert, Surveyinge, folio 59, quoted Cunningham, Growth of Industry and Commerce in the Early and Middle Ages (4th edition), pp. 527–8.
[2] v. Henry V. v. ii. 44.   [3] v. Tempest IV. i. 60.
[4] Timon of Athens IV. iii. 193.
[5] Quoted by T. E. Scrutton, Commons and Common Fields, p. 82.
[6] v. Irene [Works, 1711], 164.
[7] Quoted Scrutton, op. cit., p. 85.   [8] Quoted Scrutton, op. cit., p. 99.
[9] v. Terra (1676), 63 ; cp. Sylvester, Du Bartas, I. vii. 392 : ' A field, left lay for some few years, will yeeld The richer crop when it again is till'd ' (1591), quoted in Oxford Dictionary.
[10] v. W. Folkingham, Feudigraphia (1610), I. ii. 36.
[11] v. The English Dialect Dictionary [ed. Joseph Wright], vol. iii (Oxford, 1902), p. 547.

In the parliamentary surveys of Grafton the obscurity of meaning attaching to the word is considerable. Wherever 'leys' are separately valued in these surveys their value per acre is the same as that of the arable on the same holding and considerably less than that of the pasture or meadow. In one case, however, under the heading of meadow belonging to a certain holding, we read of one parcel 'in Ashton mead' and one parcel 'of Leeyes', each parcel being an acre in extent, and the two together have a much higher value per acre than that of arable land on the same holding, but, unfortunately, the meadow and ley land are not separately valued.[1]

It is significant that the 'leys' are sometimes spoken of as lying in the common field,[2] or in the three fields,[3] or reckoned under the head of 'arable land in common field',[4] while in another place we are told of a parcel of 'arable land called Nan [or Nun ?] leyes',[5] and in another of two parcels of leyes 'in old dam furlong'.[6]

On the other hand, as I have already pointed out, meadows and leys are classed together in one case,[7] and in another place a list of various parcels of land, which concludes with a piece 'in Broad Meadow lying within the seven acres' and 'one lott in Ash meadow', has the area of all its items summed up as 'total of arable lands and leys'.[8] Elsewhere we read of a parcel of 'Lea Ground or pasture ground',[9] and of 'Leaze or Pasture Ground called the Styes or the Cowe Pasture'.[10]

That certain lands were permanently classed as leys—perhaps because they were periodically put under grass or had been so treated at some time for a considerable period—is shown by the appearance of the word as a field name in the principal survey of Grafton. Mention is made of 'Ledgers leyes' and the 'More leyes',[11] of 'Pollecutt leyes',[12] and 'Holme leyes'[13]; and if the names 'meade leyes'[14] and 'Oxe

---

[1] v. P. S. Northants, 20, folio 87.   [2] v. ibid., folio 10.

[3] v. ibid., folio 76 and P. S. Northants, 21, folios 1–5.

[4] v. P. S. Northants, 20, folio 33, cp. folio 89.

[5] v. ibid., folio 57.

[6] v. ibid., folio 69. In the Hartwell Survey of 17 Henry VIII [v. Treasury of Receipt, Misc. Bks. 179, folios 21–9]. *A tenet B acras terre arabilis et leylande et C acras prati* is a common form of entry. In the Grafton survey of 1619 [v. Land Revenue, Misc. Bks., vol. 221] we read: *Jacobus Jenkens tenet . . . Terram arrabilem et lezuram jacentes in campis.*

[7] v. P. S. Northants, 20, folio 87.

[8] v. ibid., folios 38–9.   [9] v. P. S. Northants, 24, folio 1.

[10] v. P. S. Northants, 21, folio 22; cp. 'Ley' pasture' in Land Revenue, Misc. Bks. vol. 201, f. 13 (1605).

[11] v. P. S. Northants, 20, folio 41.   [12] v. ibid., folio 46.

[13] v. ibid., folio 33.   [14] v. ibid., folio 55.

Leyes '[1] betray the affinity of leys with grassland, the names ' Corne Crafte lea ',[2] ' the tenn leyes ',[3] and ' nyne leyes ',[4] as well as the entry ' Six leyes in Caswell '[5] seem to show their connexion with corn-growing and with the strips of the open fields. A particularly puzzling entry is that which, in a list of open field strips, mentions a parcel of land ' called Ley Close being 7 ridges lying N. of willow furlong '.[6] Ought we to suppose that seven arable strips have here been enclosed and subjected to convertible husbandry, or that an enclosure known as Ley Close has been thrown open and ploughed up and incorporated with the strips of the common field ? The name ' hanke (?) leyes hedge '[7] also suggests that leys were sometimes enclosed, though the occurrence of the name ' acre hedge '[8] should perhaps deter one from basing much upon this evidence. Similarly interesting and puzzling is the name ' New laide furlong '.[9]

The fact that on more than one holding the leyes are said to consist of three grounds, one ' in the ffen ', one ' att Gogmire Leyes ', and one ' att Well Spring Leyes '[10] makes one suspect that the dampness of the soil may have had something to do with its treatment as leys in these cases.

It is hard to know how to interpret several entries which occur early in the survey and speak of ' arable land ... lying in that ffeild called the Towne ffeild by severall pcells well knowne the whole ffeild being Lease land '.[11] Though it is impossible to regard the difference in spelling as significant because of the definite equation of ' Lease ' and ' Leyes ' in another entry,[12] I am inclined to think that the surveyor only intended to indicate that the ' Towne ffeild ' was lying fallow, perhaps for a longer period than usual, at the time when the survey was made. At all events I have classed this land as arable in all the statistical tables, and have treated similarly the ' pcell of arable land called Nan leyes '.[13]

In general it seems probable that on the leys some kind of convertible husbandry or ' Feldgraswirthschaft ' was practised.

---

[1] v. P. S. Northants, 20, folio 76.   [2] v. ibid., folio 55.
[3] v. ibid., folio 64.   [4] v. ibid., folio 75.   [5] v. ibid., folio 89.
[6] v. ibid., folio 29.   [7] v. ibid., folio 63.   [8] v. ibid., folio 64.
[9] v. ibid., folio 76.   [10] v. ibid., folio 15, for example.
[11] v. ibid., folio 15, for example.   [12] v. ibid., folio 13.
[13] v. ibid., folio 57.

APPENDIX II

PAYMENTS MADE FOR FAVOURABLE LEASES

THE practice of raising money on the Crown lands by selling leases at a low rent is illustrated by an entry in the Parliamentary Survey of Grimscott in the parish of Coldhigham.[1] It runs as follows :—

Wee whose names are underwritten authorised by Comission from the honoʳable Trustees for survey' of the late King's lands Lying and being in the County of Northton : doe certifie, yt. upon much importunity and bemoanings of the seuerall ᵽties here inserted who have showed us their Accquittances and made Oath of the truth thereoff : that these seuerall sũmes have beene truely paid to Sr George Binnion Knight then Receivor : whose Accquittances are ready to show under his hand for 31 yeares in Reuersion and knowing the very poore and low estate of these ᵽties that declare : if your Honoʳˢ be not mercifull in allowing these Moneyes they will be many of them undone : which we leave to yoʳ Honorˢ consideration.'

This is followed by a list of names and sums under the heading Roade, which begins : ' Mrs Mary Fleetwood for A Contract for 31 yeares 100 . 0 . 0 '. Then for similar contracts it seems that William Blunt paid £33, Richard Lightwood £21, John Tomlinson £7, John Stokes £6, Thos. Read £7, John and Jeffry Conn £7, John Clarke £20, Nicholas Lawson [' for halfe his fine for a Contract ' of 31 years] £25, Robert Consor £2 5s., Thomas Smith £25, John Wayt £10. For Potterspury we have the name Richard Sriuener senior who paid £140 for a 31 years' contract, while under the heading of Grafton Regis occur the names of William Smith alias Caues, £66 3s. 4d. ; William Smith (again), £45 ; and Ann Goodman, £40—all for 31-year contracts. Lastly under the heading of Cold Higham and Grimscott are eight names, of whom six it appears paid £37 and two £57 for a 31-years' contract. Then the entry concludes with the signatures of the surveyors William Fuory, Richard Sadler, and Thomas Baynard.

The real nature of the transactions mentioned above becomes clearer if we look at two cases in detail. The lands occupied by William Blunt at Roade in 1650 were valued at £19 5s. 6d. a year, but the rent payable for them under the lease of 31 August, 8 James I, to Eldred and Whitmore was only £2 0s. 4d. This lease had still 26 years to run.[2] Thomas Smith, to take another instance, held 15½ acres at Roade in

---

[1] v. P. S. Northants, 29, folio 48.   [2] v. P. S. Northants, 20, folio 42.

1650 and the holding was valued at £3 18s. 4d. a year, but the rent which he paid under a lease of 16 July, 21 James I, was only 19s. This lease had only 4 years to run on Lady Day, 1650; but it appears from a marginal note initialed by the Surveyor-General that the Committee of Obstructions by an order of September 9, 1650, allowed the reversion of the estate for another 31 years to descend to Jul. Smith—presumably in consideration of the facts stated in the survey of Grimscott.[1]

No doubt the leases of Crown lands were sometimes really 'beneficiary'. This may have been so in the case of Elizabeth's favourite, Robert, Earl of Leicester, who only paid £20 as a fine for the demesnes of Grafton in 1581.[2] But clearly efforts were made to raise large sums of ready money by the sale of leases on favourable terms.

---

[1] v. P. S. Northants, 20, folio 32.
[2] The receipt for this fine is preserved in the British Museum, v. Add. Ch. 39968 (18). It is dated July 12, 1581, and runs : *Robto. Comit. Leic. pro fine dimiss. terre. dmical. de Grafftonne de eodem fine xxli.* Perhaps this was a fine payable in advance for the reversion : certainly it appears from the Parliamentary Survey that Leicester obtained a lease of the demesne of 1 March 29 Eliz. for thirty years to commence from Lady Day, 1602.

TABLE I. THE SIZE OF HOLDINGS SEPARATELY DESCRIBED IN THE PRINCIPAL SURVEY OF GRAFTON [PARLIAMENTARY SURVEYS, NORTHANTS, No. 20]

Size of Holdings.	No.	Total area of Class.			Percentage of pasture and meadow [not counting premises of houses as pasture].	Percentage of pasture and meadow [counting premises as pasture].	Percentage of arable and leys [excluding leys definitely classed with meadow].
		A.	R.	P.			
1. 100 acres and over	1	585	2	5	100 [apparently, though 27¾ acres are not definitely stated to be pasture or meadow.]		
2. 50 acres and over but under 100 acres	4	282 [or 283]	0	3¼ [3½?]	22·4	26·3	72·3
3. 40 acres and over but under 50 acres	9	398	1	0	17·5	20·7	79·3
4. 30 acres and over but under 40 acres	2	70	2	0	15·2	25·9	74·1
5. 20 acres and over but under 30 acres	4	92	0	5	6·5	18·5	81·5
6. 15 acres and over but under 20 acres	4*	69	0	0	9·1 [25·4]†	19·6 [33·7]†	80·4 [66·3]†
7. 10 acres and over but under 15 acres	6	77	1	0	7 [8·7]‡	11·5 [12]‡	88·5 [87·7]‡
8. 5 acres and over but under 10 acres	6	46	0	0	14·9	22·3	76·6
9. 1 acre and over but under 5 acres	5	13	1	10	28·4§	50·3 [45·5]‖	28·1 [31·9]‖
10. Under one acre	15	[In none of these cases is land measured apart from the premises. Measurements of the whole area are given in 10 cases, and in 7 of these it is 10 poles or under.]					

* This is not counting one holding of 18 acres, entirely wood [folio 50].

† On one holding there is a close of 12 acres, probably pasture, but not so described. The figures in brackets are obtained when this doubtful holding is included.

‡ In this class there are three doubtful cases, where the pasture and meadow are not precisely distinguished from other land: these cases are included in the figures within brackets.

§ This figure is obtained from three of the holdings only : the two smallest are excluded, because in one case no land is distinguished from the premises of the house and, in the other, one acre is undescribed (though probably arable).

‖ The figures in brackets are obtained when all five holdings are included and the doubtful acre reckoned as arable : the figures 50·3 % and 28·1 % are for the other four holdings.

TABLE II. VALUE OF PASTURE WHERE GIVEN SEPARATELY AND APART FROM TENEMENTS IN THE PRINCIPAL PARLIAMENTARY SURVEY OF GRAFTON [P. S. NORTHANTS, 20]

No. of Folio.	Area.			Value per annum.			No. of Folio.	Area.			Value per annum.		
	A.	R.	P.	£	s.	d.		A.	R.	P.	£	s.	d.
3	3	2	0	2	15	0	53	4	0	0	2	0	0
4	86	1	10	86	5	0	57	3	0	0	1	10	0
4	85	0	0	99	3	4	60	1	0	0		10	6
4	36	1	0	48	7	4	61	1	1	0		12	8
4	13	1	0	10	13	4	63	18	0	0	7	13	4
4	9	1	0	12	6	8	75	5	0	0	3	8	0
7	3	0	0	3	0	0	77	3	0	0	1	10	0
10	10	0	0	6	10	0	79	1	0	0		13	4
18	6	0	0	7	10	8	80	1	0	0		10	0
24	1	2	0	1	10	0	89	1	0	0	1	0	0
25	1	2	0	1	5	0	95	1	2	0		15	0
27	9	2	0	2	6	8	95	4	0	0	2	0	0
28	5	0	0	1	13	4	Total	337	3	10	321	9	2
51	24	0	0	16	0	0							

Average value about 19s. an acre per annum.

TABLE III. VALUE OF MEADOW WHERE GIVEN SEPARATELY AND APART FROM TENEMENTS IN THE PRINCIPAL PARLIAMENTARY SURVEY OF GRAFTON [P. S. NORTHANTS, 20]

No. of Folio.	Area.			Value per annum.			No. of Folio.	Area.			Value per annum.		
	A.	R.	P.	£	s.	d.		A.	R.	P.	£	s.	d.
4	28	0	0	22	11	8	42	3	0	0	1	10	0
4	16	3	0	16	15	0	46	2	3	0	1	13	4
5	5	3	0	3	13	4	47	1	0	0		10	0
5	1	3	35	1	3	4	52	2	0	4	2	0	0
5	27	0	0	23	4	2	56	3	3	20	3	9	9
5	11	2	0	8	12	6	58	1	0	0		10	0
5	20	2	0	13	13	4	64		3	0		10	0
5	7	2	0	5	10	0	70		1	0		3	4
8	2	2	0	2	10	0	71		1	0		3	4
11	2	2	0	2	10	0	73		2	0		5	0
13	2	2	0	2	10	0	79	2	0	0	1	0	0
16	2	2	0	2	10	0	81	1	2	0		15	0
26	2	2	0	2	10	0	83	3	0	0	1	10	0
28	6	0	13	3	0	10	90	2	2	0	1	13	4
31		2	0		6	8	92		1.	0		3	4
32	1	2	0		15	0	96	1	0	0		10	0
33			20		1	8	Total	165	3	12	128	10	7
34		2	0		6	8							

Average value about 15s. 6d. an acre per annum.

TABLE IV. VALUE OF ARABLE WHERE GIVEN SEPARATELY AND
APART FROM TENEMENTS IN THE PRINCIPAL PARLIAMENTARY
SURVEY OF GRAFTON [P. S. NORTHANTS, 20]

No. of Folio.	Area.			Value per annum.			No. of Folio.	Area.			Value per annum.		
	A.	R.	P.	£	s.	d.		A.	R.	P.	£	s.	d.
7	36	0	0	10	16	0	61–2	8	3	0	1	12	4
12	36	0	0	10	16	0	66	5	0	0		15	0
15	36	0	0	10	16	0	71	8	0	0	1	6	8
27	13	0	0	2	3	4	73–4	7	0	0	1	3	4
27	14	3	0	2	9	7	78	33	2	0	5	6	0
27	14	0	0	2	10	8	80	10	2	0	1	14	2
32	13	0	0	2	3	4	86–7	17	0	0	2	11	0
34	3	1	0		10	10	91	16	0	0	2	13	4
36	3	1	0		9	9	95	19	0	0	3	3	4
47	13	0	0	2	3	4	Total	322	0	0	67	14	0
57	15	0	0	2	10	0							

Average value about 4s. 2d. an acre per annum.

CHAPTER III

THE ECONOMY OF THE MANORS OF GRAFTON AND HARTWELL BEFORE AND AFTER 1650

1. The Purpose and Scope of this Chapter

THE significance of social conditions at any particular period can only be appreciated fully in the light of history. A knowledge of earlier conditions and of later developments is essential to a proper understanding of any given economic structure. It is therefore necessary to consider the facts revealed by the Parliamentary Surveys of Grafton in their historical setting before comparing the economy of Grafton with that of other royal estates reported on by the parliamentary surveyors. For this purpose there is no need to trace all the details of local history from the earliest times to the present day. It will be sufficient to summarize so much of the evidence as indicates how far the conditions which obtained at Grafton in 1650 were of old standing and to what extent they were transformed by subsequent developments.

2. The Extent of 6 Edward III

Some information as to the mediaeval economy of the manor of Grafton can be obtained from an extent of the year 1332, which is preserved in the Record Office.[1] From this document we learn that the capital messuage of the manor with its immediate appurtenances was worth 6s. 8d. a year ; that there were on the demesne 120 acres of arable land worth 5d. an acre per annum ; that there were 10 acres of meadow worth 2s. an acre per annum, a *separabilis pastura* called the Wold which was worth 1s. 6d. a year, two woods, and a common pasture. There were seven free tenants on the manor who paid between them 22s. 10d. a year—half of it at Easter and half at Michaelmas—and eleven other tenants who paid between them £3 18s. 4d. by equal quarterly

---

[1] v. Ancient Extents, Exchequer Q. R. No. 84.

instalments *et nichil operantur.* There were also three tenants who paid yearly 8 capons worth 1s. 8d., and ten who paid 10 hens a year worth 1s. 3d. as well as 70 eggs worth 3d. The common oven brought in 3s., the receipts of the court 14s. a year. Thus the total value of the manor as reported on was £9 19s. 6d. a year, and this was asserted to be its value in the eleventh year of Edward II as well as in 1332.

3. The Surveys of 17 Henry VIII

It is obvious that the information provided by the Edwardian extent is not sufficiently detailed to allow any comparison to be made between the conditions of the fourteenth century and those which obtained in 1650. For material comparable with that provided by the Parliamentary Surveys it is necessary to have recourse to two surveys of the year 1526, which are in the Record Office.[1] The first of these is a rental of the manor of Hartwell : the second is a rental of the manor of Grafton. Thus it is probable that they refer in great part to the same estates as the Parliamentary Surveys analysed in the last chapter, for the chief of those surveys [2] is entitled ' A Survey of the Mannor or Lordship of Grafton being the principalle seate of the Honno' with the Mannor of Hartwell annexed '. It is, however, impossible to trace an exact correspondence between the areas reported on at the two periods. The earlier survey of Hartwell mentions a good many holdings —mostly free tenements in neighbouring parishes—without giving their acreage ; and the total area dealt with in the Parliamentary Surveys is considerably larger than that reported on in the two surveys of 1526. For purposes of comparison it will probably be best to ignore all the holdings of unspecified area mentioned in the earlier surveys, to discover the proportions of the remaining lands devoted to different uses or occupied in holdings of different sizes, and to compare these proportions with those which obtained in the middle of the next century on all the lands reported on in the various Parliamentary Surveys of Grafton.

[1] v. Treasury of the Receipt, Miscellaneous Books, vol. 179, folios 21–39.
[2] P. S. Northants, 20.

The two surveys of 1526 deal with lands of specified area,
amounting to 1,633 acres 1 rood 20 poles, of which 102¼ acres
are included in Grafton Park[1] and 29 acres in Hartwell Park.[2]
Of this area 680 acres come under the heading of arable and
leys ;[3] 592¼ acres are definitely classed as pasture; and 118¾
acres are definitely classed as meadow.   Of the remainder
100½ acres were woodland; but the precise nature of 141 acres
3 roods 20 poles is not stated, though 93¼ acres out of these
were contained in the parks and therefore probably consisted
of pasture, while 40 acres were probably arable.   Another
7½ acres of the doubtful area are accounted for by crofts
attached to houses, which may perhaps be presumed to be
grassland : half a rood is described as a ' Hemplande ' and
one acre lay in paddocks (?), probably of pasture.[4]   Now, if
these doubtful areas are assigned their probable character and
included in the calculation, it appears that the distribution
of the land described in the two surveys was : arable and
leys, 44·1%; pasture and meadow, 49·7%; woodland, 6·2%.[5]
If the doubtful areas are ignored and their acreage subtracted
from the total, the figures are : arable and leys, 45·6%;
pasture and meadow, 47·7%; woodland, 6·7%.   A certain
measure of uncertainty attaches to these figures, because the
area of the common pasture used by the tenants of Hartwell
is not stated : we are simply told that they had liberty of

[1] Besides this a pasture of 30 acres, classed with the demesne lands let
to the ' firmarius ', was called ' Little Park '.
[2] Possibly 13 acres of underwood should be added to this total ; it is
not certain, though I think it probable, that this was included in the 29 acres
over which one John Adyngton enjoyed rights of herbage (v. folios 25 and
27).   The total of 1633 acres 1 rood 20 poles does not include 3 acres of
land at Quinton held by one of the free tenants of the manor of Hartwell
along with a cottage.
[3] In the Grafton Survey leys are not mentioned at all.   In the Hartwell
Survey we generally read : ' *A. tenet N. et M. acras terre arrabilis et leylande.*'
In one case the words ' *in communibus campis* ' are added.   In one case leys
are distinguished : Richard Church ' *tenet . . . xxvi acras terre arrabilis et
sex acras leylande*'.
[4] A further element of doubt is introduced by the impossibility of
knowing in certain instances whether the area covered by buildings is
included in the acreage of adjacent closes, but the margin of error must
in any case be insignificant.
[5] That is, taking the total as 1,633¼ acres and ignoring the 20 poles of
hempland in order to simplify the arithmetic.

common in the forest of Salcey. It would, of course, be possible to make an hypothetical calculation by crediting the tenants of Hartwell with an amount of common pasture proportionate to that enjoyed by the tenants of Grafton ; but the justification of such an hypothesis depends on the assumption that the proportion which obtained at Grafton was typical, and this is extremely doubtful, for the creation of a large holding of grassland which was let to a *firmarius* Hynman may have curtailed the commons of Grafton, and the fact that the tenants of Grafton claimed common rights over some land held by one Edward Knyghtley, while no similar claim is mentioned as made by the tenants of Hartwell, in itself suggests that the common pasture was felt to be insufficient at Grafton and was believed to have been curtailed, while there is no evidence that this was the case in regard to the manor of Hartwell. On the other hand, it would be equally unfair to exclude the figures provided by the Hartwell Survey altogether and to take those of the Grafton Survey alone as typical, for the great bulk of the grassland at Grafton did not consist of common pasture, but formed the large grazing farm already mentioned, and, though the creation of this farm may have involved the appropriation of common pasture, it may also have meant a considerable conversion of arable to pasture, and, if this was so, the absence of this factor at Hartwell is a feature quite as essential to the truth of the historical picture as its presence at Grafton.[1]

The total number of tenants mentioned by name in the two surveys of 1526 is 48. Of these, 32 seem to have held land *ad voluntatem domini*, while one is described as a *firmarius*, and 17 were free tenants—two of these last being apparently identical with individuals who held land *ad voluntatem*. Besides Lord Ferrers who held the manor of Bugbrook,

---

[1] The figures provided by the Grafton Survey alone are : total area, 953 acres 1 rood 20 poles ; arable and leys, 226 acres ; pasture and meadow, 571½ acres ; woodland, 71 acres ; doubtful, 84 acres 3 roods 20 poles (of which 77¼ acres were probably pasture and 7 acres 2 roods 20 poles consisted of houses and crofts). Of the pasture and meadow, 50 acres are described as a common pasture, while the *firmarius* held 460 acres. Out of the total of 571½ acres, 96 acres were meadow and the remainder pasture.

only 7 of the free tenants are mentioned as holding any land other than gardens or crofts attached to houses. Nine of the free holdings were in places other than Hartwell or Grafton.[1]

Five surnames of tenants mentioned in 1526, and five only, recur in the middle of the seventeenth century among the names of tenants mentioned in the Parliamentary Surveys of Grafton. One Richard Churche held 54¼ acres *ad voluntatem* in 1526, besides holding *certas terras* as a free tenant, and one John Churche is also mentioned as a free tenant in the same survey. The survey of 1650 shows that over 200 acres were held by persons bearing the name of Church in the middle of the seventeenth century. In 1526 a certain John Whalley was tenant of some 56 acres besides a ruined messuage with its adjoining croft : in 1650 Anthony Whalley, Gent., was tenant of 52½ acres which he sublet to Widow Goodman, while the survey of 1656 mentions an additional 23 acres of which he had been lately tenant. Again, Richard Bryce held 40 acres in 1526 : in 1650 another Richard Bryce held just over 24 acres. Two acres were held by John Mannyng at the earlier date : rather more than 10 acres were held by his namesake at the later. On the other hand, John Adyngton appears in the Tudor survey as a fairly substantial person holding the herbage of Hartwell Park, which contained 29 acres, and farming the tithes due to the abbey of St. James at Northampton, while the chief Parliamentary Survey mentions one Cuthbert Addington who held a tenement erected on the waste and valued at 3*s.* 4*d.* per annum.

Apart from the herbage of 29 acres in Hartwell Park and the 102 acres of Grafton Park, the area of 26 holdings is given in the two surveys of 1526, one of these holdings being really a combination of three holdings.[2] Out of these 26, one

---

[1] i. e. in Bugbrook, Mursley (in Bucks), Yardley, Northampton, Quinton, and Horton. All the free tenants are mentioned in the Hartwell Survey. Only in one case is any area specified—3 acres of land held with a cottage at Quinton. I have therefore not included any of the free holdings in the agricultural statistics.

[2] It must be remembered that two of the *tenentes ad voluntatem*—one a tenant of 54¼, the other a tenant of 17¼ acres—held besides these areas *certas terras* as free tenants.

contained 460 acres and another 123 acres. The largest
farm consisted entirely of pasture and meadow, but on the
holding of 123 acres, 96 acres were arable and 'leyland'.
The farm which came next in size to these was of 95 acres,
66 of them being arable and 'leyland' *in communibus campis*.
A farm of 68 acres was held by one John Phippes. No less
than 13 out of the 26 holdings were between 30 and 60 acres
in extent—6 of them varying from 52 to 57 acres and 3 being
between 40 and 50 acres. The total area of these 13 holdings
was 590¾ acres, of which 442 acres were certainly and 482 acres
probably arable and ley.[1] There is a considerable tendency
towards uniformity in the amount of arable on these holdings.
Five of the holdings of this class mentioned in the survey of
Hartwell had from 30 to 32 acres of arable and ley : each of
the five holdings of this class mentioned in the Grafton Survey
had 45 or 46 acres of arable. Turning to the smaller holdings,
we find one of 25 acres (entirely pasture), and one of 17¼ acres
of which 15 were arable. The remaining seven holdings varied
in size from 20 poles to 3½ acres : only one of these is stated
to contain any arable land, though one other contained
20 poles of ' Hemplande '.

Besides the holdings whose area is specified, and besides
the free tenants of the Hartwell Survey—of whom 9 out of 17
are credited with land other than gardens or crofts attached
to houses—seven holdings of unspecified area are mentioned
in the two surveys. One was a mill ; one consisted of pasture ;
two were merely cottages with gardens ; and one was a ruined
messuage with a croft held by the tenant of two other holdings.

From these particulars the general position on the manors
of Grafton and Hartwell in 1526 becomes clear enough. A
mediaeval condition of things obtained on a considerable
number of medium-sized holdings, whose features approxi-
mated to those of the typical virgate as regards uniformity
and area and the supply of grazing needs by common rights.

---

[1] In the survey of Hartwell arable and ' leylande ' are usually classed
together, but on two holdings the area of the arable is given without any
mention of ley, and on one the area of the leyland (6 acres) is distinguished
from that of the arable (26 acres). In the Grafton Survey no ley is
mentioned.

On three somewhat larger holdings arable was predominant ; but the largest holding of all—one between three and four times as large as that next it in size—consisted entirely of grassland. The number of tiny holdings was considerable.

Looking more closely, one can distinguish indications of recent changes and of a movement towards engrossing, towards the creation of enclosures of pasture, and towards the suppression of common rights. At Grafton John Whalley was tenant of three distinct holdings. One was a holding of a ' virgate '. type, consisting of a messuage with its croft an acre in extent, 45 acres of arable, and 3 acres of meadow, with the common rights attached to other holdings of this class in the manor, namely, the right to graze 5 horses, 10 steers and heifers, and 40 sheep.[1] Another holding of this same tenant consisted simply of a close of pasture called Blakelande, which contained 7 acres. The entry relating to his remaining holding speaks for itself. *Idem Johannes*, we read, *tenet unum toftum quondam mesuagium edificatum et modo in decasu cum crofto adjacente ; et terre nuper dicto mesuagio pertinentes includuntur infra pasturam domini ; et reddit domino pro dicto tofto—Nichil quia in decasu et nullius valoris.*

The next tenant mentioned after John Whalley in the survey of Grafton was one Richard Holman. He held only a close of pasture called New Close, which was *juxta parcum* and contained 25 acres. In another case we find that a messuage and a croft had been severed from a holding of 47 acres (45 acres arable) : it was *nuper pertinens dicte terre in tenura Thome Lumbarde.* None of the tenants at Grafton who held very small parcels of land enjoyed any common rights, unless one may count as an exception the tenant of a cottage and a ' Hemplande ' of half an acre, of whom it is· said *nullam habet communiam nisi per licentiam tenencium.* Towards the

---

[1] Of the first tenant mentioned in the Grafton Survey it is stated : *Et potest custodire racione tenure 5 equos 10 boviculos et juvencas et 40 oves.* Of John Whalley and of three other tenants of similar holdings we read : *Et potest custodire catalla ut supra.* It is impossible to say whether the unit of 45 arable acres represents the original virgate at Grafton, or whether it arose as a result of a kind of engrossing which redistributed the land in 1½ virgate holdings.

end of the Grafton Survey are some entries in English which
are highly instructive :

Item there have bene emprowed lately within this lordship
    which is presented into the Kynges Chauncery etc.   30 li.
Item there can no ferther enprovemente there be made and
    to kepe the tenauntriez standyng.
Item the tenauntriez there be in sore decaye.

       .   .   .   .   .

Item the tenauntes there have no entercomen with no towne-
    ships.
Item the tenauntes there have no comen within themselff but
    oon comen pasture called Redehey which conteyneth
    by estimacion   50 acrez

       .   .   .   .   .

Item the saied tenauntes claymen to have comen in a
    grounde called the Styes in Aldryngton lordeship which
    is the Freeholde of Edmunde Knyghtley Èsquyer, which
    Edmunde claymeth the saied Styes to be his severall
    grounde and to be discharged of the seid comen there by
    reason of the lorde Marques graunte to hym made bifore
    thexchaunge made bytwene the kyng and the seid lorde
    Marques.

Nor is this all.   Whether Edmund Knyghtley thought that
an attack was the best defence, or whether the biter had been
bitten, or whether he had really been cozened and defrauded
throughout by the ' seid lorde Marques ', or whatever the
rights or uncertainties of the case may have been, the statement of the claim of the tenants of Grafton is immediately
followed by a claim laid by Knyghtley before the Commissioners.   A long statement in Latin declares that he and his
predecessors in the manor of Aldrington had from time imme-
morial enjoyed for themselves, their tenants, and their
' farmers ' *communiam pasture in campis et pratis de Grafton
post granam elatam et asportatam* ; and a careful topographical
description is given of the area to which this applied.   Then
the document concludes as follows :

*Et petit pro se heredibus tenentibus et firmariis suis de Aldrington
    predicta exonerari de aliqua communia sive aliquibus com-
    muniis per tenentes de Grafton in campis et pratis de
    Aldryngton percipiendis racione carte Thome Marchionis
    Dorsetie prefato Edwardo* [? Edmundo] *confecte etc.*

Next comes a note in English :

Item the saied Edmunde Knyghtley claymeth to have to him
and his heirez 5 acrez of land inclosed within the park
of Grafton by the auncestriez of the lord marques and
wrongfully withholden from the seid Edmunde and his
auncestriez by a greate space.

John Whalley too had his grievance.   The survey of Grafton
ends with a copy of a document issued by Richard Wydevile,
Earl of Rivers, in the 6th year of Henry VII, wherein he
grants certain lands at Grafton to John Whalley for his life
in return for the maintenance of an obit at the parish church
of Grafton.   This charter was apparently appealed to in
a claim which Whalley laid before the Commissioners.

Similar, though less striking, indications of the tendencies
of the time are provided by the survey of Hartwell.   The
tenants of Hartwell had liberty of common in the forest of
Salcey, for which they paid 3s. 4d. a year, and for which each
of them gave a hen.   But encroachments upon this common
had apparently taken place.   At least we find that John
Rouhed [= Roughhed ?] held with other lands a close of
24 acres of pasture called Sertlonde [= Assart-land ?], *infra
metas Foreste de Sawcy*, and that John Mersshe along with
other land held *unum clausum pasture de certlond infra Forestam
continens xxiii acras*.   Again, as at Grafton, we are told in
regard to Hartwell that ' the tenements there be in decaye ' ;
and the survey ends with the claim of one Anthony Ardys
to certain lands and tenements in Hartwell and ' Esshen '
which had come into the King's hands ' by reason of suche
Bargayn as of late is made betwne ' the Kynges Highnes &
the lorde marques Dorsett '.

4. The Surveys of the Parks of 1558 and 1564

Before the end of Henry VIII's reign, the manor of Grafton
was made the ' chief principall and capitall parte and place '
of a newly created Honour of the same name ; but the Act
of 1541–2 which effected the change contains no information
of interest with regard to social or economic conditions.[1]

[1] v. 33 Henry VIII, c. 38, in Statutes of the Realm, vol. iii (1817),
pp. 877–89.

That some significant changes had taken place since 1526 is, however, apparent from a survey of Grafton Park which was made in the year 1558.[1] The area of the park was in that year 307½ acres, and we are told that ' ye most pte thereof has beene a parke without ye remembrance of man ', but that ' ye residue of ye number of cxlvi acres has beene taken in by waye of inlargemente about anno vicesimo quarto henrici octavi & since out of ye feilds of Grafton lxxvi acrees & Alderton lxx '.[2] Actually the area added to the park since 1526 was greater than this, for in the survey of that year— as was pointed out above—the park was described as containing 102¼ acres, though perhaps the pasture of 30 acres called Little Park ought to be counted in addition. However this may be, it must not be assumed that the land ' emparked ' out of the fields of Grafton and Alderton was necessarily converted to pasture. According to the survey of 1558, Grafton Park consisted of 177¼ acres of pasture,[3] 42 acres of arable, and 88¼ acres of woodland, but it is significant that the pasture was then valued at 2s. an acre and the arable at only 8d. an acre per annum. It is very puzzling to turn from this survey of 1558 to a survey of royal parks and forests which was made in 1564 and is preserved in the British Museum.[4] Here the area of Grafton Park is given as only 80 acres, that of Pottersperry as 38 acres, and that of Hartwell as 25½ acres. It is, however, possible to explain this startling discrepancy between the two surveys on the hypothesis that the object of the later one was simply to ascertain the area of the woodland.[5]

[1] This survey is in the Record Office, v. S. P. Dom. Mary 12, No. 68, folios 136–41. Its exact date is 21 April, 4 & 5 Philip & Mary.

[2] Later in the survey the areas of certain coppices, amounting to 81¾ acres, are given, and it is just possible that these are not included in the total of 307½ acres.

[3] We are told that this was measured by a pole of 18 feet.

[4] v. B. M. Add. 34214.

[5] It will be noticed that 88¼ acres of Grafton Park were woodland in 1558, and that the area of Hartwell Park in 1526 was at least 29 acres and contained 13 acres of underwood. It seems quite impossible to suppose that Grafton Park had been reduced from 307½ acres to 80 acres between 1558 and 1564, especially as the tendency to enlarge it which obtained between 1526 and 1558 is continued at a later date, the area of the park being 622¼ acres in 1649, v. P. S. Northants, 23. There is an allusion to

5. The Hartwell Survey of 1605

In chronological order, the next document which demands consideration is a survey of the manor of Hartwell, which belongs to the year 1605 and is preserved in the Record Office.[1] This survey deals with a smaller area than that of 1526—with 543 acres 2 roods 6 poles, as compared with 680 acres. Perhaps the most remarkable fact which it reveals is the large proportion of the land still devoted to arable uses. No less than 387¼ acres, or about 71·25% of the whole area, was arable. This is an even larger proportion of arable than obtained at Hartwell eighty years earlier. According to the survey of 1526, out of 680 acres 454 were arable, which works out as 66·76%. It would, however, be unjustifiable to conclude that the arable area at Hartwell had really been increased during the intervening period, for the difference in the total area reported on in the two surveys is considerable,[2] and if the 29 acres of Hartwell Park mentioned in 1526 are excluded from the calculation on the ground that the park is not dealt with in the survey of 1605, the proportion of the remaining area which was arable at the earlier date is very little less than that which was similarly used at the later, being in fact 69·74%. None the less, it is remarkable that tillage was so well maintained on the manor during the last three quarters of the sixteenth and the first five years of the seventeenth century.

the timber at Grafton in an interesting letter addressed by Sir Charles Danvers to the Earl of Southampton on June 10, 1599. 'My Ld of Cumberland', he writes, ' hath been dealing with Sr. Ed. Carye for Grafton, and as Sr. Ed. Carye affyrmes hath offered £500. I spoke with Mr. Chamberlen and lett him knowe your Ld's desire to have it, he feares the place will not yeald you sufficient comodity of Wood, for the mayntenance of such a house as you must necessarily keepe, and that haveing no other land in it you will want many other as necessary commodetyes.' There is a copy of this letter in the British Museum, v. B. M. MSS. 6177, p. 107.

[1] v. Land Revenue, Miscellaneous Books, vol. 201, folios 1–21. It is dated 29 July, 3 James I.

[2] It should be noticed too that in the smaller area reported on in 1605 are included four holdings of free tenants, while the area given in 1526 appears to consist entirely of the farms of *tenentes ad voluntatem*. The area of the free holdings is not given in the survey of 1526, except in one instance, which I have not included in the total.

The size of the various holdings at Hartwell in 1605 is illustrated by the following table : [1]

							No. of holdings.
60 acres and over but less than 100 acres					.	.	1
30 ,,	,,	,,	60 ,,		.	.	8 (7)
15 ,,	,,	,,	30 ,,		.	.	5 (6)
10 ,,	,,	,,	15 ,,		.	.	1 (2)
5 ,,	,,	,,	10 ,,		.	.	3
1 ,,	,,	,,	5 ,,		.	.	2
Under one acre		.	.	.	.	.	4 (5)
Total number of holdings				.	.	.	24 (26)

It is interesting to compare these holdings with those reported on in 1526. If we exclude 16½ acres of woodland and the 29 acres of the park, the area dealt with at that date consisted of 634½ acres divided into 14 holdings. One of these was 123 acres in extent, 2 were over 60 but under 100 acres in extent, and 8 (as in 1605) fall into the class of holdings of between 30 and 60 acres. The remaining three holdings measured 2 acres, 2½ acres, and 17¼ acres respectively. Thus it appears that the holdings surveyed in 1605 were on the whole smaller than those surveyed in 1526.

The survey of 1605 reveals some interesting facts in regard to changes of tenancy. On the one hand, John Church claims as a free holding under a charter of 18 Henry VII a messuage and certain lands *nuper Edmundi Church patris sui et ante Johannis Church et Churches ex antiquo*.[2] On the other hand it is clear that on a holding claimed by John Myller as demised by letters patent the changes of tenants had been extremely rapid. The holding was granted on 2 July, 3 and 4 Philip and Mary, to six individuals for 21 years to date from the following Michaelmas. On the 18th of January in the 13th year of Elizabeth the reversion was granted to one Henry Ratcliffe for 30 years, and again on the 5th of August, in Elizabeth's 27th year, a further reversion was granted to Robert Constable *inter alios* for a term of

[1] In this table I have lumped together all holdings held by the same individual and have assumed the identity of John Church and John Churche and of John Millor and John Myller. The figures in brackets are obtained by supposing these persons to be four distinct individuals.

[2] v. Land Revenue, Miscellaneous Books, vol. 201, folio 2.

50 years to date from Michaelmas 1607. But this sequence of grants by no means measures the extent of the changes which actually took place. The grant of 18 January, 13 Eliz., had been made *Henrico Ratclyffe militi et assignatis suis* ; and the history of the holding between this date and the year 1605 is revealed by the following entry :

Status et interesse predicti Henrici Ratclyffe militis conceditur [sic] Thome Tydder et per ipsum datum Edwardo Tydder filio suo et Dorothee uxori eius postea uxori Ricardi Warde et per prefatum Ricardum Warde assignatur Henrico Goodricke et per ipsum assignatur Johanni Hone legium Dottori uni Magistrorum Curie Cancellarie Domini Regis et per ipsum concessum Johanni Miller.

Again, after a statement about the reversion granted to Robert Constable, we read :—

Status et interesse predicti Roberti Constable militis conceditur [sic] Ricardo Warde et devertitur [sic] prefato Johanni Myller.

So much change and traffic in rights over land had been thought worth while at this period in regard to a holding of only 25½ acres ! [1]

At first sight the contrast between this history and that of the holding which the Church family had retained for more than a century suggests the thought that we have in the latter case an instance of the obstacle afforded to change, even in an age of agrarian revolution, by the legal conditions of freehold. We are tempted to conclude that the economic forces making for traffic and change had free scope in regard to leaseholds, but that they had not sufficient power to disturb the free tenant. But generalizations based on inadequate data have long been the bane of economic history. And two facts warn us to be cautious in drawing sweeping conclusions from the evidence considered above. In the first place, it must be noticed that the grant of a reversion to Robert Constable had not in fact set a term to the tenancy of those whose rights were derived from the previous grant

---

[1] For all these facts, v. Land Revenue, Miscellaneous Books, vol. 201, folios 14–15. It appears that the rent of John Myller's farm was 17s. and its annual value £7 17s.

to Henry Ratcliffe. Secondly, the holding described in the survey next after that which the Church family had retained so long is another free holding, and this holding was claimed by '*Gasperus Owsley generosus*' under a new charter, though it had been *nuper Henrici Churche et Churches ex antiquo*.[1]

6. The Grafton Survey of 1619

The next document to be considered is one which calls itself ' An Extracte out of a Survaye of the Honor of Grafton with the members thereof, compiled by John Thorpe deputy Surveyor by warrant to him directed Anno 1619 '.[2] It appears therefore that this is not a complete survey of the Honour, and its usefulness for historical purposes is further diminished by occasional omissions to state the area of the lands surveyed, by clumsiness in the classification of the land, and by a puzzling looseness in the phraseology employed.[3] On the other hand, it deals with a larger area than any of the earlier surveys, and indeed, if we exclude the survey of Grafton and Pottersperry Parks, the Parliamentary Surveys of Grafton considered in the last chapter fall far short of it in respect of area. The lands whose area is specified in this survey amount to slightly more than 2,468 acres ; and the following table shows the uses to which they were devoted.

LANDS REPORTED ON IN THE GRAFTON SURVEY OF 1619

	A.	R.	P.
Houses and premises	54	1	33½
Arable	1,174	2	0
Pasture	658	0	0
Meadow	218	2	5
Leaze	38	0	0
Arable and Leaze (undistinguished) .	151	1	0
Wood	8	2	0
Character unspecified	165	1	20
Total	2,468	2	18½

[1] v. Land Revenue, Miscellaneous Books, vol. 201, folio 3 (?).
[2] v. ibid., vol. 221, folios 112–19.
[3] On the one hand, for example, ' Leaze ' is often distinguished from arable land ; but, on the other hand, we find such entries as *Leaze et Groves continentes per estimacionem* 10 *acras*, and *arrabil' leaze et le groves continentes per estimacionem* 18 *acras*, and *terram arrabilem et lezuram jacentes in campis*. Again, hopes of realizing the significance of the document are aroused by

It appears that the arable, which is distinguished from 'leaze' land, amounted to 47·58% of the total acreage; but if the 'leaze' and the land described as arable and leaze is included, the figure is raised to 55·25%. It is interesting to notice that, if one large grazing farm of 582 acres is excluded, the pasture and meadow only amounts to 294 acres 2 roods 5 poles out of a total of 1,886 acres 2 roods 18½ poles, though no doubt some pasture was contained in the plots attached to the houses and in the area of 165 acres odd whose character is not specified in the survey.

The classification of holdings according to size is shown in the following table : [1]

HOLDINGS IN THE GRAFTON SURVEY OF 1619

500 acres and over	.	.	.	.	.	1
100 acres and over but less than 500 acres	.	.	4
60 ,,	,,	,,	100 ,,	.	.	5
30 ,,	,,	,,	60 ,,	.	.	14
15 ,,	,,	,,	30 ,,	.	.	11
10 ,,	,,	,,	15 ,,	.	.	3
5 ,,	,,	,,	10 ,,	.	.	9
1 ,,	,,	,,	5 ,,	.	.	12
Under one acre	.	.	.	.	.	26
Total number of holdings	.	.	.	.	85

There is a great difference between the largest holding and the four which are next it in size. Sir Robert Osborne's farm consisted entirely of pasture and meadow and contained 582 acres, but the only other farms which exceeded 100 acres measured respectively 143 acres, 142 acres 2 roods 20 poles, 122 acres, and 116 acres 1 rood 6 poles. On the two largest of these the arable was of precisely the same extent—110 acres in each case—while on the third 88 acres were classed indefinitely

---

entries relating to a holding of 30 acres *vocata les yarde lande* and to *duo virgatas terre arrabilis continentes p. e.* 60 *acras*, but the confusion of tongues in the former of these entries is rivalled by the confusion of sense in the references to a holding *continentem p. e. quartam partem virgate terre videlicet* 17 *acras* and to one Thomas Moulder who held *unum tenementum et duo virgatos terre arrabilis continentes p. e.* 2 *acras*.

[1] In compiling this table I have counted distinct farms held by the same person as one holding, even in cases where that person had a partner in one tenancy though not in another. Of the holdings whose area is given in the survey six appear to have been held jointly by two or three persons. I have taken no account at all of holdings whose area is not given.

as arable and 'leaze'. The smallest of the four contained
66 acres of arable.

So far as the uncertain phraseology of the survey allows
a classification to be made, it appears that the tenants were
classified under the three heads of *Liberi Tenentes*, *Tenentes
per dimissionem*, and those who held *Tenementa ad voluntatem
domini*. Out of the total of 2,468 acres odd, some 448 were
held freely or claimed as free holdings.[1] The greatest part of
the land, however, seems to have been held by the *tenentes per
dimissionem*, but under this heading some variety of titles
was included. A marginal note marks off a few holdings as
tenementa per annum dimissa, and of the others some are described as held *per literas patentes* or *virtute literarum patentium*,
while some were held *per indenturam*, or *per assignationem
A. B.*, or *ex concessione N. et M.* The marginal note *Tenementa
ad voluntatem domini noviter erecta super vastum* precedes a list
of 12 cottage holdings in Grafton, Hartwell, and Roade.[2]

7. The documents subsequent to 1650

It is now necessary to turn to the history of the manors
of Grafton and Hartwell in the second half of the seventeenth
century, but unhappily the material for this history in the
Record Office is scanty in comparison with that which relates

---

[1] Of one tenant of a cottage who is classed among the *liberi tenentes* we
are only told that he held by charter—*tenet per chartam*—but I am inclined
to think that the word *libere* which occurs in other cases has here been
omitted by mistake. No less than ten of the free holdings contained less
than two acres each. The largest free holding whose area is given contained 91 acres, but of the free holdings of unspecified area two were
entire manors—the manor of Horton and that of Wickham and Wick-
hive (?). Four of the free tenants are described in the survey as also
holding land by another tenure.

[2] One of the cottagers, Cuthbert Addington, also appears as tenant of
a cottage 'erected on the waste' in the Parliamentary Survey of 1650.
The entry in the survey of 1619 is *Cuthbertus Addington pro uno cotagio
super vastum cum gardino continente 3 perticas 12d.—3s. 6d.* Presumably
1s. was the rent, 3s. 6d. the annual value of this tenement. Addington's
tenement was valued at 3s. 4d. per annum in 1650. The form of the entry
in the survey of 1619 is followed in four other cases and contrasts, e. g.
with that which immediately precedes it—*Johannes Tomleyne unum cota-
gium noviter erectum continens 3 perticas—12d.—4s.* One is tempted to
guess that possibly in the former cases ground had been granted for cottages
which had not yet been built.

to earlier periods. The explanation of this fact is simple. The creation of the Duchy of Grafton in 1675 involved the alienation of the Grafton estates from the Crown.

With regard to the earlier alienation of Crown lands, for which the Parliamentary Surveys were a preparation, a certain amount of information can be obtained from the ' Particulars for the Sale of Crown Lands ', which are preserved in the Record Office ; and it is worthy of notice that on April 11, 1650, Grafton and Pottersperry Parks were contracted to be sold to Robert Wakeman and Nicholas Trottman at 30 years' purchase and 16s. 3d. over.[1]

More interesting are the facts revealed by the surveys made at the Restoration. A summary abstract prefixed to a volume of these shows that, exclusive of the area which was built over, the distribution of the land at Grafton and Hartwell in 1660 was as follows : [2]

> Grafton : Arable, 237 acres 2 roods 5 poles ; Pasture, 627 acres 0 roods 22 poles ; Meadow, 12 acres 2 roods 0 poles.
> Hartwell : Arable 604 acres 2 roods 4 poles ; Pasture, 182 acres 3 roods 23 poles ; Meadow, 44 acres 0 roods 38 poles.

Thus the total area reported on in 1660 was close upon 1,709 acres, as compared with some 1,760 acres described in the Parliamentary Surveys. The arable in 1660 amounted to about 49·27% of the total area, exclusive of the parks and the land occupied with buildings. The corresponding figure for the Parliamentary Surveys is 50·34%, or some 48% if the principal survey of 1650 is alone taken into consideration. On the whole, then, it seems that the fields of Grafton and Hartwell suffered little change in the uses to which they were put during the decade of political revolution. As regards the parks, however, we have definite information that changes took place. In the survey of 1660 the following passage occurs : [3]

' Grafton and Pury Park Contains 1020 acres or thereabouts

---

[1] v. Particulars for Sale of Crown Lands, N. 5.
[2] v. Land Revenue, Miscellaneous Books, vol. 222.
[3] v. ibid., folio 151.

The Lord Mounson have cutt down and Converted all
the Trees in Pury Parke and the Greatest part of those
in Grafton Park to his own Use by selling them to the
Kings Damage £3100 And also hath Ploughed about
100 ac. of Grafton Park that were formerly Coppices to the
damage of the King £3300 more Farnando Marsham Esq.
Holdeth the seid Parks for his Life by Grant from the
late King, Sr George Strowd Mr. Duke & Mr. Saunthill
claim the inheritance by Grant from the late King of
these Two Parks paying £20 p. ann. after Mr. Marsham's
Death.'

From a marginal note it appears that the conversion of
woodland to arable described in this passage took place
' before 1658 '. Doubtless the ' Lord Mounson ' who thus
felled timber ' to the damage of the King ' was that Sir William
Monson who was created Viscount Monson of Castlemaine in
1628 and, being one of the ' regicides ', was sentenced to be
degraded from all his honours and to be imprisoned for life
in 1661. He was brother to the Sir John Monson who
undertook to reclaim some of the fens in 1638, so apparently
a tendency to look with favour upon change, either in the
agricultural or the political sphere, ran in the family.[1]
For the latter part of Charles II's reign, some information
can be obtained from a ' detailed rental ' of eight folios which
is preserved in the Record Office and belongs to the ' 32nd
year ' of the reign—presumably to the year 1680.[2] Under
the heading of Hartwell this rental mentions 20 holdings,
and under the headings of Grafton and Roade 18 more. But
only in the case of 21 out of these 38 farms are we told anything definite about the extent of the land or the use made
of it. Excluding the land occupied by houses and their
premises—the area of which is only given in three instances
—the total area reported on in the rental is 569 acres.[3] The
following table shows the distribution of this land according
to the uses to which it was put :

[1] v. Dictionary of National Biography, vol. xxxviii, pp. 195, 202.
[2] Rentals and Surveys, General Series, Portfolio 31, No. 2.
[3] The houses and premises measured account for 3 acres 2 roods 8 poles
in addition.

	Hartwell.			Grafton and Roade.			Total.		
	A.	R.	P.	A.	R.	P.	A.	R.	P.
Arable . . .	149	2	0	171	2	0	321	0	0
'Land' (probably arable)	52	0	0	38	3	0	90	3	0
Pasture . . .	101	1	0		nil.		101	1	0
Meadow . . .	35	2	0	11	0	0	46	2	0
Ley	2	0	0	7	2	0	9	2	0
Total . . .	340	1	0	228	3	0	569	0	0

Thus the arable certainly amounted to 56·41%, and probably to rather more than 72% of the whole area. But it would be a great mistake to base any important conclusion upon figures so manifestly incomplete as those provided by this rental; and there is no evidence at all to show that the arable area had been extended on the manors since 1660. The large pasture farm which had been for so long a striking feature of the economy of Grafton is clearly not included in the lands whose area is specified in the rental of 1680, and if the figures for Hartwell are taken by themselves, the arable, including the land which was probably arable, amounted there to only 59·22%, as compared with about 72·70% in 1660.

The same caution as to the incompleteness of the evidence must be given in regard to the classification of holdings. But it may be noticed that out of 21 holdings reported on in 1680, six were over 30 and under 60 acres, while six were between 15 and 30 acres in extent.[1] And even the few facts which the rental provides supply some indication of the general continuity of things agrarian on the manors during the Stuart period. In 1619 Francis Blunt held a farm of 75 acres containing 67 acres of arable : in 1680 Thomas Blunt held a farm of uncertain total area which, according to the rental, included 67 acres of arable and 3 acres of meadow. Again, William Smith in 1619 held a farm consisting of 36 acres of arable, 2½ acres of leys, and 2½ acres of meadow : in 1680 the land of Robert Smith consisted of precisely the same amount of each class of land.

---

[1] The figures do not as a rule include the area occupied by buildings. One other holding contained 20½ acres of arable, but I have not counted it among those of 15 to 30 acres because it also contained other lands of unspecified extent.

A faint suggestion of much longer continuity than this is the only interesting hint to be obtained from the last of the series of documents relating to Grafton which I have consulted in the Record Office. This is a rental of the manors belonging to the Honour of Grafton which is assigned in the official Lists and Indexes to the eighteenth century, but apparently this dating is based solely on palaeographical considerations, and I am told that the handwriting might really belong to the decade 1680–90.[1] The rental gives a list of those paying rent in the manor of Hartwell, and among them appear persons of the names of Church, Brice, Addington, and Manning. All these names are to be found among the tenants of the manor in the survey of 1526; and it may be noticed that, according to the survey of 1619, John Church of Hartwell was then holding land under a charter of 10 August, 2 Henry VII.[2]

8. Summary of the evidence

It is now necessary to review the facts collected in the preceding pages and to ask whether any conclusions can be drawn from them as to the general trend of economic developments on the manors of Grafton and Hartwell in the sixteenth and seventeenth centuries.[3] The chief uncertainty springs from the fact that the various surveys do not refer to precisely the same area of land. It is doubtful how much waste was attached to these manors, and impossible to be sure whether the neighbourhood of Salcey Forest provided an outlet for economic forces that otherwise would have produced

---

[1] v. Rentals and Surveys, Exchequer, Portfolio 26, No. 4.

[2] A few other instances of families remaining tenants for a long period may be given. The names Wiltesey and Rouhead occur among the tenants of 1526. I am inclined to recognize these names in the names Whittlesey and Roughead which are found in the Rental of 1680. Whalley and Thornton [or Thorneton] certainly are found as names of tenants both in 1526 and in 1680, and it will be remembered that certain lands at Grafton had been granted to one John Whalley so early as the 6th year of Henry VII. The name Boughton occurs in 1526 and in 1619.

[3] I regret that I have not been able to trace the history down to a later period; but an inquiry which I addressed to the Duke of Grafton, with a view to discovering whether his Grace possesses any eighteenth-century documents relating to these manors, has not been favoured with a reply.

large internal changes. But in spite of this, a few striking facts emerge from the puzzling details of the surveys.
Already by 1526 the profitable nature of grazing had been
perceived at Grafton, and a farm of 460 acres of pasture and
meadow even then dwarfed all the other holdings. Both at
Grafton and at Hartwell tenements were decayed and rights
over land were in some cases uncertain and were being chal-
lenged with a sense of grievance. And clearly considerable
changes took place after 1526. The largest farm at Grafton
grew larger, and was reckoned at 582 acres in 1619 and at
about 585½ acres in 1650. At the same time 'emparking'
was carried on on a large scale. Between the 24th year of
Henry VIII and the year 1558 no less than 146 acres had
been taken out of the fields of Grafton and Alderton and
incorporated in Grafton Park. In the survey of 1526 it is
stated that the 'saied park conteyneth 102 acrez and oon
rode ', but in 1558 the area of the park was 307½ acres, and
in 1649 it contained 622¼ acres.[1] The appearance in the
survey of 1619 of landless cottages newly erected upon the
waste marks another feature of the changes which had been
taking place. And even in the middle of the seventeenth
century there was still doubt and dispute about the exercise
of rights of common over a pasture called the Styes which
had been the subject of a similar dispute in 1526.[2]

Yet, though the signs of change are manifest in the surveys,
the surprising thing, to any one who has been accustomed
to regard the Tudor and early Stuart periods as an age of

---

[1] It is true that a survey of 1564 only assigns 80 acres to Grafton Park;
but, as I have pointed out above, this survey may only refer to actual
woodland.
[2] v. P. S. Northants, 21, folio 22. The memories of countryfolk, especially
in regard to grievances, are astonishingly long ; and the traditions of history
linger in a strange way. The little band of Oxfordshire villagers who tried to
upset the social order and introduce the millennium in 1596 were encouraged
by distorted traditions of the rising of the Communes in Spain more than
70 years before. The ringleader, a carpenter named Stere, affirmed that
' the Commons, long sithens in Spaine did rise and kill all the gentlemen
in Spaine, and sithens that time have lyved merrily there '. It is true that
in Valencia the revolt had been of the nature of a social war. v. S. P. Dom.
James I, vol. 28, No. 64, printed by E. F. Gay: Transactions Royal Hist.
Soc. (New Series), vol. xviii, pp. 238–9. cp. ibid., p. 212 ; also E. Armstrong,
The Emperor Charles V (1902), vol. i, p. 97.

agrarian revolution, is rather the permanence of so many
features of the older economy during the century and a half
subsequent to the date of the Henrician surveys. The
enlargement of the Park at Grafton seems to have caused
little disturbance, if indeed the surveys tell us anything
approaching the whole truth. Though the large grazing farm
extended its boundaries, and though the value of pasture
was still in the middle of the seventeenth century more
than 4½ times as great, on an average, as that of arable, the
tendency to convert arable into pasture was far from being
so strong as one might expect, and arable farming was on the
whole singularly well maintained.[1] The survey of 1558,
which tells us that within the last quarter of a century 76 acres
of land had been abstracted from the fields of Grafton and
included within the park, also states that 42 acres of arable
lay inside that park. A century later, when the sale of the
Crown lands might be expected to free economic forces from
the restraints of traditional administration, we find Lord
Monson ploughing up a hundred acres of Grafton Park. On
the whole, the proportion of the land under plough—apart
from the parks—varied little throughout the period. The
following table shows this in the case of Hartwell :

Date.	Total acreage surveyed.	Percentage of arable.
1526	651	69·74[2]
1605	543½	71·25
1660	831½	72·70
1680	340¼	59·22[3]

If the two manors are taken together, and it is almost impossible to distinguish them in the surveys of 1619 and 1650—

[1] It will be remembered that in 1558 the pasture of Grafton Park was
valued at three times as much per acre as the arable, but it is not until we
come to the Parliamentary Survey of 1650 that we get sufficient information
to be the basis of a general statement as to the average values of arable
and pasture on the two manors.
[2] This includes some leys which are not distinguished from the arable in
the survey.
[3] This includes land which is probably but not certainly arable. But in
any case no importance can be attached to the figures for 1680, as the
survey of that year covers only a small area of land compared with the
others.

and if the area of the parks and so far as possible the lands built over are excluded, we get the figures shown in the next table :

Date.	Total acreage surveyed.	Percentage of arable and leys.	Percentage of arable.
1526 .	1,502	45·27	
1619 .	2,468½	55·25	47·58
1650[1] .	1,598½	50·08	48·14
1660 .	1,709	—	49·27

Again, as regards the type of holding, the evidence suggests that farms of from 15 to 60 acres maintained themselves at Grafton and Hartwell in spite of all the forces which made for engrossing, though there was, it is true, a distinct tendency for them to get fewer in number. In 1526 we find that 15 out of 26 holdings belonged to this class, and in 1605 at Hartwell the number was 13 out of 24 ; but on the larger area surveyed in 1619 only 25 out of 85 farms were between 15 and 60 acres in extent, and in the Parliamentary Surveys considered in the last chapter the corresponding figure is 11 out of 52. It is true that the rental of 1680 mentions 12 farms out of 21 as being of from 15 to 60 acres ; but the small area covered by this document removes all significance from this fact, for clearly several of these holdings may have been in the hands of men who were also tenants of farms not mentioned in the rental. I have already shown that certain families managed to retain a hold upon the land in these manors throughout the whole of the period.

[1] The figures given are those for the principal survey of 1650 only.

CHAPTER IV

THE ECONOMY OF THE CROWN ESTATES IN NORTH-AMPTONSHIRE, OTHER THAN THE MANORS OF GRAFTON AND HARTWELL, AS DESCRIBED IN THE PARLIAMENTARY SURVEYS.

1. The scope and purpose of this chapter

In the last two chapters an attempt has been made, firstly, to analyse the Parliamentary Surveys of the manors of Grafton and Hartwell, and, secondly, to reveal the historical setting of the economic conditions described in those surveys. It is now necessary to examine the other Parliamentary Surveys of royal manors in Northamptonshire with the object of discovering whether the economy of Grafton and Hartwell was normal or unusual, and what range of variation in economic structure obtained on the Crown estates within the county. For this purpose a statistical abstract dealing with all the manors together would obviously be inadequate, since the same average figures might represent either a uniform type everywhere in evidence or a balance struck between sharply contrasted economic organizations. Hence, in this chapter, the more important facts will be set forth with regard to each manor separately—or, rather, an abstract of each survey will be given—before any attempt is made to present a summary for the whole county.

2. The Manor of Aldrington

The first fourteen Parliamentary Surveys in the North-amptonshire series, according to the numbering of the Augmentation Office collection, are merely surveys of Hundreds and contain no information of value for the purposes of this monograph, so the first survey to be considered here is the fifteenth, which deals with the manor of Aldrington.[1] This survey was made in August and September 1650, and

[1] v. P. S. Northants, 15.

concerns lands of specified area amounting to 874 acres, of
which 36 acres 20 poles were occupied by houses and their
premises. The land classed as arable or as arable and leys
amounted to 387 acres 1 rood, and 127 acres were of unspecified
character. It is interesting to compare these figures with
those for the year 1660. The area then reported on at
Aldrington was 750 acres 1 rood 20 poles, exclusive of the
land occupied by houses, and out of this total 356 acres
1 rood 13 poles were arable, 352 acres 3 roods 8 poles were
pasture, and 41 acres 39 poles meadow.[1]

The land definitely described as arable in the Parliamentary
Survey of Aldrington contained 166½ acres, and this was valued
at £41 3s. 6d. per annum, or about 4s. 11d. an acre on an
average.[2] The most valuable piece was a *close* of two acres
valued at 24s. a year : the least valuable arable was eleven
acres which lay in scattered strips in the three fields and was
estimated to be worth just 4s. 6d. an acre per annum. One
acre out of these eleven was made up of five distinct parcels
of land in one of the great fields.[3]

The pasture consisted mainly of closes and amounted to
253 acres 3 roods, which were valued at £224 2s. 8d., or nearly
17s. 8d. an acre per annum.[4] One close called the ' parsonage
close' was worth 31s. 8d. an acre : this was the most valuable
bit of pasture. The least valuable pastures were three closes
containing 10¼ acres, which were valued at £4 7s., or not quite
8s. 6d. an acre. It is perhaps significant that of these three
closes of pasture one was called ' neather Leyes ' and another
' the upper leyes '.

The pasture closes at Aldrington varied greatly in size.
Colonel Edward Cooke held two whose combined area was

---

[1] v. Land Revenue, Miscellaneous Books, vol. 222, prefatory abstract.
[2] This does not include the land described as arable and leys.
[3] How far the difference in value between the best and the worst arable
is to be explained by the *consolidation* of the former and how far by its
enclosure remains doubtful. The case of Mrs. Fleetwood's farm at Roade
(dealt with in the Grafton Survey) suggests that consolidation of strips did
not do much to enhance the value of the land when it did not mean its
withdrawal from common of shack, v. *supra*, p. 57.
[4] Probably some other pasture was to be found among the 127 acres
whose character is unspecified, and also in small closes attached to the
houses and not separately valued.

120 acres, and Thomas Hezzlerigge had one of 30 acres. On the other hand we find on one holding 21¼ acres of pasture divided into seven closes, and on another 11½ acres divided into three closes.

The meadow amounted to 69 acres 3 roods 20 poles, worth £63 14s. 0d. a year, or nearly 18s. 3d. per acre. The most valuable piece of meadow contained 2¼ acres and was valued at £2 6s. 0d., or slightly more than 20s. 5d. an acre: the least valuable was reckoned to be worth slightly more than 17s. 1d. an acre.

Eighteen holdings are separately described in the survey, but two pairs of these were held together. Of the sixteen farms held by different tenants one contained 184 acres 1 rood 20 poles, of which 109½ acres were arable, while another consisted of 120 acres which were entirely pasture. Six farms contained from 50 to 55¼ acres each, and two others contained 44 and 48½ acres respectively. Six holdings were between 20 and 30 acres in size. On the whole these facts suggest that the general economic condition at Aldrington did not differ greatly from that which obtained in the estates described in the Parliamentary Surveys of Grafton, but that the forces making for change had not impaired the mediaeval economy so much at Aldrington as at Grafton. At Aldrington as at Grafton there was a large pasture farm, but it was not a giant which dwarfed all the other holdings and in fact was smaller than one predominantly arable farm. The fact that half the farms were between 30 and 60 acres in extent recalls a similar condition which was noticeable in the earlier surveys of Grafton and Hartwell. On the other hand the absence of tiny holdings at Aldrington suggests a contrast which is really quite deceptive, for the survey starts by mentioning three small tenements in the township of Foxcote which were built on the waste, and three other tenements in Aldrington, but it does not state the area occupied by these, so I have not counted them in the total analysed above. It should be noticed too that three of the holdings at Aldrington contained no house,[1]

---

[1] Or four, if we include a holding of 3 acres of pasture held by the tenant of another farm.

and that four of them contained one and one of them two
farm-tied cottages besides the farmhouse. Again, the fact
that the names of four of the tenants of surveyed holdings
occur in the list of free tenants makes it probable that these
persons held other lands besides those surveyed.

It may be noted that in nearly every case the arable is
described as lying in 3 fields or 3 common fields, though on
one holding the arable and leys lay in 2 fields, while another
holding contained a close of arable. Lots in the common
meadow are mentioned, and ' Lammas closes ', and in one case
we read of 6¼ acres of meadow being dispersed in 16 parcels.
The Bailiff, we are told, was paid 40s. a year—exactly the
amount of his fee at Grafton—and the freeholders paid as
a relief at every change of tenancy double their rent. As
regards the leases, it seems best to reckon all leases made on
the same day and for the same period as one lease, and if this
method is adopted we have mentioned in the Aldrington
survey 4 leases of the reign of Elizabeth, 12 of the reign of
James I, and 4 of the reign of Charles I. Of those belonging
to Elizabeth two were for 3 lives and two—the latest in date—
for 21 years. Of James's leases, two are for 3 lives, one for
90 years or 3 lives (whichever should determine first), three for
60 years, four for 40 years and two for 31 years. The latest
of the leases for lives—that for mixed lives and years—belongs
to the 8th year of the reign : the earlier of the two leases for
31 years belongs to the 18th year. All the leases for 60 years
are of the 8th year, while those for 40 years date from the 3rd
to the 8th year. All the leases of Charles's reign are for 31
years.

3. The Manor of Ashton

The next survey to be considered is that of the manor of
Ashton, which was annexed to the Honour of Grafton.[1] It was
made in September 1650, and deals with lands of specified
area amounting to 1,168 acres 2 roods 10 poles, of which
65 acres 1 rood 10 poles were occupied by houses and their
premises, for in this survey an unusual amount of land is
described along with the buildings, in a way which makes it

[1] v. P. S. Northants, 16.

impossible to estimate the cultivated area at all exactly. Apart from these doubtful plots, the land described as arable amounted to 371½ acres, while 284½ acres more were classed as arable and leys, and a parcel of 120 acres was described simply as 'Ley ground'. The pasture accounted for 51¾ acres and the meadows for 51 acres, while 111½ acres were woodland and 113 acres consisted of 'assarts' of unspecified character. These figures may be compared with those given in the survey of 1660, which refers to 1,109 acres 9 poles exclusive (so it seems) of the land occupied by buildings. Of this total, 195 acres 3 roods 15 poles were classed as pasture and assarts, 49 acres 3 roods 25 poles[1] as meadow, and 863 acres 1 rood 9 poles as arable.[2] These figures suggest that the leys of the Parliamentary Survey ought to be classed with the arable and that possibly some of the assarts were also under the plough. At all events it is clear that arable farming still predominated at Ashton.

In the Parliamentary Survey the 371½ acres definitely classed as arable were valued at £75 0s. 4d. per annum, which works out at slightly more than 4s. an acre. On one holding, 39¼ acres were valued at £7 16s., or a trifle less than 4s. an acre; on another, 12 acres were valued at 5s. 3¼d. an acre. All the rest was reckoned to be worth exactly 4s. an acre. Most of the arable clearly lay in three common fields, though that on one holding seems to have lain in four fields.[3] There is, however, one fragment of evidence which suggests that some of this land may have been enclosed without being withdrawn from common of shack. We read of a parcel of 'arrable land lying in yᵉ common ffeild called the Lords Close'. Unfortunately this parcel of 8 acres is not valued separately from a cottage which was built upon it.

The 51¾ acres of pasture were reckoned to be worth £34 1s. 4d., or nearly 13s. 2d. an acre per annum on an average; but if the arable varied little, the pasture varied a good deal

---

[1] The writing of the MS. is here a little indistinct, and this figure may be 23 and not 25.

[2] v. Land Revenue, Miscellaneous Books, vol. 222, prefatory summary.

[3] Probably this may be explained by the surveyor's failure to distinguish clearly between 'fields' and 'furlongs'.

in quality. The best—a close of 3 roods—was valued at the rate of 26s. 8d. an acre, and another close of 3½ acres was valued at 23s. 4d. an acre. The poorest was only worth 6s. 8d. an acre. Most of the pasture is described as enclosed.

The 51 acres of meadow were valued at £40 2s. 9d., or nearly 15s. 9d. an acre. In most cases the meadow was valued at 16s. an acre. The lowest rate was 15s. and the highest 18s. Much of the meadow clearly lay in scattered lots or doles : even the most valuable lay in small parcels—5¼ acres in 13 parcels—though all held by one tenant.

Sixteen holdings are separately described in the survey; but, if we count as a single holding all farms which belonged to the same tenant, and exclude one holding which consisted merely of a tenement of unspecified area, this number is reduced to eleven.[1] Out of the eleven one was 512 acres 2 roods 10 poles in extent, and another 204 acres 2 roods 20 poles. The first of these seems to have consisted partly of clearings made on the edge of Salcey Forest : 113 acres are described as assarts bounded by that forest on the east, and 95 acres more were woodland, while the 120 acres described as ' Ley Ground ' were called ' Ashwood leys '. Apart from the areas of doubtful character, arable seems to have predominated on this large farm, for 132 acres are said to consist of arable and leys lying in diverse parcels in three common fields. On the farm which is second in size, 61½ acres were arable, and besides this 112½ acres out of the total of 204½ acres odd consisted of arable and leys in three fields. The next farms to these in size were of 95 and 82¾ acres, with 82 and 71 acres of arable respectively. Then comes a farm of 72 acres 2 roods 6 poles with 40 acres of arable and leys, in addition to a parcel of arable which is not separately measured but together with a cottage was 8 acres in extent. Four holdings were between 30 and 60 acres in extent. Of the remaining two holdings, one contained 18 acres 4 poles (of which 12 acres were arable), and one was a wood of six acres.

Thus it appears, as the most noteworthy characteristic of

[1] Or ten if ' John Marriott of the Spout ' was the same person as ' Mr. John Marriott ' and ' John Marriott gent '.

the economy of Ashton, that engrossing had gone far there, though grazing had hardly been developed at all. Besides the size of the farms, evidence of engrossing appears from the facts that the largest farm contained, besides the capital messuage, no less than 12 other tenements or cottages, one of which is said to have been built on the waste. The second largest farm consisted of three separately described holdings, and, besides a farmhouse or cottage which formed the nucleus of each of these, it contained 8 subsidiary cottages or tenements. Two other farms contained, besides the farm house, 4 and 2 subsidiary tenements respectively, and yet another two holdings included one farm-tied cottage each besides the farmhouse.

The leases for the most part seem to have been for shorter terms at Ashton than they were, for example, at Grafton. Reckoning all leases of the same day and for the same term as one lease, we find one lease of 31 Henry VIII for 40 years, two leases of Elizabeth's reign (of which one was for 30 years and the other probably for 31), and seven leases dating from the reign of James I, out of which five were for 15 years, one for 17 and one for 60. Ten leases of Charles I are mentioned, and of these one was for 16, three for 17, five for 31, and one for 53 years. It should be noticed that all the leases for 15 years belonged to the 21st year of James I, while those of Charles's reign which were for 16 or 17 years belonged to the 2nd or 3rd year of the reign. Three of the leases for 31 years dated from the 14th year of Charles I : the lease for 53 years belonged to his eleventh year.

4. The Manor of Brigstock

The Manor of Brigstock, which was surveyed in October 1650,[1] is chiefly remarkable for the fact of 'the manor being intyrely demised to the Inhabitants of Brigstock'. The manor and its demesnes had been leased on March 27 in the 10th year of James I to Samuel Linton, William Turlby, and others for 60 years 'for the only use and behalfe of the said tenants for the manor of Brigstock'. The rent to be paid was £66 13s. 4d. ;

[1] v. P. S. Northants, 17.

but the value of the lands granted under this lease, including
quit rents and royalties amounting to £21 8s. 4d.,was estimated
at £181 7s. 10d. per annum, while we are told that ' the free
Rents before mentioned are noe psell of the grant with the
Coppie hould lands which are by themselves p. ann. 33s. 1d.'

Besides two corn mills of unspecified area which were under
one roof and were ' in the tenour and occupation of the
demeane tenants of the manor of Brigstock', the lands
described in the survey amounted to 310¼ acres. Of this
area 15¼ acres were arable in the common fields of Stanion,
195 acres were arable and leys in three fields, 55 acres consisted
of closes of pasture, and 34 acres were meadow, while the
precise nature of a close of 11 acres is not specified.

The land definitely described as arable was valued at just
over 6s. an acre ; and the average value of the meadow was
nearly 16s. 6d. an acre per annum—the best of it being valued
at £1 an acre and the rest at 16s. The pasture was worth on
an average nearly 12s. 9d. an acre—the values of different
closes ranging from 10s. to just over 16s. 11d. an acre. All the
pasture seems to have been enclosed.

The survey contains an interesting statement about the
rights and obligations of the copyholders. ' The Coppie
houlders of the aforesaid manor of Brigstock', we read,
' houlding of the said manor by fine certaine pay for every
suit house foure shillings att Allination and for halfe a suit
two shillings and soe porshonably but if any land be Allinated ;
with the halfe suit or quarter suit lett the quantytie be neuer
soe grate there is noe fine payable for it but if any land be
Allinated without the suit seuered from them then it payeth
for a fine two pence the acore and upon desent foure pence the
acore and for tenants that are noe psells of the suits two
shillings upon Allination and foure shillings upon desent.
The Cusstum of the Coppie hould tenants is that upon the
first purchas being not surrendered the Estate ffallett two
the Eldest sonn ; but after the first desent not being surrendered it falleth to the youngest sonn after the death of
the Ancestor.' We are also told that the copyholders might
cut down timber upon their copyholds without licence or

forfeiture, might let their copyholds for a whole year 'without surrender of forfeiture', and might get timber for the repair of their houses out of the forest of Rockingham. In that, forest, too, they had right of common for their great cattle. No heriots were payable on the manor ; and the copyholders had full liberty to grind corn or malt where they pleased. A somewhat mysterious sentence informs us that the copyholders could take down other copyhold 'souses' without licence. Can it be that this word is a penman's mistake for 'houses', and that it was actually permissible for an engrossing tenant who became possessed of more than one copyhold to pull down houses which he did not need ?

5. The lands of Chacombe Monastery

The next survey on the list deals with some lands of Chacombe Monastery which had been annexed to the Honour of Grafton, and were surveyed in October 1650.[1] These lands amounted to $57\frac{1}{2}$ acres, of which 43 acres were arable, $5\frac{3}{4}$ acres meadow, and $1\frac{1}{4}$ acres pasture, while $7\frac{1}{2}$ acres were occupied by houses and their premises. All the arable was valued at the rate of 5s. 6d. an acre, the pasture at £1 an acre, and all the meadow at 18s. an acre per annum. The land was divided into three holdings of $35\frac{3}{4}$ acres, 11 acres, and $10\frac{3}{4}$ acres respectively. There were 27 acres of arable on the largest holding and 8 acres on each of the others. Four distinct and dated leases are mentioned. Three of them belonged to the reign of James I, two being for 60 and one for 40 years. One lease of 31 years dated from the reign of Charles I.

6. Chelveston cum Caldecott

The survey of Chelveston cum Caldecott, which is described as parcel of the manor of Higham 'Ferries', was made in December 1649, and refers to an area, as it seems, of 619 acres 2 roods 27 poles.[2] The arable amounted to $528\frac{1}{2}$ acres, the pasture to 9 acres 3 roods 20 poles, while the area of the meadow appears to have been 65 acres 35 poles. The houses

---

[1] v. P. S. Northants, 18.   [2] P. S. Northants, 19.

and their premises occupied 8 acres, and the character of 8 acres 12 poles is unspecified. The one doubt about these figures concerns the meadow on three holdings, which amounted apparently to 55 acres 32 poles. In the case of these three holdings the meadow is measured in a peculiar way. Instead of giving its area in square measure, the surveyor describes the meadow as being 66 poles long and 6 broad, 148 poles long and 28 broad, and 148 poles long and 29 broad, respectively. The obvious interpretation of these figures, which yields the total given above, becomes doubtful when we notice that the value of these pieces of meadow is on this supposition abnormally low. On the other holdings where the meadow is measured in the ordinary way its average value is nearly £1 an acre : on the three holdings in question we have apparently 55 acres 32 poles worth only £6 4s., or scarcely more than 2s. 3d. an acre.[1]

The arable land was valued at £86 13s. 9d. a year, or a little over 3s. 3d. per acre, the values of the different lots varying from just over 2s. 8d. to nearly 3s. 6d. an acre. All the arable lay in three fields. Most of the pasture was worth £1 an acre, but one close of an acre was valued at 18s. 9d., and the value of the total of 7¾ acres separately valued was £7 13s. 9d., or about 19s. 10d. an acre. All the pasture appears to have been enclosed.

There were nine holdings. One was 116 acres 30 poles and another 113 acres 2 roods 38 poles in extent. Four were over 60 but under 100 acres, the largest of the four being a farm of 94 acres 2 roods 12 poles. Two holdings were between 30 and 40 acres in extent, and there was one small holding of 7¾ acres.[2] On every one of the nine holdings arable largely predominated. On one farm, which is described as ' One

---

[1] On account of this uncertainty I have not included any of the Chelveston meadows in the general statistical table at the end of this chapter, which gives the values of the different kinds of land ; but in the tables dealing with the size of holdings and the proportions of the land subjected to different uses I have included them at their apparent area, as the amount of error thus introduced must be insignificant.

[2] The doubt about the meadows makes these figures uncertain ; but in any case six of the holdings must have been between 60 and 120 acres in extent, two between 30 and 40, and one just 7¾ acres.

pightle and one yardland ' and was 35 acres 2 roods 36 poles in
extent, there was no farmhouse, while in regard to another
holding of 37 acres 3 roods 24 poles we are told that the houses
were much decayed and that the last tenant had fled and was
unable to make satisfaction. Three farms contained a subsidiary tenement besides the farmhouse and the subtenant's
name is given in two cases.

Seven distinct leases are mentioned in the Chelveston Survey
as belonging to the reign of Elizabeth. Of these four are for
31 years, two for 21 years, and one for 50 years. Out of four
leases of James I two were for 40 and two for 31 years. Three
leases of Charles I are mentioned. One was for 20 years, one
for 60, and one for 60 years or three lives, whichever should
determine first. In a few cases we are informed that the lessee
' is not allowed either Houseboote, Plough Boote, or ffire
Boote '.

7. The Manor of Greens Norton

If we omit six surveys of Grafton which were analysed in
the second chapter, the next surveys on the list are three of
the manor of Greens Norton, which was annexed to the Honour
of Grafton. The principal survey was made in May and June
1650, and deals with lands in the parishes or townships of
Greens Norton, Whittlewood, Paulerspury, Darlescott (in the
parish of Pattishall), Grimscott, Cold Higham, Maidford, and
Blakesley.[1] The other two surveys were made respectively
in October 1650 and September 1653, and concerned some
lands which were claimed either as glebe or freehold, or as
held in free socage like the manor of East Greenwich.[2] The
area surveyed amounts to 3,358 acres 1 rood 26 poles, of which
1,636½ acres are definitely stated to be pasture, while 176 acres
1 rood 20 poles were meadow, 408 acres 1 rood 20 poles arable,
451¼ acres arable and leys (undistinguished), and 29 acres
3 roods 20 poles leys. The woodland amounted to 95½ acres,
the houses and their premises to 119¾ acres, and the area the

---

[1] v. P. S. Northants, 26. This does not pretend to be a complete list: it
is almost impossible to determine exactly what parishes and townships
all the fields were in.   [2] v. P. S. Northants, 27 and 28.

character of which is not stated to 378 acres 2 roods 30 poles. In addition, 4½ acres were described as pasture *or* meadow, 57½ acres as grassland lying in the common fields in numerous parcels, and 16 poles as hemplands.

Obviously the most remarkable feature in the economy revealed by this survey is the great development of pasture farming. The area definitely described as pasture, large as it is, does not measure the real extent of this development. Among the lands classed above as 'houses and their premises' there are a pasture called the Town Close, which together with a tenement measured 10 acres, 3 closes of pasture and a tenement measuring 29 acres, and another close of pasture, 'now divided into three closes', which with the tenement and its premises measured 30 acres.[1] Again nearly all the land of unspecified character is definitely stated to have been enclosed, and I suspect that the greater part of it was pasture. Nine acres of it made up what is described as a 'close of pasture or Arrable Land lately enclosed'.

The predominance of pasture on the Greens Norton estates is equally evident in the survey of 1660, which states that out of a total of 3,174 acres 1 rood 5 poles no less than 2,108 acres 13 poles were pasture, while the meadow amounted to 112 acres 32 poles and the arable to just 954 acres.[2]

The total amount of pasture separately valued in the Parliamentary Surveys is 1,512 acres, and its total value was £998 16s. 6d. per annum, which works out at nearly 13s. 3d. an acre. The rate at which the different closes and plots of pasture were valued varied from 8s. to £4 an acre—the highest figure being for a tiny close of 20 poles.

Of the arable, 381½ acres were separately valued, and the

---

[1] As a general rule I have classed as 'houses and their premises' all lands which are not measured in the surveys apart from dwellings ; but a field containing a barn I class with the kind of land to which the field belongs, even in the case (which occurs in this survey) where a tenant was living in the barn. I have been careful to omit such cases from the particulars from which the average value of the different sorts of land has been calculated. In analysing this survey I have departed from my usual practice in one case. A tenement and a close of pasture together measured 123 acres, and this area I have classed along with the pasture, not with the area of houses and their premises.

[2] v. Land Revenue, Miscellaneous Books, vol. 222, prefatory abstract.

total value of this area was £100 3s. 11d., or about 5s. 3d. an
acre. The rates for the different lots vary from 3s. 4d. to 10s.
an acre.[1]

The meadow separately valued amounted to 174 acres
3 roods 20 poles, and it was estimated to be worth £155 17s. 7d.,
or just over 17s. 10d. an acre. The rates vary from 15s. to £1
an acre.

Of the land described as grass-ground in common fields,
51½ acres were separately valued—the rate being not quite
4s. 7d. an acre on an average. On one holding 19 acres of
this land lay divided into 53 distinct parcels.

Out of the total area dealt with in the Parliamentary Surveys
of Greens Norton 2,235 acres are described as enclosed. Two
entries throw a little light upon the process of enclosure and
conversion. In one case we read of a ' closse of pasture Ground
or arrable land called Corne Closse : with A tenement called
the Shepherds house ', and in another of a ' closse of pasture or
Arrable Land lately enclosed '.

The land was divided into 38 holdings held by 35 tenants.[2]
If we count as a single holding all the land held by a single
tenant, we find that of the 35 holdings one contained 1,715 acres
2 roods 20 poles, one 208 acres, one 200 acres, and a fourth 109
acres, while nine contained between 60 and 100 acres, eleven
between 30 and 60 acres, two between 15 and 30 acres, three
between 5 and 10 acres, and one between 1 and 5 acres. Five
holdings were less than an acre in extent.[3]

On the largest holding 1,179¼ acres were certainly pasture,
and 129½ acres meadow, while 265 acres consisted of enclosures
the character of which is not stated, and 3 acres were described
as meadow *or* pasture.

The holding of 208 acres consisted entirely of pasture except
for the area actually covered by the farmhouse and its
premises. The holding of 200 acres, which the Committee
of Obstruction decided to be the freehold inheritance of

[1] The most valuable arable was that claimed as glebe, and its high value
is partially explained by the fact that it was tithe free, v. P. S. Northants, 27.
[2] This is including the land claimed as freehold.
[3] This is including a holding which consisted of a cottage, though its
area is not stated.

Sir Peter Wentworth, also consisted entirely of enclosed pasture. The holding of 109 acres was made up of 60 acres of wood, 6 acres of meadow, and 43 acres of enclosure whose character is not specified. On the other hand, arable or arable and leys formed more than half the area of each of the holdings of 60 to 100 acres, and in most of these cases a great deal more than half.[1] Again arable or arable and leys predominated on a majority of the holdings of between 15 and 30 acres.

Four distinct and dated leases are mentioned in the survey which belonged to the reign of Elizabeth. Three of them were for 3 lives and one for 50 years. There are 22 distinct leases of James I mentioned. Of these, four were for 3 lives and one for 2 lives. Two were for mixed lives and years—for 70 and, in the other case, for 90 years or 3 lives, whichever should determine first. Four of James's leases were for 60 years, two for 50 years, one for 41 years, four for 40 years, and four for 31 years. From the reign of Charles I we have 15 distinct leases. One was for 3 lives and one for 80 years or 3 lives, whichever should determine first. Nine were for 31 years, one for 21 years, one for 20 years, and two for 18 years.

8. Grimscott

The next survey to be considered is that of some lands which had belonged to the monastery of Dunstable and afterwards to one John Mantle, but had, it seems, come into the possession of the Crown on his attainder. These lands were situated in the township of Grimscott and in the parish of Cold Higham, and they were annexed to the Honour of Grafton. The survey was made in June and July 1650,[2] and deals with 501 acres 3⅓ poles of land. This total consisted of 291 acres 20 poles of arable land, 117 acres 1 rood 10 poles of leys, 16 acres 3 roods 33⅓ poles of meadow, 10 acres 3 roods 20 poles of meadow and leys (undistinguished), 3 acres of pasture, 41 acres of land described as grass-ground, 5 acres of

---

[1] On one holding of 65 acres odd the arable only amounted to 29 acres 2 roods 20 poles, but the leys amounted to 23 acres 1 rood 20 poles. In all the other cases the bulk of the land is made up either of land definitely described as arable or of land described as arable and leys without distinction.   [2] v. P. S. Northants. 29.

bushey ground, and 15¾ acres which were occupied by houses and their premises.

The arable, leys, and grass-ground are not separately valued in the survey, but the pasture was valued at 15s. an acre, and the 16 acres 3 roods 33½ poles of meadow were estimated to be worth £13 9s. 6d. a year, which works out at nearly 15s. 11d. an acre. The best meadow was worth about 16s. 6d. an acre, the poorest 15s.

Eight holdings are separately described in the survey, but two of these were in the hands of one tenant, and if we reckon these two as a single farm, we find that of the seven farms the largest was 120 acres 3 roods 20 poles in extent, while four farms were over 60 though under 100 acres, and the remaining two 35¾ and 41¾ acres respectively.

Two distinct leases of Elizabeth's reign are mentioned : both were for three lives. Of three distinct leases of James I's reign, two were for 60 and one for 40 years. All three belonged to the 8th year of the reign.

9. The Manor of Higham Ferrers

If we omit the survey of a small holding at Hartwell,[1] which has been dealt with in the second chapter, and also a ' survey ' which is nothing more than a certificate concerning a grant of Heathencote Farm, made in the reign of Henry VIII, and contains no information useful for the purposes of this monograph,[2] the next surveys on the official list are three which deal with the manor of Higham Ferrers and Higham Park.[3] The principal survey was made in January 1650, that of the park in February of the same year, and the subsidiary survey of certain lands attached to the manor in December 1652. The total specified area dealt with in the three surveys is 2,070 acres 3 roods 11½ poles, but of this 714¾ acres were contained within Higham Park and the premises of Higham Lodge, and 96 acres were reported on in the survey of 1652 as either claimed by the town of Higham Ferrers, or by the executors of one Richard Child, or as being out of lease

---

[1] v. P. S. Northants, 30.   [2] P. S. Northants, 31.
[3] P. S. Northants, 32, 33, and 34.

and in the ' present possession ' of the Commonwealth. Of the lands dealt with in the principal survey 946 acres 2 roods 11⅓ poles appear to have been let on lease, but the survey concludes with a list of 22 free holdings and 7 copyholds, and in the case of these the description of the land is lacking in precision and no measurements are given of 13 of the free holdings. The area which is measured amounts to 181½ acres in the case of the freeholds, and probably the omissions were insignificant, for 5 of the unmeasured freeholds seem to have consisted merely of houses, one other consisted of ' a back syde ', and yet another of a single close. The copyholds included 132 acres, besides some meadow and pasture the extent of which is not stated. All the copyholds except one of 10 acres were situated in Chelveston cum Caldecott.

If we exclude the area dealt with in the survey of Higham Park, we are thus left with a specified area of 1,356 acres 11⅓ poles, of which 600 acres 13⅓ poles were arable, 24 acres ley, 109 acres 2 roods 6 poles pasture, and 158 acres 20 poles meadow, while 3 acres 22 poles clearly consisted of houses and their premises. Of the remainder, 62 acres 2 roods 20 poles were described as ' every yeere's land ',[1] and 398 acres 2 roods 10 poles were of unspecified character. If we include the park and the premises of Higham Lodge, we must add to these figures 31¼ acres of meadow, 2 acres covered by the Lodge and its premises, and 681½ acres the character of which is not stated, though they probably consisted of pasture and woodland.[2]

Of the arable land, 596 acres 3 roods 13⅓ poles were separately valued, the estimate being £116 1s. per annum, or not quite 3s. 11d. an acre on an average. The values of the different plots varied from just over 3s. 2d. to 12s. an acre.

[1] Some of this land is described as ' More arable land called Euery yeeres lād ', and some more on the same holding as ' One pcell three leyes lamas '. On another holding we come across a parcel of every year's ground ' consisting of fower acres of Arable land '. Perhaps by ' every year's land ' is meant arable land which had been withdrawn from common of shack and from the obligation to lie fallow at customary intervals.

[2] We are told that the park contained 190 deer and 3,327 timber and other trees.

Most of the arable lay, it seems, in scattered strips in three common fields, but in some cases the strips were consolidated.[1] The 'every year's land' varied in value from 8s. 4d. to 15s. 6d. an acre—the leys from less than 2s. 11d. to as much as £1 an acre.

The pasture—amounting to 109 acres 2 roods 6 poles—was valued at £69 9s. 9d., or about 12s. 8d. an acre per annum. The different lots were valued at rates from just under 10s. to £2 an acre—this high value being reached in the case of a tiny piece of 20 poles. Of the pasture, 46 acres 3 roods 26 poles was definitely described as enclosed.

The total value of the meadow, which it will be remembered amounted to 158 acres 20 poles, was £179 4s. 2d. per annum, which is just £1 2s. 8d. an acre. The poorest was worth 10s. and the best almost exactly £2 11s. 5d. an acre per annum, but only one acre was valued at the lowest and only 7 acres—divided into 3 closes—at the highest figure. A great deal of the meadow was reckoned to be worth just £1 an acre.

It is impossible to determine the size of holdings in the manor of Higham Ferrers with real precision, for the freeholds and copyholds are not precisely measured in the principal survey, and among the lands let on lease we find some which are stated to be in the occupation of several individuals, though it is not clear whether these were joint occupiers or how the land was divided between them. But if the more doubtful cases are excluded, it appears that out of 33 holdings one was 491 acres 2 roods 6 poles in extent,[2] and another 151 acres 1 rood 5⅓ poles in extent,[3] while a third contained 94 acres 1 rood 20 poles. Six holdings contained 30 acres or

---

[1] On one farm the arable—amounting to 10 acres—is described as ' One pcell on Chappell hill called eighteen sellion of land ; one other pcell in yᵉ same called twelve sellion '. These ten acres were valued at £3 6s. 8d. per annum.

[2] Besides these lands Thomas Rudd, the tenant, held a bakehouse, and, as a freeholder, 4 messuages and some land called ' Buscott land '. None of these holdings is measured. Of the 491 acres 2 roods 6 poles, 100 acres were freehold. In addition to all this Rudd was *tenant* of 67¼ acres which were occupied by three other men.

[3] The tenant of these lands was also, it seems, joint tenant of 11¾ acres.

more, but under 50 acres, and six contained between 15 and 30 acres.[1] There were five holdings of 10 acres or more, but less than 15 acres in extent, and two between 5 and 10 acres.[2] Ten contained one acre or more, but less than 5 acres. One was less than an acre in extent. In addition to these 33 measured holdings, six others, of which five were freeholds, appear to have consisted of landless houses, so these ought really to be added to the class of holdings containing less than one acre.

But a further amendment of these figures is necessary. Five freeholds of unspecified extent and six of the copyholds mentioned in the principal survey of Higham Ferrers are distinctly stated to be situated in Chelveston cum Caldecott, and the lands dealt with in the survey of Chelveston[3] are there described as forming part of the manor of Higham Ferrers. On comparing the two surveys, we find that 3 names occur in both, and if we count as one and the same holding all lands held by the same individual—in whichever survey they are mentioned—we find that the measured holdings in the manor (including Chelveston cum Caldecott) were 39 in number. Their classification is shown in the following table :

Over 400 acres	.	.	.	.	.	1
150 acres and over, but under 200 acres	.	.	.	2
100 ,, ,, ,, 150 ,,	.	.	.	1
60 ,, ,, ,, 100 ,,	.	.	.	5
30 ,, ,, ,, 60 ,,	.	.	.	7
15 ,, ,, ,, 30 ,,	.	.	.	6
10 ,, ,, ,, 15 ,,	.	.	.	5
5 ,, ,, ,, 10 ,,	.	.	.	3
1 acre and over, but under 5 ,,	.	.	.	8
Under one acre	.	.	.	.	.	1 (7)[4]

In spite of the various uncertainties mentioned above, one general fact emerges clearly from a study of the holdings

[1] One tenant of 34 acres odd was also joint (?) tenant with two others of a farm of 67¼ acres. Another farmer, whose measured holding contained 16 acres odd, was one of the partners in this farm and also possessed a tenement as a freehold.

[2] A freeholder, whose holding consisted of a tenement and 6 acres of land, had in addition a share as joint (?) tenant in 6¾ acres of land.

[3] i.e. P. S. Northants 19, v. *supra*, pp. 97-9.

[4] The figure in brackets is obtained by including the landless houses, whose area is not stated in the survey of Higham Ferrers. None of the figures given above includes Higham Park.

on the manor of Higham Ferrers. Engrossing had taken place without interfering with tillage. On the farm of 491 acres odd, 223¼ acres were certainly arable, and there is no reason to doubt that some arable was also included within the area of 139½ acres whose character is not stated. The second largest farm contained 86¼ acres of arable and 46 acres which were probably arable[1] out of a total of 162 acres 30 poles. On the only other farm whose area exceeded 150 acres, 121 acres odd out of 151 acres 1 rood 5⅓ poles were arable. Again, on a farm of 113 acres 2 roods 38 poles at Chelveston we find 83½ acres of arable; and on two other farms of 94 acres odd the arable amounted to 87¼ acres in the one case and 77½ acres in the other.

The formation of large farms by a process of engrossing finds ample illustration in the principal survey of Higham Ferrers. Thomas Rudd's farm of 491 acres odd was made up of six holdings separately described in the survey.[2] And three at least of these six holdings were themselves composite. One of them appears to be a combination of three very similar holdings, and one of the three is referred to as ' this 2 yard land '. Another holding out of the six included, in addition to 119 acres odd of various kinds of land, some land which is described as two yardlands and included 41¼ acres of arable.[3] Lastly, the hundred acres of land which Rudd held as a freeholder went along with four messuages. To take other cases, Freeman's farm of 151 acres odd was made up of five separately described holdings, and Vincent's farm of 162 acres 30 poles consisted of two such holdings.

---

[1] We are told simply that this copyhold consisted of 46 acres of land with some meadow and pasture.

[2] This is not including the unmeasured bakehouse which Rudd held, nor an unmeasured freehold, nor the farm of 67¼ acres of which he was tenant, though others occupied it. The survey of the bakehouse contains an interesting note : ' Memorandum the Custome of the said backehouse is to backe ye bread well for Two pence the bushell and likewise yᵉ leaseholders are bound to bake all there bread at the said backehouse.'

[3] Another separately surveyed holding of Rudd's—one of the six—is described as ' one yard-land '. It contained 23½ acres of arable, 3¼ acres of every year's land, and three acres of meadow. The ' 2 yard land ' on the holding described in the text as made up of three holdings contained 47½ acres of arable, 4¼ acres of every year's land, and 6 acres of meadow. The other two parts of this holding contained 38¾ and 43½ acres of arable respectively, each with meadow and every year's land attached.

In the consideration of the Higham leases, it will be best
to take them along with those mentioned in the survey of
Chelveston cum Caldecott and to treat as one lease all leases
which were of the same day and for the same term.[1] Following this method, we have for this manor (including Chelveston
cum Caldecott) 36 distinct or presumably distinct leases.[2]
Of these, 13 belonged to the reign of Elizabeth and 8 of them
were for 31 years, 3 for 21 years, one for 50 years, and one
for 3 lives. From the reign of James there are 15 leases, one
being for 3 lives, one for 60 years, 4 for 40 years, 8 for 31 years,
and one for 30 years. Six leases of Charles I's reign are mentioned. One of them was for 60 years if any one of 3 lives
should survive so long ; one was for 60 years without qualification, and three were for 21 and one for 20 years. Under
the Commonwealth, two leases had been issued for one
year in accordance with the requirements of the Act of
July 16, 1649.

10. The Manor of Holdenby

The Parliamentary Survey of the lordship and manor of
Holdenby [3] deals with 1,700¼ acres of land, of which 500½ acres
were contained within Holdenby Park. Of the remainder,
847 acres were pasture,[4] 161¼ acres meadow, 9½ acres wood,
while 36 acres were of unspecified character and 146 acres
were not distinguished from the premises of houses.[5] There
is nothing to show that there was any arable at all on the
estate. With regard to the park, we are only told that it
was ' impaled ', that it contained some 200 deer, 11 cows, and
3 calves, and that there were 2,817 timber and other trees
within it. Besides this, 609 acres of the pasture land are
stated to consist of closes,[6] so that there is definite evidence
that 1,109¼ acres out of 1,700¼ were enclosed and no evidence

---

[1] I have in this way combined the Chelveston and Higham Ferrers leases
in the summary at the end of this chapter.

[2] Some leases are not precisely dated.   [3] v. P. S. Northants, 35.

[4] This is including 124 acres which contained a house.

[5] One house together with a field of unspecified character amounted to
102 acres, and the mansion and its gardens account for another 38¼ acres.

[6] Some of these closes were very large : one of 217 acres and another of
148 acres are mentioned.

at all which suggests that any of the remainder was not
enclosed. The total value of the 723 acres of pasture land
which were separately valued is £513 16s. 8d., or on an average
nearly 14s. 3d. an acre per annum. The poorest was worth
10s., the best £1 an acre. The 161¼ acres of meadow were
valued at £136 12s., or about 16s. 11d. an acre per annum.
The values of the different pieces varied from 12s. to £1 an
acre.

It is unfortunate that the size of holdings at Holdenby
cannot be determined from the survey, for though the names
of some tenants are mentioned, it is by no means clear how
the land was divided between them, and it is therefore impossible to estimate the extent to which engrossing had been
carried on the manor. But the fact that only six tenants'
names occur, and the fact that only five houses besides the
mansion are mentioned, seem to suggest that the mediaeval
order of things had been almost completely swept away.[1]
It is just possible that a trace of the indignant conservatism
of the peasantry may be found in a note which is appended
to the description of the park. ' There are lately two Hedge
Rowes Cutt ', we are told, ' for which Major Bingley is ready
to be accomptable to the State for [sic] & were done for the
p'servation of them they having bin Hacked & spoiled by
the adjacent poore.' On the whole, however, I am more
inclined to see in this hacking and spoiling the dire need for
firewood which is an accompaniment of landless penury, than
to regard it as the outcome of an attempt to destroy the hated
enclosures. Two leases are mentioned in the survey, both
of the reign of Charles I. One was for 17, the other for
21 years.

11. The Manor of Irchester

The next survey on the official list is that of the manor
of Irchester, which was made in March 1650,[2] but it seems
that the lands of the manor consisted almost entirely of free-

---

[1] A good many holdings without houses appear in the survey of Higham
Ferrers ; but perhaps this may be explained by the hypothesis that the
farmers lived in the houses within the borough.
[2] v. P. S. Northants, 36.

holds and copyholds which were not surveyed, for the only
lands described in the survey are two parcels of meadow—
one of two roods valued at 11s. and one of one rood valued at
5s. per annum. But the following note, which occurs in this
survey, is of considerable interest :

'Memorandū we find by a decree made betwene King
James on yᵉ one ptie baring date yᵉ 26th of November 1618
in Miklls terme yᵉ 16th yeare of his Rayne. And ye cus-
timary tenants of yᵉ mānoʳ of Irchester in yᵉ county of North-
amtō on yᵉ other pty : wherein yᵉ said King James hath
ordered and decreed that for and in consideratiō of yᵉ sum
of seuen hundred twenty three pound of currant English
mony : one moytie therof was payd to yᵉ Receuer generall
at yᵉ pasing of this decree : And yᵉ other moyetie there
beinge 361li 10ˢ to be payde wᵗʰin three months next after
the decree shalbe confermed and estableshed by Actt of
pliamēnt to make there fines certaine libberties to Incloasse
&c wᵗʰ divers other pfeits pʳuiledge and ffreedoms as it is
more att large expressed in yᵉ said decree. The sayd decree
is not yet confermed by Actt of Parlement.'

It is stated in the survey that the fines ' upon Alination or
desent are certen according to yᵉ custom one years Antient
rent.'

12. Lands in Kettering

The next survey on the list [1] may be ignored by the student
of rural economy. It simply concerns some lands in Kettering
which, on May 17, 1626, had been granted in trust for the
maintenance of a grammar school for 17 years or the life of
Sir Lewis Watson. The estate consisted almost entirely of
houses, and no statistical information of any value can be
extracted from the account of a few tiny parcels of land which
were included. Indeed, only 2 acres of land altogether are
distinguished in the survey from the premises of houses. One
acre was a close of unspecified nature worth 35s. a year :
one acre consisted of 3 leys and was worth 12s. a year.[2]

[1] v. P. S. Northants, 37.
[2] Where the figures given in a survey are obviously quite incomplete,
as in this case and at Irchester and Kingscliffe, I have thought it best to
exclude them altogether from the summary at the end of the chapter.

13. The Manor of Kingscliffe

The survey of the manor of Kingscliffe,[1] which was made in October and November 1650, is also of little value as a document for economic history. The lands described in it only amounted to 38 acres 4 poles in addition to 3 tenements of unspecified area, two of which had been ' erected upon the wast '. Of the measured lands, 20 acres were a close of pasture valued at £10, 10¼ acres were meadow, and 4 acres arable and leys, while ½ an acre is simply described as 'ground'. The remainder of the 38 acres 4 poles consisted of houses and their premises—three acres being covered by a corn mill and 1 rood 4 poles consisting of six apparently landless tenements. The total value of the meadow was £7 5s., or nearly 14s. 2d. an acre—six acres of it being worth 10s. and the rest £1 an acre. One lease is mentioned. It belonged to the reign of James I and was for 60 years. It is obviously impossible to draw any conclusions from this survey as to the size of holdings at Kingscliffe. Apparently the lands of the manor consisted almost entirely of copyholds which are not described. The customary rents amounted to £40, and at Raundes, where these rents reached a total of £45 2s. 8d. there were nearly 200 copyholds.

The only information of real interest in the survey of Kingscliffe is contained in a note about the custom of the manor. We are told that the copyholders held by a certain fine, which was twopence an acre for arable, pasture, or meadow land, and in the case of cottages half a year's rent. Any customary tenant might surrender his estate into the hands of the lord ' for the use of any pson or psons for euer '. Copyholders had the right to fell trees, and copyhold estates descended to the eldest son, or, if male heirs failed, were equally divided among the female.

14. The Manors of Moorend and Potterspury

Three surveys deal with lands in the parish of Potterspury. The first is a survey of the manor of Moorend, which lay in that parish.[2] It was made in April and May 1650, and

---

[1] v. P. S. Northants, 38.   [2] Ibid., 39.

contains a description of the demesne farm, which amounted to 170¾ acres besides a cottage and close of unspecified extent. Of the measured area, 2½ acres were occupied by the manor house and its premises, 59½ acres consisted of pasture in 3 closes, 98¾ acres were arable and leys in 3 fields, and 7 acres were meadow. The remaining 3 acres consisted of a close ' called the greene Asart ', which was bounded on one side by the forest of Whittlewood. The arable and leys lay in strips, but some progress had been made in the work of consolidation, for 8 acres lay together in one field and 5 acres in another. The pasture was valued at £24, or nearly 8s. 1d. an acre on an average—the best being worth 13s. 4d. and the rest 6s. 8d. an acre. The meadow was worth £5 5s., or 15s. an acre.

The second survey is that of the manor of Potterspury, which was made in May 1650,[1] and the third is a survey of some lands in the manor which had once belonged to the monastery of St. James, Northampton.[2] This survey was made in October 1650. Together these two surveys deal with 264¾ acres of land, of which 139¾ acres were arable, 32¾ acres arable and leys, 18 acres pasture, 12 acres 1 rood 20 poles meadow, 30 acres wood, 16 acres 1 rood 20 poles unspecified, and 15½ acres occupied by houses and their premises. The arable, nearly all of which is described as lying in three common fields in strips, was valued at £57 3s. 2d., or just over 8s. 2d. an acre on an average. The best was worth about 9s. 4d., the poorest 4s. an acre. The pasture was worth £13 11s. 2d., or nearly 15s. 1d. an acre—the rates for the different lots varying from 10s. to £1 7s. 4d. an acre. The total value of the meadow was £11 18s., which works out at nearly 19s. 3d. an acre. The least valuable meadow was worth 18s., and the rest £1 an acre.

If the demesnes of the manor of Moorend are counted as one holding, there were nine holdings in all on the lands described in the three surveys. One contained 170¾ acres ; two were between 60 and 100 acres in extent ; and the rest measured respectively 37 acres, 30 acres, 19 acres 1 rood

---

[1] v. P. S. Northants, 40.   [2] Ibid., 41.

20 poles, 9 acres 20 poles, and 3 acres.[1] Arable predominated
on the 4 largest holdings. In the three surveys taken
together we find mention of 9 distinct leases. Of these,
4 belonged to the reign of Elizabeth, one being for 3 lives, two
for 50 years, and one for 21 years. From James I's reign there
were 3 leases, one being for 40 and two for 60 years. Both
the remaining leases, which date from the time of Charles I,
were for 31 years. Besides the lands described in these surveys, there were 22 copyholds in the manor of Moorend and
9 copyholds in the manor of Potterspury. There are some
interesting memoranda in the surveys about the affairs of
the copyholders. At Moorend, we are told, the copyholds
were for two lives and one assign, and ' the longer liver of the
two lives may nominate before his death any one to be his
assigne and that assigne is to holde the estate dureinge his
naturall life paying the Lord of the Mannor his rents '. If
the ' longer liver ' neglected to nominate, the estate fell in
to the Lord, but the next of kin could redeem it by paying
4 years' rent. A heriot of 2s. was payable at the death of
every tenant. The survey embodies the following complaint
which the copyholders seem to have made :

' O^r rentes are certaine our herriotts are certaine and o^r
ffines have alway bene certaine untill within this fo urty
yeares, but haueinge manie times change of Stewards are
[sic : = our ?] Customes are broken for when any tennant
was to renew his estate the Steward would call him aside
into a corner and there contract for the fine whereas it should
have bene in open Court before the Jury that we might have
justified o^r Customes, and concerninge o^r assigne we value
worth one twentie yeares for by the assigneinge it one to
another wee can keepe o^r estates from forfeiture and falling
into the Lorde hands & therefore we thinke we cannot value
it at the worth for wee cannot heare of such another holde
againe in England.'

---

[1] Some of the tenants seem to have held lands elsewhere, if we may argue
from an identity of names. Mrs. Marthana Wilson, who had 87¼ acres at
Potterspury, also held 7 acres at Grafton. Thomas Hezzlerigg, who appears
at Potterspury as the modest tenant of 19 acres 1 rood 20 poles, held
184 acres odd at Aldrington. Again, Mrs. Mary Butler, who held 30 acres
of wood at Potterspury, had 2½ acres at Stoke Bruerne, 27¼ acres at
Aldrington, and 8¼ acres at Pury.

The opinion of the surveyors with regard to these contentions is expressed in the following passage :

' Memorandum whereas we find most of the copie holders of the aforesaide manno^r have brooke their ancient Customes and beinge to us doubtfull which way to state their tenures we therefore thought it o^r safest way to returne the anuall improuem^t to yor hono^{r}d viewe to contract as yor wisedomes see cause

If they be found Arbitrary The ffines and herriotte Combz Annis will amount to a greater proportion.'

In spite of this uncertainty, however, the survey states that the copyholders of Moorend paid as a fine twice a year's rent.

A similar memorandum about breach of custom and the doubts of the surveyors occurs in the survey of Potterspury ; and there also the copyholders had a grievance, as appears from the statement in which they say, according to the survey, ' our ffines have always formerly beene Certaine, as doth appeare by o^r Ancient coppies : But some of us have paid great ffines of late yeares, by reason of some cruell sharpe stewards : for our custome is to pay two yeares Rent of the ancient Rent for A fyne for one life : But they have forced some of us to pay three yeares value of the Racke for one life.' It is noted in the survey that the heirs of freehold tenants paid a double rent as relief, and that the copyholders held for three lives but no assign, though the next of blood could redeem the estate when it fell in by paying four years' rent. Two years' rent was payable ' for the setting in of one life ', and 2s. were paid as heriot at the death of every tenant.

The survey of 1660 seems to have included the copyholds at Moorend and Potterspury within the measured area. Certainly it refers to a much larger extent of land than the Parliamentary Surveys of these manors—to no less than 1,353 acres 23 poles in fact, of which 1,061 acres 3 roods 30 poles were arable, 192 acres 3 roods 13 poles pasture, and 98 acres 1 rood 20 poles meadow.[1]

[1] v. Land Revenue, Miscellaneous Books, vol. 222, prefatory abstract.

15. The Manor of Pury

The next survey which deserves consideration is that of the Manor of Pury,[1] for the one which comes next in the list to the surveys of Potterspury is merely a certificate correcting the date of a lease which is mentioned in the survey of the lands of Chacombe Monastery.[2] The survey of Pury was made in September 1650, and deals with 169 acres 3 roods 20 poles, of which 30 acres 20 poles were arable, 102½ acres arable and leys, 9¼ acres pasture, 12 acres 20 poles meadow, 8 acres wood, and ¼ acre of unspecified character, while 7 acres 1 rood 20 poles were occupied by the premises of houses and ¼ acre by a pond.

The arable was valued at £8 6s. 1d., or about 5s. 6d. an acre —the values for different lots ranging from about 5s. to about 5s. 9d. an acre. The total value of the pasture was £8 11s., or about 18s. 6d. an acre on an average—the best being worth £1 an acre and the poorest 16s. The total value of the meadow was £10 18s. 3d. : it was all valued at 18s. an acre.

A good deal of the land described in the survey is lumped together and assigned to a number of tenants without distinction, so that it is impossible to determine how much each held. But apart from this, two tenants are credited with holdings of between 15 and 30 acres,[3] seven with holdings of between 5 and 10 acres, and two with holdings of between 1 and 5 acres.

Three distinct leases of the reign of James I and two of Charles I's reign are mentioned. The former were all for 15 years, and of the latter, one was for 17 and one for 31 years.

16. The Manor of Raundes

The survey of the Manor of Raundes, which was made in March 1650,[4] does not contain any description of lands. It seems that, with the exception of one house—presumably the manor house—all the lands of the manor consisted of freeholds and copyholds. The rent-roll in the survey mentions

[1] v. P. S. Northants, 43. [2] v. P. S. Northants, 42, cp. ibid., 18.
[3] The tenant of the largest holding (23¼ acres) also held some of the 73¼ acres which five other tenants shared. [4] v. P. S. Northants, 44.

2 freeholds and 196 copyholds, but no information is given as to the size of these nor as to the uses to which the land was put. The quit rents were £22, and the rents of the customary tenants who held by certain fines were £45 2s. 8d. According to a statement in the survey, James I had by a 'decree' of Nov. 28, 1618, agreed with the customary tenants of the manor (in consideration of £1,640, half of which was paid when the decree was issued while the remainder was to be paid on its establishment by Act of Parliament) that these tenants 'should have hould and injoye all and singuler there customery Estates, with liberty of inclosing and Exchanging his or there customary Estates and thay likewise hold by coppie of court Role and there fines are certaine that is euery of the said customary tenantes shall paye one hole yeeres Aincent Rent for the same'. This decree, we are told, had not been confirmed by Parliament.

The Reeve of the manor received for his services meadow and leys worth £4 per annum and £1 5s. 9½d. in money.

On the whole it seems clear that the Manor of Raundes was a refuge of mediaevalism. This is shown not only by the absence of leaseholds but by the fact that 4,700 acres of land at Raundes remained to be enclosed by Act of Parliament in 1797.

17. The Manor of Rushden

The survey of Rushden, which was made in February 1650, resembles that of Raundes and contains no more information.[2] Here too all the land other than the demesne seems to have consisted of freeholds or customary holdings and none of it is described. There were 36 freeholds and 123 'copiehould and customarie' holdings. Two leases of the demesne lands are mentioned—one of Elizabeth for 41 years and one of James I for 31 years ; but no description of the demesne is given and we are told that the 'demeasnes lands belonginge to this Mannor were by the whole inhabitants of the said Manor taken by lease of Sir Peter Yonge Knight'.

---

[1] v. Gilbert Slater, The English Peasantry and the Enclosure of Common Fields (1907), p. 293. The present parish of Raunds appears to contain 4,287 acres.   [2] v. P. S. Northants, 45.

As at Raundes, the old order of things had not been maintained in unchallenged security. On Nov. 28, 1618, the Attorney-General of the Duchy of Lancaster had ' exhibited a bill ' against the ' customary and copyhold ' tenants which they could not answer, and they had then compounded with the King for £2,165 19s. 10d. (half paid when the decree was passed and half to be paid within three months of its confirmation by Parliament) ' to make theire fines upon alienation or descent certaine, to uphould theire antient customes, with libertie to inclose etc' with divers other prveleges and ffreedoms '. Again, we are told that this decree had not been confirmed by Act of Parliament ; but nevertheless the survey states that the fines of the copyholders were certain—being one year's ancient rent. And whether the tenants obtained the ' libertie to inclose ' or not, enclosure here as at Raundes was long delayed, for an Act of 1778 provided for the enclosure of 3,500 acres.[1] The Bailiff at Rushden was allowed meadow land worth £1 3s. 4d. a year.

18. The Manor of Stoke Bruerne

The next surveys to be considered are two of the Manor of Stoke Bruerne, the principal one of which was made in August 1650.[2] They deal with 1,104 acres 1 rood 21 poles of land, of which 349¼ acres were arable, 325 acres arable and leys, 155¾ acres pasture, 90 acres meadow, and 117¾ acres wood, while 46 acres 21 poles were occupied by the premises of houses and 20½ acres were of unspecified character.

Of the arable, 324¼ acres were valued at £83 15s. 3d., or about 5s. 2d. an acre.[3] The poorest was worth 5s., the best 5s. 6d. an acre. The pasture—amounting to 155¾ acres—was valued at £136 7s. 9d., or 17s. 6d. an acre, the best being worth £1 an acre and the poorest 11s. 10½d. The meadow was valued at £80 19s., or nearly 18s. an acre, one lot of 2 acres being valued at 17s. 6d. an acre and the rest at 18s. The distribution of the land according to different uses may be

---

[1] v. Gilbert Slater, op. cit., p. 292. The present parish of Rushden appears to contain just 3,500 acres. [2] v. P. S. Northants, 46 and 47.
[3] This is excluding one lot of 25 acres arable, the value of which is not clearly legible.

compared with that revealed by the survey of 1660.   According
to that survey there were in Stoke 847 acres 1 rood 39 poles
of arable, 235 acres 1 rood 22 poles of pasture, and 99 acres
2 roods 30 poles of meadow.   Thirty holdings are separately
described in the surveys of Stoke, but if we reckon as a single
holding all farms which were occupied by one tenant, this
number is reduced to twenty-two.   Of these, one was 157 acres
3 roods 6 poles in extent and two were between 100 and
150 acres.   Five were between 60 and 100 acres ; five between
30 and 60 acres, two between 15 and 30 acres, one between
5 and 10 acres, one between 1 and 5 acres, and five under
1 acre.   On the largest farm there were 100¾ acres of arable
and leys ; but the holding which comes next in size consisted
entirely of wood.   The third largest farm contained 104¼ acres,
and 79 acres of this total were arable and leys.   Thirty-two
distinct and dated leases are mentioned in the Stoke Bruerne
surveys.   Eleven of them belonged to the reign of Elizabeth,
and except one for 31 years, all these were for 3 lives.   Of
the ten leases of the reign of James I, two were for 60 years,
five for 40 years, two for 31 years, and one for 21 years.   Nine
leases of Charles I's reign were for 31 years, and of the two
remaining leases of his reign one was for 60 years and the
other for 80 years, provided in each case that one of three
lives should survive so long.

19. The Manor of Little Weldon

The survey of the Manor of Little Weldon,[1] which was made
in December 1652, deals with 247 acres of land, of which
185 acres consisted of coppices, while the demesne farm contained 57 acres of arable, 2 acres of pasture, and 3 acres of
meadow.   The arable was valued at £14 16s. 8d., or about
5s. 2d. an acre, the poorest of it being worth about 4s. 8d.
and the best 5s. 6d. an acre.   The meadow was valued at
£2 11s., or 17s. an acre ; the pasture at £1 an acre.   We are
told that the coppices were enclosed by the Lord for 7 years
after felling, but were then thrown open—the tenants having
common rights.   Besides the lessee of the demesne, the only

1 v. P. S. Northants, 48.

tenants appear to have been copyholders.   There were, it seems, 36 copyholds within the manor, and all the copyholders were copyholders of inheritance, but upon death or alienation they paid a fine ' at the will of the Lord '.   One lease is mentioned in the survey.   It belonged to the reign of Charles I and was for 31 years.

20. Porters Wood

The only remaining survey of the series under consideration is that of a wood called Porters Wood in the parish of Whittlebury.[1]   It was made in November 1650.   The wood covered 38 acres and was valued at £19 per annum.

21. Summary and Conclusions

It is easy to compile a merely statistical summary of the more important facts revealed by the Parliamentary Surveys of Northamptonshire.

The following table shows the total amount of land of different kinds described in all these surveys taken together : [2]

	A.	R.	P.
Houses and premises	547	3	1
Arable	3,525	1	33½
Arable and leys	2,091	0	0
Leys	301	1	30
Pasture	3,774	0	36
Meadow	1,041	2	20⅔
Wood	957	1	0
Miscellaneous and unspecified	3,253	0	8
Total area	15,491	3	9

The next table summarizes the evidence as to the value of the different kinds of land in so far as they are separately valued in the surveys :

Description of Land.	Amount separately valued.			Total value.			Average value per acre per annum.[3]		Highest value per acre.[3]			Lowest value per acre.[3]	
	A.	R.	P.	£	s.	d.	s.	d.	£	s.	d.	s.	d.
Arable	2,986	0	33½	669	4	10	4	6	12	0		2	8
Pasture	3,299	1	16	2,393	19	9	14	6	4	0	0	4	11
Meadow	963	3	25½	863	13	10	17	11	2	11	5	10	0

[1] v. P. S. Northants, 49.
[2] This is including the surveys of Grafton dealt with in Chapter II.
[3] These values are calculated to the nearest penny.

The size of the various holdings mentioned in the surveys is shown in the following table:[1]

1,500 to 2,000 acres	1
400 to 600 acres	3
200 acres and over but under 400 acres . . .	3
150 ,, ,, ,, 200 ,, . . .	5
100 ,, ,, ,, 150 ,, . . .	6
60 ,, ,, ,, 100 ,, . . .	29
30 ,, ,, ,, 60 ,, . . .	33
15 ,, ,, ,, 30 ,, . . .	20
10 ,, ,, ,, 15 ,, . . .	4
5 ,, ,, ,, 10 ,, . . .	20
1 acre ,, ,, 5 ,, . . .	12
Under one acre	24
Total number of holdings	160

Lastly, the information which the surveys provide as to the length of the leases made in the reigns of Elizabeth and the first two Stuarts is summarized in the following table:[2]

Length of Lease.	Elizabeth.	James I.	Charles I.	Total number.
3 lives . . .	34	7	1	42
2 lives . . .	0	1	0	1
Mixed lives and years	0	4	5	9
60 years . . .	0	25	1	26
53 years . . .	0	0	1	1
50 years . . .	5	5	0	10
41 years . . .	1	2	0	3
40 years . . .	0	27	0	27
31 years . . .	11	22	42	75
30 years . . .	2	2	0	4
21 years . . .	8	2	6	16
20 years . . .	0	0	2	2
18 years . . .	0	0	2	2
17 years . . .	0	1	6	7
16 years . . .	0	0	1	1
15 years . . .	0	8	0	8
Total numbers .	61	106	67	234

Such, then, are the chief statistical results of an examination of the Parliamentary Surveys of the Crown Estates in

[1] These holdings do *not* include several parks which are mentioned in the surveys.

[2] The table does not include a lease of Henry VIII's reign for forty years or one or two leases of the Commonwealth for a year. It is possible that some of the 234 leases may not have been really distinct; for lands in different manors may have been granted out under a single lease. Leases of the same date and for the same period I have treated as one lease when they are mentioned in the same survey or belong to the same manor.

Northamptonshire. Unfortunately, the road which leads from statistical information to historical truth is hard to find and difficult to traverse, and all the short cuts are perilous. It is so easy to suppose that figures prove more than they do. And it is therefore important to remember the precise limitations of the statistics collected in the preceding tables.

In the first place, the figures only refer to the Crown lands in a single county.[1] It would be rash to argue from them to the conditions which obtained on the estates of other landowners or in other counties. For example, the tendency to grant leases for years rather than for lives, which shows itself under the first two Stuarts, and the common occurrence of leases for 31 years in the reign of Charles I, may merely indicate a change in royal policy; and we must not assume that private landlords followed the same fashion. Again, the proportion of arable to pasture or the size of holdings, even if typical of Northamptonshire, may be peculiar to that county.

Secondly, there are certain special defects attaching to the different tables, which must not be ignored if they are used as material for economic history.

On the whole, I am inclined to regard the figures which give the average values of the different sorts of land as being the most satisfactory for historical purposes of all those which can be extracted from the surveys. But even these figures

[1] I have examined several of the Lambeth Parliamentary Surveys in the hope that they would provide material for a comparison between the ecclesiastical estates in Northamptonshire and those of the Crown. But so far as Northamptonshire is concerned, these surveys only seem to deal with tithes and with pieces of glebe too small for statistical purposes. The only noteworthy entry which I came across was one referring to a ' close ' of pasture ' lyinge open with the feild ' [v. Lambeth Parl. Surveys, vol. xiv, p. 75]. This suggests that the word ' close' was sometimes used very loosely and did not necessarily imply enclosure. But as I have not noticed any similar entry in the Parliamentary Surveys of the Augmentation Office, I have assumed that in these the word was used in a more exact sense. In case any one wishes to compare the economy of the Crown Estates in Northamptonshire with that of other counties, I may remind my readers that the Parliamentary Surveys of the Crown Lands in Sussex have been transcribed and published by J. R. Daniel-Tyssen in the Sussex Archaeological Society's Collections, vols. xxiii, xxiv, and xxv [reprinted in one volume at Lewes in 1878]. Three Surrey surveys have also been published by W. H. Hart, Surrey Archaeological Society, v. pp. 75 et seq.

cannot be used without caution.   Clearly the average values
of pasture, meadow, and arable in a particular district are
affected by other factors besides the general condition of the
market for different agricultural products.   Local peculiarities
of soil and climate count.   Again, differences in agricultural
policy affect the relative values of the land.   Where the conversion of arable to pasture has been carried out with energy,
we should expect to find the average value of the pasture less
and that of the arable greater than in more conservative
districts.   It is possible to find some indications of this by
comparing the figures of individual surveys.   Arable largely
predominated at Chelveston cum Caldecott, and its average
value there was only 3s. 3d. an acre, while the average value
of the pasture was 19s. 10d.   On the other hand, at Greens
Norton, where pasture farming had been developed to a great
extent, the average value of the pasture was 13s. 3d. an acre,
and that of the arable 5s. 3d.   At the same time, while these
considerations must not be forgotten, it is not without interest
to compare the general averages obtained from all the Parliamentary Surveys of Northamptonshire with Gregory King's
statement of the value of different sorts of land in England
and Wales in 1696.   King values arable at 5s. 10d. an acre,
and pasture and meadow at 9s.[1]   The corresponding figures
for the Crown lands in Northamptonshire in the middle of
the century are 4s. 6d. and 15s. 3d.[2]
With regard to the table which tells of the size of holdings,

---

[1] v. Natural and Political Observations [edited George Chalmers, 1810],
p. 52.   Charles Davenant, who professes to quote King's figures, puts the
average value of arable at 5s. 6d. an acre and that of pasture at 8s. 8d.
v. An Essay upon the Probable Methods of making a People Gainers in
the Ballance of Trade by the Author of the Essay on Ways and Means,
1699, p. 70.   Chalmers observes that Davenant garbled King's conclusions.
v. op. cit., p. 22.

[2] On the demesnes of forty-one monasteries the average values of the
various kinds of lands, according to the Paper Surveys which belong to
the years 1536–40, were, for arable, 7d. an acre, for pasture 1s. 1¾d. an acre,
and for meadow 1s. 8¼d. an acre.   v. Savine, English Monasteries on the
Eve of the Dissolution [in Oxford Studies, vol. i.], p. 173.   Thus it appears
that the pasture was then on these estates worth twice as much as the arable.
But according to the Parliamentary Surveys of Northamptonshire it was
in the middle of the seventeenth century worth more than three times as
much as the arable.   v. supra, p. 119.

certain warnings must also be given. The surveys do not as a rule give the size of freeholds or copyholds, so the table refers almost entirely to farms let on lease. Thus it reveals the more modern aspects of the economic organization on the manors to which it refers. On the other hand, it probably underestimates the amount of engrossing which had taken place on the land let on lease. Some tenants—as has been noticed in one or two cases in the preceding pages [1]—held farms in more than one manor ; but in the table different farms held by the same tenant have only been treated as one farm when they were in the same manor or were reported on in the same survey. But if these qualifications are borne in mind, it is possible to compare the figures with statistics previously collected. Rather more than half the holdings were between 15 and 100 acres in extent. On the manor of Forncett in Norfolk in 1565 it appears that only 49 out of 178 holdings belonged to this class ; [2] and in four other Norfolk villages in the period 1586-8 there were 32 holdings out of 88 of this size.[3] According to the figures collected by Mr. Tawney for a large number of manors in many different counties—figures which belong mainly to the sixteenth century, though some date from as late as 1649—out of 1,664 customary holdings 675 were between 15 and 100 acres in extent, while out of 390 freeholds only 61 come within this class.[4] Unfortunately, the table which Mr. Tawney gives of leasehold farms does not enable farms of this particular class to be isolated, though it appears that out of 67 such farms 7 were between 50 and 99 acres in extent, while 6 were under 50 acres.[5] If we take separately those of Mr. Tawney's figures which refer to Northamptonshire, we find that farms of between 15 and 100 acres numbered 84 out of 255 customary holdings and 21 out of 116 freeholds.[6] It is perhaps worth while to make

[1] v. *supra*, p. 48.
[2] v. F. G. Davenport, Economic Development of a Norfolk Manor (1906), pp. xvi–xviii (Appendix VI).
[3] v. W. J. Corbett, Transactions of Royal Hist. Soc. (New Series), vol. xi, pp. 76-7.
[4] v. R. H. Tawney, Agrarian Problem in the Sixteenth Century (1912), pp. 32-3, 64-5.
[5] v. R. H. Tawney, op. cit., p. 212.   [6] v. ibid., pp. 32-3, 64-5.

comparison in regard to the larger farms also. The following table shows the results :

Source of Information.	Date.	No. of Farms of 100 acres and over.	Total number of holdings.
Davenport (Forncett)	1565	2	178
Corbett (4 Norfolk Villages)	1586–8	7	88
Tawney (various)	1450–1650	91	2,121
Parliamentary Surveys of Northamptonshire	c. 1650	18	160

The largest farm at Forncett in 1565 was 131 acres 2 roods 20 poles in extent, or 164$\frac{1}{4}$ acres if we include land which its tenant held within the vill but outside the manor.[1] The largest farm of those described by Mr. Corbett was 280 acres in extent. Apparently none of the farms described by Mr. Tawney exceeded 900 acres, and his table of large farms only gives four farms of more than 550 acres. But the Parliamentary Surveys of Northamptonshire reveal one farm of 1,715$\frac{1}{2}$ acres odd and three other farms of over 400 acres.

In considering the table which shows the different uses to which the land was put on the Crown Estates in Northamptonshire, it is most important to remember that as the Parliamentary Surveys were made with a view to the sale of the lands, they do not as a rule contain any precise description of the freeholds and copyholds. Thus the manors on which the old order had been preserved almost intact are hardly represented at all in these figures. It is possible, however, that this defect may only counteract another, and that in consequence the table is more typical of rural England, or rather of rural Northamptonshire, in general than it otherwise would be. For it may be argued that, except as regards the form of enclosure which was known as ' emparking ', the Crown had set itself against the forces which made for agrarian changes in the sixteenth century, that the management of the royal estates was probably more conservative than that of private estates, and that therefore the more modernized royal manors were more typical of rural economy in general than any type which might be deduced by a process of

---

[1] I am not quite sure whether this is what Miss Davenport means by the two columns of her table.

averaging from all the royal estates, if the figures happened to be available.[1] Another doubt envelops the statistics because it is impossible to know whether the manors surveyed included large common pastures in addition to the lands which are measured and described. In some cases, as for example in the principal survey of Grafton, we are definitely told that the value of common rights was included in the value of the several holdings, so that this uncertainty really attaches to the values of the various kinds of land as well as to the proportion obtaining between them. It is therefore far from easy to use the figures as a basis for comparison. If we exclude the land covered by houses and their premises, we find that the land definitely described as arable together with that described as ' arable and leys ' amounted to 37·58% of the whole, or if we also exclude the area of the parks at Grafton, Potterspury, Higham, and Holdenby, to 44·14% of the remainder.[2] This last figure may be compared with that for the surveys of 1660. On ten of the Crown manors in Northamptonshire which were surveyed in that year, it appears that 6,030 acres 2 roods 20 poles were arable, 4,329 acres 2 roods 6 poles pasture, and 471 acres 3 roods 7 poles meadow.[3] Thus the arable amounted to 55·67% of the total cultivated area reported on. I am inclined to think that the higher proportion of arable found in these surveys may partly be explained by the inclusion of freeholds and copyholds, and partly by the more definite description given in them of lands whose character is not specified in the Parliamentary Surveys, but it must also be noticed that the manor of

---

[1] As regards parks, it is true that emparking was one of the subjects of inquiry set before the commission of 1517, but parks were expressly excepted from the complaints made against enclosures in the articles drawn up at Doncaster at the time of the Pilgrimage of Grace, and deer parks were excluded from the provisions of the Act of 1552 [5 and 6 Edward VI, c. 5], v. English Economic History, Select Documents [edited Bland, Brown and Tawney, 1914], p. 247; Gilbert Slater, op. cit., p. 325; cp. T. E. Scrutton, Commons and Common Fields (1887), p. 83; R. E. Prothero, op. cit., p. 60.

[2] The land described simply as arable is only 23·59 % of the whole area exclusive of the land associated with houses.

[3] v. Land Revenue, Miscellaneous Books, vol. 222, prefatory abstract. The manors surveyed were Grafton, Hartwell, Moorend, Potterspery, Blisworth, Greens Norton, Stoke Bruerne, Aldrington, Ashton, and Paulerspury.

Blisworth, which is included in this series of surveys, though
it is not included among the Parliamentary Surveys, contained
894½ acres of arable, but only 405 acres 3 roods and 30 poles
of pasture and no meadow. Again, the manor of Holdenby,
where grazing had been largely developed, is not among those
reported on in the abstract of 1660.

It will perhaps be convenient to set down a few other
figures for comparison with those given above. Gregory
King estimated that throughout England and Wales in 1696
the amount of arable land stood to the amount of pasture and
meadow in the ratio of eleven to ten,[1] and Charles Davenant
a few years later put it at nine to twelve.[2] In the parishes
of Forncett St. Mary and Forncett St. Peter in Norfolk, Miss
Davenport has reckoned the arable in 1565 at 1,837 acres
out of a total area, exclusive of houses, crofts, and gardens,
of 2,598 acres.[3] On a series of demesne farms surveyed
during the sixteenth and early seventeenth centuries,
Mr. Tawney found that out of a total area of 16,866 acres,
8,302 acres, or 49·2%, were arable, while on the customary
holdings on 16 manors in the same period the arable amounted
to 6,841 acres out of a total of 7,786 acres, or no less than
87·7%.[4] On the demesne lands of 41 monasteries surveyed at
the time of the Dissolution, Dr. Savine has calculated that out
of 16,780 acres, 6,235¾ acres, or 37·1% were arable.[5] Lastly,
an examination of the Feet of Fines for Staffordshire has
revealed the fact that on lands which were transferred in the
decade 1577–86 the arable amounted to 59,582 acres and the
pasture to 60,514 acres.[6]

The Parliamentary Surveys of Northamptonshire do not
throw much light upon the vexed question of the progress of

[1] v. Natural and Political Observations and Conclusions upon the State
and Condition of England, 1696, by Gregory King [edited George Chalmers,
1810], p. 52.
[2] v. Charles Davenant, Works [ed. Charles Whitworth, 1771], vol. ii,
p. 216.
[3] v. F. G. Davenport, op. cit., pp. 5–6.
[4] v. R. H. Tawney, op. cit., pp. 225–6.
[5] v. A. Savine, op. cit., pp. 171–3, quoted by R. H. Tawney, op. cit.,
p. 225.
[6] v. F. G. Davenport, Quarterly Journal of Economics, vol. xi (1896–7),
p. 208.

enclosure and conversion in the Midlands during the sixteenth
and seventeenth centuries. We know that the percentage
of the land reported on, as subjected to illegal changes which
involved enclosure, was in Northamptonshire higher than in
any other county except Oxfordshire in 1517, and highest of
all in 1607; while the county was prominent in the prose-
cutions under the Act of 1563 which Dr. Gay has noted, and
it is classed with Buckinghamshire and Oxfordshire as suffer-
ing from the development of sheep-farming, in the tract
called ' Certayne causes gathered together ', which apparently
belongs to the reign of Edward VI.[1] Again, evidences of
changes during the seventeenth century abound. The tendency of sheep-farming to produce depopulation in Northamptonshire was complained of in 1615 by the writer of the
' Geographical Description of England and Wales ', who uses
words that recall those used a century before by Sir Thomas
More.[2] In 1630 the Council sent a letter to the justices of
Northamptonshire and four other counties calling attention
to the enclosure and conversion which had been going on
and requiring them to remove all enclosures which had been
made during the last two years. Reports made in answer
to this letter show that in Leicestershire nearly 2% of the
entire area of the county had been enclosed during the two
years 1628–30. This figure may be compared with that
revealed by the Commission of 1607, which showed that
2·32% of the area of Leicestershire had been enclosed in the
far longer period from 1578 to 1607.[3] And though similar
reports for Northamptonshire do not seem to have been preserved, a letter issued from the Council in March 1631, after
the reports had been received, seems to class the enclosures
which had taken place in Northamptonshire along with those
of Leicestershire. In 1635 was published Joseph Bentham's

[1] v. E. F. Gay, Quarterly Journal of Economics, vol. xvii (1902–3),
pp. 581, 591 ; and for Certayne Causes, Early English Text Society, Extra
Series XIII (1871), p. 96.
[2] v. Gonner, op. cit., p. 159.
[3] The rapidity of enclosure in Leicestershire in 1628–30 is best appreciated when one notices that the highest percentages reported on in 1517
and 1607 were 2·45 % (Oxon, 1517) and 4·30 % (Northants, 1607). Both
these figures refer to periods of over 30 years.

' Christian Conflict ', which, Miss Leonard tells us, ' contains sermons preached at Kettering ', and in this book the author ' refers to the inclosures of several towns adjoining Kettering '. In the four years 1635–8 fines amounting to £8,678 were levied from depopulators in Northamptonshire.[1] A controversy about the merits of enclosure which raged between John Moore, Joseph Lee, and an anonymous writer in the years 1653–6 began, according to Professor Gonner, 'with the inclosures in Leicestershire, Northamptonshire, and the counties adjacent'. Again, Miss Leonard quotes four cases of enclosure in Northamptonshire which were carried out by agreement between 1646 and 1669. Three of these—dating from 1659 to 1669—involved altogether 3,864 acres. But on the other hand, Morton, writing in 1712, spoke of Northamptonshire as still mainly unenclosed ; and it is indisputable that 54% of its area was enclosed by Acts of Parliament in the eighteenth and nineteenth centuries.[2]

On the whole it seems clear enough from this evidence that the progress of enclosure in the county, though by no means steady and continuous, went on for four hundred years without any long interval of quiescence. With this conclusion the evidence of the Parliamentary Surveys and the earlier surveys examined in the second chapter of this essay does not conflict. Enclosure, conversion, and decay of houses had occurred at Hartwell before 1526, while land was taken out of the fields of Grafton and incorporated in the park sometime between the 24th year of Henry VIII and 1558. Between 1558 and 1649 Grafton Park had doubled in size, and in 1619 we find that cottages had been newly erected upon the waste at Grafton, Hartwell, and Roade. In 1618, at Irchester, at Raundes, and at Rushden, the customary tenants had been willing to pay large sums of money on the one hand that their fines might be certain, and on the other hand that they might themselves have liberty to enclose. On the manors of Moorend

---

[1] v. Gonner, op. cit., p. 167.

[2] For nearly all these facts I am indebted either to Miss E. M. Leonard's essay on The Inclosure of Common Fields in the Seventeenth Century [Trans. Royal Hist. Soc., New Series, vol. xix, pp. 101–46] or to Gonner, op. cit., pp. 153–86, 255–8.

and Potterspury the customary tenants are in 1650 complaining of harsh stewards, of secret breaches of custom, and of the augmentation of fines which used to be certain, in a manner which recalls the petitions and pamphlets of the reigns of Henry VIII and Edward VI. Occasionally in the Parliamentary Surveys we come across entries which speak of land 'lately enclosed'. And at the same time it is clear that a good many of the estates surveyed were still in an almost mediaeval condition.

There remains an important question to be considered. If, so far as Northamptonshire is concerned, we must learn to regard the transformation of the manorial economy into the modern economy as a process long drawn out, and not as a change which was accomplished by two storms of agrarian revolution occurring under the Tudor kings and the Hanoverians respectively, what was the character of the forces that governed the chronology of this slow development? Was the change driven forward by overwhelming economic forces? Were market conditions and geological conditions the inevitable determinants of its progress at different dates and in different districts? Can we recognize in its history the intelligent and irresistible advance of the economic man winning victory over the stubbornness of nature? I am inclined to think that some recent writers exaggerate the responsiveness of English rural society and of English agricultural methods to the needs of urban markets and the chances of gain. The various changes, which we class so roughly under the name of enclosures, cannot have been carried out in each decade or even in each half-century so far as would have been profitable. The movement was one by which time-honoured habits and methods were slowly broken down. It often involved oppression, often aroused bitter hostility, and for a long period was opposed by the legislature. Local differences in custom, the kindness of an individual here, the stupidity of another elsewhere, and sometimes haste or cruelty involving loss, hardship, and reaction—these were the kind of factors which determined in detail the chronology and geography of enclosure. The strong economic forces must of course be taken account of, but the history of rural England will never be understood fully unless due allowance is made for the inertia of rural conditions which have been long established. The noisy outcry and the bitter lamentations which enclosures aroused in the Tudor period are too often heard by the historian merely as indications that economic revolution was at hand. But it might be argued that we have here a sure proof that strong forces were resisting change. No doubt it was different in the latter half of the eighteenth and the early years of the nineteenth century, when the great landlords, using Parliament in the work, finished off the movement with relentless intelligence. Then, indeed, those who suffered suffered almost in silence. There was no outburst of eloquent rage. But in earlier periods local hindrances to change were greater. And of this we have, I think, some evidence in the Parliamentary Surveys of Northamptonshire. The difference between the average value of the arable and that of the pasture on the different manors varies from 6s. 9d. to 16s. 7d. an acre. This seems to suggest that the work of conversion was far from being carried everywhere to the same ' margin '.

In general, too, I am inclined to think that the most interesting fact which emerges from a study of these surveys is the great variety of conditions which obtained, even though the manors surveyed were all within a single county and all belonged to the Crown. There is variety in tenures and variety in agricultural arrangements. At Irchester and Kingsliffe, at Raundes, and at Rushden, leaseholds had hardly been developed at all, and nearly all the lands within these manors were held as freeholds or as customary estates. At Brigstock and at Rushden the community of the tenants had sufficient corporate feeling to lease the demesne. In the manors of Grafton, Hartwell, Greens Norton, and Stoke Bruerne, on the other hand, I have not noticed any signs of the existence of copyholders, and a large area of land other than the demesne farm was let on lease. As regards the size of holdings and the uses to which the land was put, it may be pointed out that at Grimscott we find holdings of moderate

size and a predominance of arable, that in the manor of
Higham Ferrers, apart from the park, evidences of engrossing
abound, though tillage was very well maintained even on the
largest farms, and that at Ashton, too, large farms had
developed without producing conversion of arable to pasture.
At Grafton yet another variety appears. The surveys of
Grafton and Hartwell not only reveal a large park which had
grown from small things during the past hundred years:
they also show us a grazing farm of nearly 600 acres; and yet
along with this we find a number of moderate sized holdings
consisting for the most part mainly of arable. And finally, at
Greens Norton and at Holdenby we have a state of things
such as might well alarm the small farmers of half a county
and fill them with fear of enclosure and hatred of large
graziers. On the former manor a huge grazing farm of
1,700 acres dwarfs all the other holdings, and two other
farms of 200 and 208 acres respectively consist entirely of
pasture. On the other hand, even here 20 holdings of between
30 and 100 acres remain, and arable or arable and leys pre-
dominate on a large majority of them. At Holdenby, however, the survey reveals no trace of arable cultivation. Out
of an area of 1,700¼ acres, 500½ acres consisted of the park,
and besides this, 1,008¼ acres were certainly pasture or
meadow. Only six tenants' names and only five houses
besides the mansion are mentioned.

INDEX

OF PLACES AND CHIEF TOPICS